Clinical Doppler Ultrasound

Commissioning Editor: Michael J. Houston
Production Controller: Helen Sofio

Clinical Doppler Ultrasound

EDITED BY

PAUL L. ALLAN,
PAUL A. DUBBINS,
MYRON A. POZNIAK
W. NORMAN McDICKEN

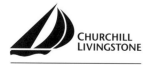
CHURCHILL
LIVINGSTONE

LONDON EDINBURGH NEW YORK PHILADELPHIA ST LOUIS SYDNEY TORONTO 2000

CHURCHILL LIVINGSTONE
An imprint of Harcourt Publishers Limited

© Harcourt Publishers Limited 2000

⚓ is a registered trademark of Harcourt Publishers
Limited

First published 2000

ISBN 0 443 055491

Cataloguing in Publication Data:
Catalogue records for this book are available from the
British Library and the US Library of Congress.

Note
Medical knowledge is constantly changing. As new
information becomes available, changes in treatment,
procedures, equipment and the use of drugs become
necessary. The editors, authors, contributors and the
publishers have, as far as possible, taken care to ensure
that the information given in this text is accurate and up
to date. However, readers are strongly advised to confirm
that the information, especially with regard to drug
usage, complies with the latest legislation and standards
of practice.

The
publisher's
policy is to use
**paper manufactured
from sustainable forests**

Printed in China

Contents

CONTENTS

Contributors

Paul L. Allan, BSc DMRD FRCR FRCPE
Consultant Radiologist
University of Edinburgh and Royal Infirmary
Edinburgh, UK

Paul A. Dubbins, BSc MBBS FRCR
Consultant Radiologist
Department of Radiology
Derriford Hospital
Plymouth, UK

Peter R. Hoskins, BA MSc PhD FIPEM
Principal Physicist
Department of Medical Physics and Medical
Engineering
University of Edinburgh and Royal Infirmary
Edinburgh, UK

Fred T. Lee Jr, MD
Associate Professor, Chief of Abdominal
Imaging
Department of Radiology
University of Wisconsin School of Medicine
Madison, WI, USA

W. Norman McDicken, PhD FIPEM
Head, Department of Medical Physics and
Medical Engineering
University of Edinburgh and Royal Infirmary
Edinburgh, UK

Myron A. Pozniak, MD
Professor, Abdominal Imaging
Department of Radiology
University of Wisconsin School of Medicine
Madison, WI, USA

David J. Rowlands, MRCOG
Consultant Obstetrician and Gynaecologist
Department of Obstetrics and Gynaecology
Wirral Hospital
Wirral, UK

Preface

The Doppler effect was first described over 100 years ago, while clinical ultrasound was developed in the 1960s and real-time ultrasound in the 1970s. Although Doppler ultrasound techniques had been investigated for many years, it wasn't until the development of duplex Doppler in the late 1970s and early 1980s that the technique started to become an increasingly important component of ultrasound examinations generally. Colour Doppler and, more recently power Doppler, second harmonics and echo-enhancing agents have arrived and further expanded the value of Doppler techniques in relation to both ultrasound examinations in general and vascular assessments in particular.

Modern ultrasound systems are complex assemblies and whilst many of the functions are now automated, or can be preset, there is still a need for those undertaking Doppler studies to be aware of the basic principles of the techniques they are using. In addition, the technique of examination and the interpretation of

the results require knowledge and understanding of the criteria being used together with an awareness of the advantages and disadvantages of these.

This book has been written to provide a guide to those taking up Doppler techniques who wish to obtain an understanding of these techniques, their major applications and their role in patient management. The authors have written their contributions based on a background of many years' experience with Doppler ultrasound and an appreciation of what does and does not work, what is or is not valuable and an appreciation of the role of Doppler ultrasound in relation to other imaging techniques. The benefit of this experience is given in the following chapters.

Paul L. Allan
Paul A. Dubbins
Myron A. Pozniak
W. Norman McDicken

Physics: principles, practice and artefacts

W. NORMAN McDICKEN and PETER R. HOSKINS

A number of techniques have been developed which exploit the shift in frequency of ultrasound when it is reflected from moving blood. This frequency shift is known as the 'Doppler effect'[1]. Five types of diagnostic Doppler instrument are usually distinguished:

1. Continuous wave (CW) Doppler
2. Pulsed wave (PW) Doppler
3. Duplex Doppler
4. Colour Doppler imaging (CDI; colour velocity imaging)
5. Power Doppler imaging

The characteristics of an ultrasound beam, the propagation of ultrasound in tissue and the design of transducers as found in B-mode imaging are all relevant for Doppler techniques[2–6].

THE DOPPLER EFFECT AND ITS APPLICATION

For all waves such as sound or light the Doppler effect is a change in the observed frequency of the wave because of motion of the source or observer. This is due either to the source stretching or compressing the wave or the observer meeting the wave more quickly or slowly as a result of their motion. In basic medical usage of the Doppler effect, the source and observer (receiver) are a transmitting and a receiving crystal usually positioned next to each other in a hand-held transducer (Fig.1.1a). A continuous cyclic electrical signal is applied to the transmitting crystal and therefore a corresponding CW ultrasound beam is generated. When the ultrasound is scattered or reflected at a moving structure within the body, it experiences a Doppler shift in its frequency and returns to the receiving (detecting) crystal. Reflected ultrasound is also detected from static surfaces within the body but it has not suffered a Doppler shift in frequency. After the reflected ultrasound is received, the Doppler instrument separates the signals from static and moving structures by exploiting their different frequency.

Motion of the reflector towards the transducer produces an increase in the reflected ultrasonic frequency, whereas motion away gives a reduction. The system electronics note whether the detected ultrasound has a higher or lower frequency than that transmitted, and hence extracts information on the direction of motion relative to the transducer.

When the line of movement of the reflector is at an angle θ to the transducer beam, then the Doppler shift, f_D, is given by:

$$f_D = f_t - f_r = \frac{f_t.2.u.\cos\theta}{c}$$

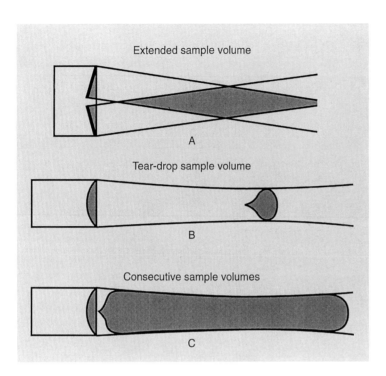

Extended sample volume

A

Tear-drop sample volume

B

Consecutive sample volumes

C

Fig. 1.1 Sample volumes in Doppler techniques. (a) For dual crystal CW Doppler unit. (b) For PW Doppler unit. (c) Neighbouring sample volumes along a beam for imaging Doppler units.

where f_t is the transmitted frequency, f_r is the received frequency, c is the speed of ultrasound and $u\cos\theta$ (i.e. $u \times$ cosine θ) is merely the component of the velocity of the reflecting agent along the ultrasonic beam direction. For a typical case of blood flow in a superficial vessel:

Transmitted frequency, f_t =
5 MHz = 5×10^6 Hz
Velocity of sound in soft tissue, c =
1540 m s^{-1}
Velocity of blood movement, u = 30 cm s^{-1}
Angle between ultrasonic beam and direction of flow, θ = 45°

The Doppler shift is therefore:

$$f_D = (5 \times 10 \times 2 \times 30 \times \cos45)/154\,000$$
$$= 1372\ Hz$$

The shift in frequency is small and within the audible range. In an ultrasonic Doppler instrument, the electronics are designed to extract the difference in frequency, $f_D = f_t - f_r$ (the Doppler shift frequency). The instrument can therefore feed a signal of frequency f_D to some output device such as a loudspeaker, or frequency analyser as discussed later.

So far we have considered an ultrasound beam being reflected from a structure moving at a fixed speed and hence generating a Doppler shift of one particular frequency. In practice, there are many reflecting blood cells and their speeds are different. The ultrasound signals returned to the detector from the different cells therefore have suffered different Doppler shifts and add together to give a complex signal containing a range of frequencies. The Doppler shift frequencies are extracted from the detected complex signal and can be fed to a loudspeaker where they can be interpreted by listening. High-frequency (high-pitch) components in the audible sound are related to high speeds, whereas low-frequency components correspond to low speeds. Strong signals, that is of loud audible volume, correspond to strong echoes that have received a Doppler shift. Strong signals could be due to the detection of many blood cells, say in a large vessel, or to echoes from tissue. Later it is noted that an output display called a spectral display or spectrogram is often used to portray the frequency content of Doppler signals.

In the PW Doppler technique, the electrical excitation signal is applied to the crystal as pulses, each containing say 10 cycles, at regular intervals and therefore a corresponding train of pulses of ultrasound are transmitted. For example, 10-cycle pulses can be transmitted, separated by non-transmission intervals of duration 20 times that of each pulse. Regularly spaced echoes are then received back from a reflector and they can be regarded as samples of the signal which would be received if a continuous wave had been transmitted as discussed above. If the reflector is moving the system electronics can extract a Doppler shift signal from the samples. The Doppler equation again applies to this Doppler shift and can be used to calculate the speed of the reflector[7].

A bonus of PW Doppler is that since pulsed ultrasound is employed, the range of the moving target may be measured from the echo-return time, as well as its speed from the Doppler shift. The range can be measured from one echo signal; however, the calculation of the Doppler shift and hence speed typically requires 50–100 echoes. As for the CW case, a group of blood cells moving with different velocities produce a range of Doppler shift frequency components in the output signal.

It was noted above that the frequency of reflected ultrasound is shifted upward or downward depending on whether the motion of the reflector is toward or away from the transducer. A numerical example illustrates this point and emphasises the small changes in frequency that the instrument must distinguish. When 2 MHz ultrasound is reflected from an object travelling at 30cm s^{-1} toward the transducer, it returns to the receiver with a frequency of 2.00078 MHz, a shift of +0.00078 MHz. If the object moves at 30 cm s^{-1} away from the transducer, the ultrasound returns with a frequency of 1.99922 MHz, a shift of −0.00078 MHz. Virtually all Doppler instruments which measure velocity preserve this direction information.

CONTINUOUS AND PULSED WAVE DOPPLER INSTRUMENTS

Doppler blood flow instruments are required to be extremely sensitive and to be capable of detecting weak signals from moving blood in the presence of much stronger signals from static or moving tissues; the latter give rise to low-frequency Doppler shift 'clutter' signals. The magnitude of the scattered signal from blood is typically 40 dB below that received from soft tissues. Blood flow signals may be detected even though the vessel is not clearly depicted, for instance in the fetal brain, or the renal artery of the neonate.

The transducer of a basic CW Doppler unit has two independent piezoelectric crystals. Since the transmitting crystal is continually driven to generate a continuous wave of ultrasound, a second crystal is used to detect the reflected ultrasound. When a CW Doppler mode is implemented as part of an ultrasound system which uses array transducers, separate groups of array crystal elements are used for transmission and reception. On extraction of the Doppler shift frequency a filter, the 'wall thump' filter, is often used to remove large, low-frequency components from the signal, such as those from slowly moving vessel walls. Typically in a Doppler unit operating at 5 MHz, Doppler shift frequencies below 100 Hz are removed by filtering. Basic CW Doppler instruments are small and inexpensive; CW Doppler mode facilities are incorporated into many array systems to allow them to detect high velocities.

The transmitted ultrasound field and the zone of maximum receiving sensitivity overlap for a particular range in front of the transducer (Fig.1.1a). Any moving structure within this region of overlap will contribute a component frequency to the total Doppler signal. The shape of the region of overlap (the beam shape) can be considered as having a crude focus which depends on the field and zone shapes and on their angle of orientation to each other. In practice, the beam shapes are rarely well known for CW Doppler transducers. A 5 MHz blood flow instrument might be focused at a distance of 2 or 3 cm from the transducer and a 10 MHz device at a distance of 0.5–1 cm. CW Doppler instruments normally have ultrasonic output intensities (I_{spta}) of less than 10 mW cm^{-2} although they may be significantly higher when used in conjunction with duplex systems to measure high velocities.

A PW Doppler instrument, operating with 5 MHz ultrasonic pulses, may have a pulse repetition frequency (PRF) of 10 000 per second, i.e. 10 kHz. The highest velocity that the instrument can measure is directly proportional to its PRF (see aliasing artefact), therefore the PRF is made as high as possible while still avoiding overlap between successive echo trains. Echo signals, i.e. trains of echoes, are produced as a transmitted pulse passes through reflecting interfaces and regions of scattering targets. After amplification, successive echo signals from a specific depth are selected by electronic gating and the Doppler shift frequency is extracted as described above.

Pulsed Doppler devices can be used on their own by altering slowly the beam direction or the gated range depth while listening to the output, for example in transcranial blood flow studies. Identification of vessels is made easier by combining the PW Doppler mode with a real-time B-scan mode to form a duplex system; however, this obviously adds to the cost and complexity.

Since the ultrasound is pulsed and the excitation time is short, a stand-alone PW unit uses a single crystal transducer for transmission and reception (Fig.1.1b). On setting the electronic gate to select a signal from a specific range, reflectors within a volume, known as the sample volume, contribute to the signal. The shape and size of the sample volume are determined by a number of factors: the transmitted pulse length, the beam width, the gated range length, and the characteristics of the electronics and transducer. The sample volume is often described as a tear drop in shape (Fig.1.1b). Sample volume lengths are usually altered by changing the gated range length. In a blood flow unit for superficial vessels, the sample volume length may be as short as 1 mm, whereas in a transcranial device it can be 1 or 2 cm; however, the precise lengths are rarely known.

The ultrasonic output intensity of pulsed Doppler instruments varies considerably from unit to unit. The intensity (I_{spta}) may typically be a few hundred mW cm^{-2} but can be as high as 1000 mW cm^{-2}, particularly when they are required to penetrate bone, as in transcranial Doppler. At present the most common use of stand-alone PW units is in transcranial examinations of cerebral vessels.

Technical factors in the use of CW and PW Doppler

1. Doppler beams are subject to the same physical processes in tissue as B-mode beams, i.e. attenuation, refraction, speed of sound variation, defocusing, etc.
2. Since the stand-alone CW and PW units are used blind, the beam direction and also the sample volume in the PW case must be systematically moved through the region of interest to maximize both the volume and pitch of the audible Doppler signal.
3. PW Doppler is subject to the aliasing artefact in the measurement of high velocities, CW Doppler is not.
4. The sensitivity (gain, transmit power) of the Doppler unit should not be so high that noise detracts from the signal quality.

5. The instrument should be assessed on normal vessels where the blood flow pattern is known and the expected Doppler signal well understood.

6. The wall-thump filter should just be high enough to remove the strong low-frequency signal from vessel walls and any other moving tissue.

7. The final result in many cases should be a distinct display, called a 'sonogram', with a clearly defined maximum-velocity trace.

8. Since the beam–vessel angle is unlikely to be known, the sonogram cannot be calibrated in velocity and the vertical axis remains as Doppler shift frequency.

9. Care should be taken to ensure good acoustic coupling between the transducer and the patient. Since there is no associated image it is not always apparent that a weak signal may be due to a lack of coupling agent.

10. If possible, information should be obtained on the shape of the sample volume for both CW and PW beams. The sample volume size can then be related to the size of the vessel under study. With CW Doppler there is very little depth discrimination. With PW Doppler the sample volume depth and size are set by the user.

IMAGING AND DOPPLER

There are three types of imaging used with Doppler techniques. The first, known as 'duplex Doppler', uses a real-time B-scanner to locate the site at which blood flow is to be examined then a Doppler beam interrogates that site. The second type creates an image from Doppler information, i.e. an image of velocities in regions of blood flow[8]. Known as 'colour Doppler', 'colour Doppler imaging' or 'colour velocity imaging' (CVI), it is normally combined with a conventional real-time B-scan so that both tissue structure and areas of flow are displayed. The third type of Doppler

imaging is similar to colour Doppler but generates an image of the power of the Doppler signal from pixel locations throughout the field of view and is known as 'power Doppler imaging' (power Doppler)[9]. A power Doppler image depicts the amount of blood moving in each region, i.e. an image of the detected blood pool.

Duplex instruments

Duplex systems link CW or PW Doppler features and real-time B-scanners so that the Doppler beam can interrogate specific locations in the B-scan image (Fig 1.2). CW duplex is normally only used where very high velocities have to be measured without the aliasing artefact, for example in the estimation of the velocity of a jet through stenosed heart valves. The direction of the CW beam is shown as a line across the B-scan image. In the case of PW Doppler, a marker on the beam line shows the position of the sample volume. The same transducer is usually employed for both imaging and Doppler but two separate ones may be linked together. The Doppler beam is often directed across the field of view so that it does not intersect the blood flow at 90°.

In practice it is difficult to run the B-mode display and the Doppler facility simultaneously, as pulses from one unit are picked up by the other. A time-share solution is employed by many manufacturers, whereby most time is spent in the Doppler mode and the B-mode image is only refreshed at short time intervals. The operator can then check that the ultrasound beam is still intersecting the site of interest. Another option is to switch off the imaging mode once the Doppler beam direction has been fixed and to maximize the PRF for the PW Doppler.

In duplex systems, the transmitted ultrasound frequency in the Doppler mode is often lower than that for the B-mode. The low Doppler beam frequency is to enable higher

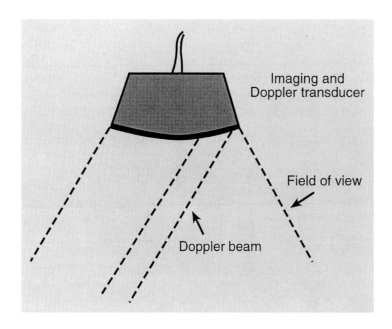

Fig. 1.2 Duplex system combining real-time B-mode and a Doppler beam of variable position across the B-mode field of view.

velocities to be handled before aliasing occurs, while the high B-scan frequency is to optimize resolution in the image. An example could be 5 MHz for Doppler and 7 MHz for B-mode when studies of superficial vessels are undertaken.

Technical factors in the use of duplex Doppler

1. The factors quoted for CW and PW Doppler may also be relevant.
2. A spectrogram can be obtained from a known vessel and a known location within the vessel.
3. The Doppler beam may be refracted and not pass along the line shown in the B-mode image.
4. The beam–vessel angle may be measured manually, allowing blood velocity to be estimated.
5. Simple estimates of blood flow may be obtained from the measured diameter and mean velocity.
6. Spectral broadening due to the use of wide aperture transducers to give good focusing can cause large errors in the measurement of maximum velocity.
7. Since the Doppler beam is held fixed and the PRF is high, particular attention should be paid to the outputs of PW units in relation to safety.

Colour Doppler imaging

Pulsed Doppler techniques require between 50 and 100 ultrasonic pulses to be transmitted in each beam direction for the determination of velocities of blood in a sample volume. It is therefore not possible to move the beam rapidly through the scan plane to build up real-time Doppler images of velocity of flow. Such imaging became possible when signal processing was developed which could quickly produce a measure of mean blood velocity at each sample volume from a small number of ultrasonic echo pulses. A technique called 'autocorrelation processing' of the signals from blood quickly gives the mean velocity in each small sample volume along the beam (Fig. 1.1c). This real-time colour Doppler imaging processes between 2 and 16 echo signals from each sample volume. In addition, the direction of flow is obtained by examining the signals for the direction of the shift as for CW and PW Doppler devices. Each image pixel is then colour-coded for direction and mean Doppler shift (Fig. 1.3a).

B-scanning and Doppler imaging are carried out with the common types of real-time transducer. Echo signals from the blood and tissues are processed along two signal paths in the system electronics (Fig. 1.4). Going along one path, the signals produce the real-time B-scan image; going along the other path, autocorrelation function processing and direction flow sensing are employed to give a colour flow image. An important exclusion circuit in the autocorrelation path separates large-amplitude signals which arise from tissue and excludes them from the blood velocity processing. The B-mode and mean velocity images are then superimposed in the final display. Strictly speaking, the flow image is of the mean Doppler shift frequency and not the mean velocity, since the beam–vessel angles throughout the field of view are not measured. Colour shades in the image can indicate the magnitude of the velocity, for example light red for high velocity and dark red for low velocity. Turbulence, related to the range of velocities in each sample volume, may be presented as a different colour or as a mosaic of colours.

Doppler images typically contain about 64 genuine lines of information and 128 consecutive sample volumes along each line. The frame rate varies from 5 to 40 frames per second, depending on the depth of penetration and the width of the field of view. As in B-scanning, the appearance of the image is usually improved by inserting additional lines or frames whose data are calculated from the genuine lines, a process known as interpolation. Alteration in flow can occur rapidly over the cardiac cycle, therefore a cine-loop store of up to the last 128 frames is of value for review purposes. Doppler spectro-

grams can be made by selecting the appropriate beam direction and sample volume location in the image and then switching to the PW or CW mode. PW and CW Doppler techniques provide more detailed information on blood velocities than colour Doppler, so spectral information is still of value.

Technical factors in the use of colour Doppler imaging

1. The mean Doppler frequency is the quantity which is presented in a colour-coded form in each pixel. When the colour bar is labelled in velocity the beam–vessel angle has been assumed to be zero throughout the image.
2. The velocity component along the Doppler beam is heavily dependent on the angle between the direction of flow and the beam direction (the cosine θ dependence). The colours depicted in the image are therefore heavily angle dependent.
3. The flow pattern on the colour Doppler display can be related to the structures shown in the B-mode image.
4. CDI is a pulsed technique so aliasing is a problem.
5. A good CDI machine is one which discriminates well between signals from tissue and those from blood.
6. The CDI field of view box should be adjusted to cover only the region of interest and therefore maximize the frame rate.
7. The velocity range covered by the colour scale should be carefully matched to the velocities expected in the study.
8. A cine-loop is useful for the review of fast-changing blood flow patterns.
9. A change in the direction of flow, say from toward to away from the transducer, and hence a colour change, need not mean a change in the direction of flow along a vessel. It may merely mean the beam–flow angle has changed from less than 90° to more than 90°.

(a)

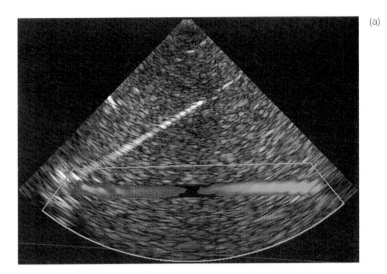

(b)

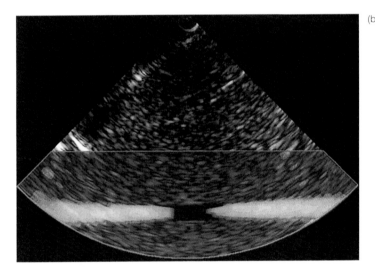

Fig. 1.3 (a) Colour flow image of flow in a straight tube. When the flow velocity component is along the beam towards the transducer it is colour-coded red, when the component along the beam is away from the transducer it is coded blue. (b) Power Doppler image of flow in a straight tube. Direction of flow is not measured so it is not colour-coded.

Power Doppler imaging

The power of the Doppler signal from each small sample volume in the field of view may be displayed rather than the mean frequency shift (Fig. 1.3b). The power of the signal from each point relates to the number of moving blood cells in that sample volume. The power Doppler image may be considered to be an image of the blood pool. The power mode does not measure velocity or direction and therefore the image shows little angle dependence, neither does it suffer from aliasing;

however, it obviously presents less information about blood flow. The attraction of power Doppler images is that they suffer less from noise than velocity images, as the power of the background noise for any sample volume with no blood flow signal is less than the power of the background noise plus Doppler signal when blood flow is present. The background noise may be used to set a threshold above which signals are accepted for Doppler flow. Noise from sample volume regions lacking blood flow is therefore reduced in the power image by a threshold

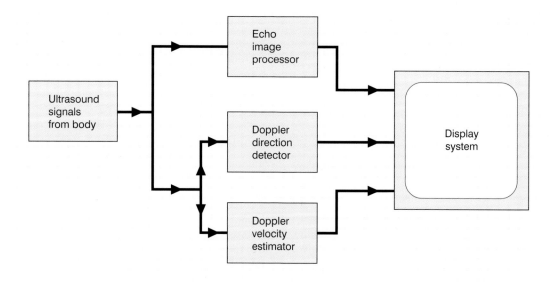

Fig. 1.4 B-mode and Doppler imaging signal processing paths in a scanning machine.

detector. However, when the same signal is used in the velocity imaging mode, the noise will produce a mean velocity value which the machine will treat as a genuine blood velocity and which will therefore appear in the image. The power Doppler mode is therefore less prone to noise and hence more sensitive and can be used to detect small vessels. Further sensitivity can be obtained by averaging power images over several frames to reduce spuriously distributed noise even more. In velocity imaging there is interest in showing quick changes in blood flow and hence less averaging is used.

Power Doppler imaging is fairly easy to use and often provides a more complete image of the vasculature than velocity imaging. This has made it popular in clinical use and it is commonly used initially to locate regions of interest prior to investigation by colour Doppler or duplex methods. It is also possible with some equipment to use the direction information in the colour Doppler image to colour-code the corresponding power image.

Technical factors in the use of power Doppler imaging

1. In the power Doppler image, the power of the Doppler signal at each pixel is colour-coded.
2. No velocity information is displayed.
3. Most power Doppler systems are direction insensitive; i.e. the display is the same regardless of whether the blood is flowing toward or away from the transducer. However, some machines do display different colours depending on the direction of blood flow by including some directional Doppler information.
4. The power Doppler image is insensitive to angle except near 90° where the Doppler signal may fall below the clutter filter, which cuts out low Doppler shifts, and no signal is displayed.
5. There is no aliasing, because the frequency information is not estimated from the Doppler signal.
6. The power Doppler image is very sensitive to movement of the tissue or probe (the flash artefact). Some machines incorporate a flash filter to try to reduce this effect.

1

ULTRASONIC CONTRAST AGENTS

A number of agents have been considered which can enhance the scattering of ultrasound from blood and hence could be employed as echo-enhancing or contrast agents. Ophir and Parker[10] have reviewed contrast agents. From this review and more recent experience it has become obvious that agents in the form of encapsulated microbubbles are by far the most likely to be successful echo-enhancing agents in the immediate future. This is due to the large difference in acoustic impedance between the gas in the bubbles and the surrounding blood. In addition, bubbles of a few microns in diameter have a fundamental resonance frequency of a few megahertz. For example, 4 μm diameter bubbles resonate at 4 MHz, which is well within the range of medical ultrasound systems. Bubbles of these dimensions are important since, even with only very thin wall encapsulation, they are able to pass through the capillaries of the lung into the systemic circulation. An investigation by a committee of the American Society of Echocardiography concluded that contrast echocardiography carried a minimal risk for patients and that there were few residual or complicating side-effects[11]. More recent individual studies have confirmed these conclusions; however, more work is required on new agents as they become available[12].

The development around 1990 of contrast agent microbubbles that can be used by percutaneous venous injection was the breakthrough which gave rise to the current high level of activity in this field. Table 1.1 gives examples of agents which are currently under commercial development. The 'Echogen' agent is different from the others in that it undergoes a phase change from liquid to gas as a result of the increase in temperature following injection into the bloodstream. Large gas molecules are encapsulated in some agents to reduce the rate of diffusion and so increase the lifetime of the bubbles. Typically the lifetime in blood ranges from 2–3 min up to 20–30 min. An attraction of contrast agents is the ability to increase the

Table 1.1 Properties of some common intravenous, lung-crossing contrast agents. Produced courtesy of C. Moran.

Left heart agent	Manufactured by	Type of agent	Capsule	Gas	Bubble size (μm)	Dose/conc.
Levovist	Schering	Lipid-stabilized bubble	Palmitic acid	Air	3–5	0.8–3.2 g
ShU 563A (Sonovist)	Schering	Solid microspheres	Cyano-acrylate	Air	Mean 2	0.1–1 μl kg^{-1} (200 × 10^8 μ.bubbles ml^{-1})
Definity (DMP-115)	ImaRx/ Du Pont	Encapsulated bubble	Lipid	Perfluoro-propane	Mean 2.5	3–5 μl kg^{-1} (10 × 10^8 μ.bubbles ml^{-1})
Quantison™	Quadrant Healthcare	Rigid microsphere	Albumin	Air	Mean 3.2 (<2% >6)	Infused at 1 ml min^{-1} (5 × 10^8 μ.bubbles ml^{-1})
Optison	Mallinckrodt	Encapsulated microsphere	Albumin	Octafluoro-propane	Mean 3.7	1 ml @ fundamental 0.5 ml @ second harmonic (5–8 × 10^8 μ.bubbles ml^{-1})
BRI (Sonovue™)	Bracco	Stabilized bubble	Phospho-lipids	SF$_6$	2–3 (90%<8)	(1–5 ×10^8 μ.bubbles ml^{-1})
Albunex (Infoson in Europe)	Nycomed (Europe) Mallinckrodt (USA)	Encapsulated bubble	Albumin	Air	Mean 4 Range 2–10	0.025–1.0 ml kg^{-1} (3–5 × 10^8 μ.bubbles ml^{-1})

signal obtained from small blood vessels which are difficult to detect by conventional Doppler methods, e.g. cerebral or renal vessels. There is also interest in perfusion studies, for example to observe and measure the wash-in and wash-out of agent in the myocardium in a manner analogous to nuclear medicine studies.

Enhanced scattering is obtained if a bubble is insonated with ultrasound of a frequency equal to that of the fundamental resonance frequency of the bubble. At low power the oscillations of the bubble are about the centre of the bubble and are directly in proportion to the size of the pressure fluctuations in the ultrasound wave. However, at higher powers the oscillations become distorted and ultrasound at frequencies different from that of the incident wave are generated by the bubbles. These frequencies are known as harmonics and are simply related to the fundamental resonance frequency of the bubble, e.g. the second harmonic frequency is twice the fundamental frequency. There is considerable interest in detecting and using the second harmonic, since tissue does not produce this effect to any great extent and the second harmonic signal comes predominantly from the echo-enhancing agent in the blood vessels. Both pulse–echo and Doppler systems have been designed to pick out the second harmonic component in the ultrasound returned to the transducer and use it to enhance the signal from the agent in blood, possibly by as much as 20–30 dB. These systems are being evaluated in clinical practice[13].

The scattering from contrast agents can also be enhanced if the acoustic pressure fluctuations in the beam are large enough to damage the microbubbles, causing them to leak. An unencapsulated gas bubble then forms next to the original one; however, since it has no outer shell, the scattering from it is undamped and can be around 1000 times higher than that from the encapsulated bubble. This effect has been exploited in a technique known as 'intermittent' or 'transient' imaging, which allows time for the damaged bubbles to be replaced between sweeps of the ultrasound beam[14].

Technical factors in the use of echo-enhancing agents

Contrast agents are still very much in the developmental stage. Nevertheless, some technical points of importance are becoming apparent.

1. Check the age and shelf life of the agent.
2. Microbubble contrast agents are fairly fragile. The handling instructions should be carefully followed and indeed with experience some additional precautions may be identified.
3. The ultrasonic beam may be capable of destroying some microbubbles; higher transmit power will therefore not necessarily produce a stronger echo signal.
4. Several contrast agents require to be insonated at high acoustic pressures to give enhanced backscatter due to bubble destruction. This phenomenon is also known as 'acoustically stimulated emission'. Aspects of its safety still need to be fully evaluated.
5. Determine the physical phenomena which are expected to be present under the operating conditions and which will enhance the echo signal, e.g. harmonic scattering, free bubble creation and bubble destruction.

INFORMATION FROM DOPPLER SIGNALS

When the Doppler signal which contains information on blood velocities and haemodynamics is being produced it is necessary to interpret it. It is essential to obtain good-quality signals in order to be able to detect disease.

The spectrum analyser

A Doppler signal may be analysed into its frequency components in order to give a display of the velocities of the blood cells at each instant (Fig. 1.5)[2]. Short time intervals of the Doppler signal are analysed, for example a

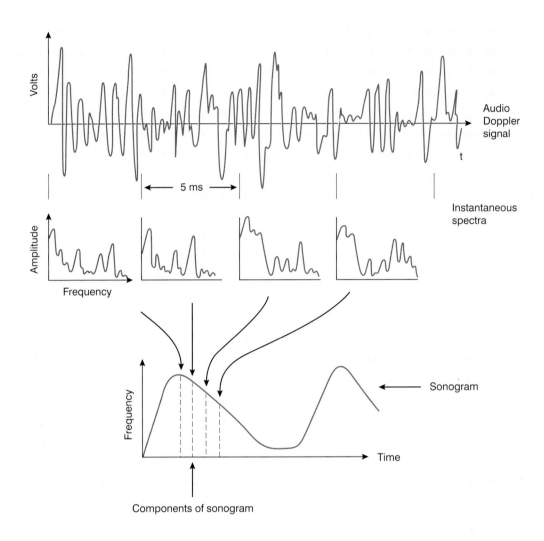

Fig. 1.5 Schematic representation of the analysis of a Doppler signal to form a sonogram (spectrogram). Reproduced with permission from W.N. McDicken[2].

segment of 5 ms duration. This produces an instantaneous spectrum of the frequencies in the sample volume. If an angle correction is then applied, this spectrum will represent the range of velocities in the sample volume. The range of frequencies in each spectrum is displayed on the vertical axis and the power of each frequency component is presented as a shade of grey. The consecutive velocity spectra are then displayed as side-by-side grey-shade lines. In this way a spectral display,

or spectrogram, is built up (Fig. 1.6). Note the difference between the instantaneous velocity spectrum which tells us about the pattern of velocities in the sample volume at that instant and the spectral display or spectrogram, which shows how the velocity pattern varies with time. Spectrograms are generated in real time during the clinical examination and it is usually possible to store a few seconds of the trace in an analyser for subsequent review.

The temporal resolution in a spectrogram,

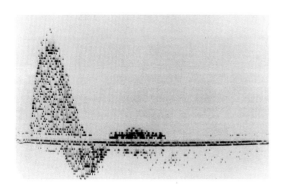

Fig. 1.6 An enlarged sonogram to illustrate pixel structure and speckle pattern.

line and sweep speed.

2. Arrange the grey tones, or colours, of the spectral display to give the best 'image' quality by adjusting the Doppler gain.

3. Treat with caution information from weak signals in a noisy background.

4. A clear spectrogram is required before the maximum frequency can be traced.

5. It is usually best to make measurements over at least five heart cycles. However, if this is not possible, perhaps due to respiratory movement, useful information can be obtained from one or two cardiac cycles.

6. Make use of the total storage capacity of the analyser to make a full recording from which the most suitable part of the spectrogram can be selected, using the scroll facility, in order to make measurements.

7. Check thoroughly the reliability of automatic tracing techniques for maximum and minimum velocity.

8. Note whether the vertical axis has been calibrated in velocity by allowing for the beam–vessel angle.

9. To obtain reproducible results, try to use the same beam–vessel angle for all examinations, e.g. 60°.

that is the smallest discernible time interval, equals the length of the portion of Doppler signal used to produce each instantaneous spectrum and is typically 5–10 ms. The frequency (or velocity) axis of the sonogram usually has about 100 scale intervals, a total frequency range of 10 kHz, and therefore has intervals of 100 Hz. The Doppler signal is therefore resolved into frequency components separated by 100 Hz, the frequency resolution of the spectrogram.

It is often desirable to make measurements on a spectrogram, for example an estimate of the time between two events or of the maximum velocity during systole or diastole. Measurement is performed by placing a cursor on the relevant points of interest; a variety of calculations can be performed by the system computer. Indices related to the sonogram shape and hence to normality or abnormality of flow velocities can be calculated within the analyser and displayed on its screen. These are discussed later in this chapter. The oscillatory shape of a spectral trace is often referred to as a waveform.

Technical factors in relation to spectral analysis

1. Arrange the frequency and time scales to best display the detailed information in the sonogram by adjusting velocity scale, base-

SPECTROGRAMS AND INDICES

A good-quality audible Doppler signal will result in a good quality sonogram. Degradation of a sonogram is due to electronic and acoustic noise which should only be a problem when the gain of the Doppler unit or analyser is very high for the detection of weak signals. Noise in sonograms creates considerable difficulties for the automatic calculation of quantities and they should therefore be used with caution. It is sometimes possible to check traces drawn automatically on a sonogram to see if they have been corrupted by noise. If the automatic mode cannot deal with the noise, then the traces should be drawn manually making use of the eye's ability to distinguish noise from true signal. It should also be remembered that the vertical axis of a sonogram can only be labelled as velocity after the beam–vessel angle has been measured.

Waveform indices

Waveform indices are derived from a combination of a few dominant features of the waveform[3]. Indices that have the same or similar names in the literature are occasionally defined differently, so a first step is to check the definition of any index to be used. In practice only two classes of index are used to any great extent, those related to the degree of diastolic flow and others related to spectral broadening. The variation in time of the maximum velocity displayed in a spectrogram is commonly used as a source of data for the derivation of an index (Fig. 1.7a). Since the maximum velocity is not always clearly apparent in a spectrogram, some analysers produce a trace which is closely related to the maximum velocity trace. One example is a trace showing the upper velocity boundary below which the velocity components contain seven eighths of the power of the Doppler signal.

The mean velocity waveform (average velocity waveform) is also employed (Fig. 1.7b). To calculate the mean velocity at each instant, the values of velocity and the intensities of the signal for each velocity component in the instantaneous spectrum are used. The mean velocity is used together with the vessel cross-sectional area to calculate blood flow rate. However, it is difficult to measure mean velocity accurately and there are several other problems associated with calculating flow rates; these are discussed further in Chapter 2.

Since the beam–vessel angle may not always be known, the waveforms or spectrograms will not be corrected for angle. Indices are therefore defined involving ratios of velocities. In such a ratio, the angle factors appear on both the top and bottom and hence cancel each other out, so that the index is independent of beam angle.

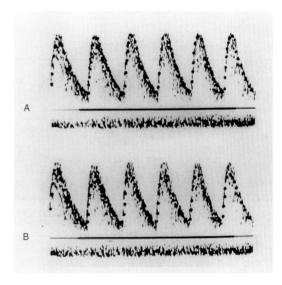

Fig. 1.7 (a) A maximum-velocity trace on a sonogram. (b) A mean velocity on a sonogram.

Errors are also reduced by averaging the calculated indices over several heart cycles.

A number of the most commonly encountered indices are briefly discussed below:

A/B ratio

The A/B ratio is defined as the ratio of two specified velocities, e.g. maximum velocities, at two points in the cardiac cycle (Fig. 1.8). It is usually employed where there is no reverse flow in the waveform.

Resistance index (RI)

In Fig. 1.8:

$$RI = \frac{S-D}{S}$$

High resistance in the distal vessels produces low diastolic flow in the supplying artery and results in a high value for this index; a low resistance results in a low value as there is higher diastolic flow. It is also known as the Pourcelot index.

Pulsatility index

The pulsatility index (PI) is defined as:

(a)

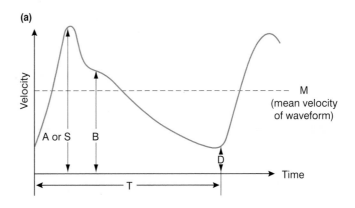

(b)

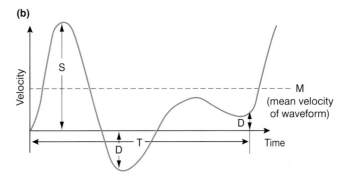

$$RI = \frac{S\text{-}D}{S}$$

S/D ratio (umbilical and uterine arteries)

A/B ratio (carotid arteries)

$$PI = \frac{\text{Maximum velocity excursion}}{\text{Mean velocity}}$$

$$= \frac{S\text{-}D}{M} \text{ in (a)}$$

$$= \frac{S+D}{M} \text{ in (b)}$$

Fig. 1.8 Waveform indices, normally calculated from a maximum velocity waveform, but the mean velocity waveform can also be used. Reproduced with permission from W.N. McDicken[2].

$$PI = \frac{\text{maximum velocity excursion}}{\text{mean of the velocity}}$$

It is used in vessels where reverse flow may occur, for example in the lower limbs (Fig. 1.8). The PI may typically have a value of 10 for the normal common femoral artery but be around 2 when proximal disease severely dampens the waveform.

As defined above, the PI index is heart rate dependent. To avoid this, PI can be calculated over a specified time from the start of systole, e.g. for the first 500 ms. The pulsatility index is then labelled 'PI(500)'.

Damping factor

The damping factor is defined as the ratio of pulsatility indices at two sites along an artery. It quantifies the damping of the waveform downstream along a diseased vessel.

$$\text{Damping factor} = \frac{\text{PI(proximal site)}}{\text{PI(distal site)}}$$

The numerical value of this index increases as disease becomes more severe, a value of 2 being typical of a high degree of damping. This index is mentioned for completeness, it is not widely used.

Spectral broadening

Turbulence increases the range of blood cell velocities in a vessel. One index to quantify this broadening of the spectrum of velocities is

Spectral broadening index (at systole)

$$= \frac{\text{maximum velocity}}{\text{mean velocity}}$$

Conclusions with regard to the presence of turbulence should be made with caution and only after familiarity has been gained with the patterns for laminar and plug flow for the particular instrument being used. Other technical factors can cause spectral broadening; for example 'geometrical spectral broadening', which results from the range of Doppler angles with which ultrasound can insonate a sample volume in the vessel from points on the face of the transducer.

Transit time

The time for the pulse pressure wave to travel along a length of artery can be measured by placing a Doppler probe at either end of it. From this time and knowing the length, the pulse wave velocity (PWV) is calculated. Alternatively, using the electrocardiogram (ECG) and one Doppler unit the transit time can also be measured, the QRS of the ECG giving the time when the pressure pulse leaves the heart. The time is first measured for the pulse to travel from the heart to the proximal artery site; a second time is then measured for the pulse to go from the heart to the distal site. Subtracting these two times gives the transit time and, if the length of the artery is known, the PWV can be calculated. Any error associated with the assumption that the QRS represents the time at which the pulse leaves the heart is removed by the subtraction.

A normal aorta has a PWV of around 10 m s^{-1}. The transit time along 0.5 m is then 50 ms. Pulse wave velocity depends on disease states of the artery wall and blood pressure. This index is also mentioned for completeness, it is not widely used.

Technical factors in the application of waveform indices

1. Use good-quality spectral data to calculate indices.
2. Most indices are calculated using the maximum Doppler frequency as this is relatively insensitive to beam–vessel alignment and sample volume size.
3. Mean Doppler frequency shift is very sensitive to alignment and sample volume size and is not widely used to estimate indices.
4. Indices of waveform shape are insensitive to the beam–vessel angle except near 90° where the end-diastolic component may disappear below the high-pass filter.
5. For obstetrics use, the wall-thump filter must be set low, typically 50–100 Hz, in order that absent end-diastolic flow may be ascertained unambiguously.
6. The most suitable index or measurement for each application can be determined from the literature. Indices are useful in that they allow velocity patterns to be classified and related to disease state. However, they do not extract any more information than can be deduced by direct observation of the whole sonogram.

ARTEFACTS IN DOPPLER TECHNIQUES

The most important artefacts are mentioned here and methods of dealing with them are suggested. Further details can be found in other texts[2, 5]. Artefacts are usually dealt with by explaining their origin or by recognizing that they occur fairly frequently and are not of significance.

Attenuation

The reduction in echo signal size due to attenuation of the beam in tissue is very familiar from B-mode imaging. The same attenuation processes occur for Doppler techniques, hence stronger signals are detected from superficial vessels than from deep ones. With CW Doppler units this imbalance cannot be compensated. With PW stand-alone and duplex Doppler devices, the signals are from a sample volume at a selected depth and the gain can therefore be adjusted to optimize the signal. In colour Doppler and power Doppler imaging, time gain compensation (TGC) could help to compensate for attenuation but it is more usual just to process all signals that are above the noise level; obviously those from deep vessels will be closer to the noise level and hence will be more likely to be affected by noise.

Refraction

Refraction deviates a beam as it crosses at an angle the interface between two tissues in which the speed of sound is different. The direction of the transducer axis may not, therefore, coincide with the actual beam path. With duplex systems a weaker signal than expected from a well-imaged vessel is probably due to refraction of the Doppler beam. This is less of a problem with colour or power Doppler imaging instruments, since the presence of a signal is noted first in the image before any spectral analysis is attempted.

Shadowing and enhancement

Attenuation of a Doppler beam at a structure may be so large that blood flow behind it cannot be detected, for example at a calcified plaque on a vessel wall. Microbubble contrast agents can also give rise to shadowing problems behind them. Signal enhancement occurs where the beam passes through a medium of low attenuation to reach the vessel, such as a collection of amniotic fluid, or the full bladder.

Beam width

A wide beam can cause contributions to the Doppler signal from moving structures well off the central axis. This is most likely to be due to a strong reflector such as a heart valve leaflet, but it could also be due to a large blood vessel. A narrow beam may result in only partial insonation of a vessel with the related errors in the Doppler signal; for example, overemphasis of the high-velocity flow at the centre of a vessel occurs when a narrow beam is directed into a vessel but does not encompass the slower-moving blood at the side.

Spectral broadening

Spectral broadening is another artefact resulting from beam shape. As noted in the discussion on the spectral broadening index, this arises due to ultrasound insonating a sample volume over a range of angles.

Speckle and the spectral display

The speckled appearance of a sonogram results from fluctuations in the power levels of the velocity components in neighbouring pixels (Fig. 1.6). These fluctuations are due to fluctuations in the ultrasonic signal received from the random distribution of blood cells. Due to this speckle noise the power level in a pixel cannot be directly related to the number of cells moving with a particular velocity. Averaging the power levels in neighbouring pixels gives a more accurate measure of the number of cells moving with each velocity.

Inadequate coupling

Weak Doppler signals can be attributed to a lack of coupling liquid between the transducer and the skin. In CW and PW Doppler applications this artefact is not as evident as in imaging techniques, where poor penetration is readily seen.

Electrical pick-up

Doppler devices are required to be highly sensitive and are therefore prone to electrical pick-up of stray signals. Some such signals can be recognized by their pattern in the sonogram. The spectrum analyser unit may allow the operator to attempt to clean up the sonogram by deleting spurious signals.

Compression of the spectral display

When a sonogram is compressed, either in its grey shades or in its scale of presentation, information is lost. A sonogram should be treated as a type of image and thus presented with optimum grey-shade contrast and spatial detail. The latter means that the velocity and time axis scales should be selected to show detailed structure in the sonogram. The accuracy of measurements from the sonogram will also be affected by poor presentation.

Erroneous direction sensing

The direction-sensing circuitry does not always function correctly since its design and implementation are difficult. Flow will then be presented in the wrong direction, either in a sonogram or in a colour Doppler image; if this is suspected then the set-up of the system can

be checked by examining a normal artery in which the direction of flow is known.

Filtering

Filters are used to greatly reduce low frequencies, such as those obtained from arterial walls. Filters also remove information on slow-moving blood but this is not usually a serious problem unless it is desired to measure mean velocity accurately or slow flow specifically (Fig. 1.9).

Harmonic generation by large signal distortion

The harmonics of a frequency are higher multiples of that frequency; for example, harmonics of 100 Hz are 200 Hz, 300 Hz, etc. If a signal is too large to be handled by the electronics it becomes distorted and then contains additional harmonic frequency components. When such a distorted signal is analysed, the harmonics appear at regular frequency intervals in the spectral display. Strong blood flow signals exhibit harmonic components as a

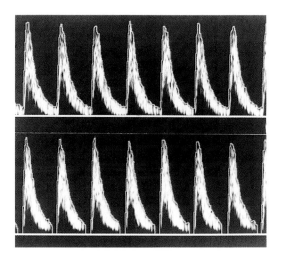

Fig. 1.9 Filtering. Raising the high-pass (wall-thump) filter as in the lower sonogram removes low-velocity signals.

higher frequency part of the sonogram above that which would probably be obtained if the gain were reduced (Fig. 1.10).

High or low sensitivity

In colour Doppler and power Doppler imaging, setting up the system with too low a sensitivity causes blood flow signal to be lost. Too high a sensitivity causes spurious echoes to be colour-coded as blood (Fig. 1.11).

Aliasing

Pulsed Doppler and colour Doppler units have to reconstruct the complete Doppler shift signal from regularly timed samples of information, rather than the complete signal as used in CW units. The sampling rate is equal to the PRF of the Doppler unit. If the sampling rate is too low, the frequency of the reconstructed Doppler signal is also too low and the direction of flow is presented wrongly. In a spectral display or flow image, this is known as an 'aliasing' artefact (Figs 1.12 and 1.13).

The aliasing artefact is encountered when high-frequency Doppler shift signals are produced, usually by high-velocity flow. It also occurs when sampling deeper vessels, as the PRF is reduced to allow time for the echoes from a pulse to return before the next pulse is transmitted. If the PRF is too low for the Doppler shift frequencies from the blood in the vessel, aliasing will occur. An approach to raising the velocity level at which aliasing becomes a problem is to use a high PRF (the high-PRF mode), even although the echoes from deep structures have not died out before the next pulse is transmitted. If the deep echoes are strong enough, Doppler signals from deep vessels may then be superimposed on those from a more superficial site. This uncertainty with regard to the source of the signal is referred to as 'range ambiguity'. The high-PRF mode must therefore be used with care.

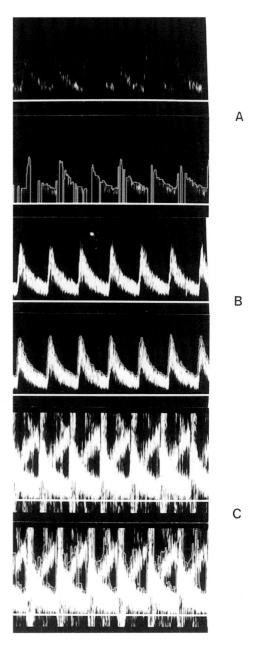

Fig. 1.10 Increasing gain from (a) to (c). Very high gain distorts the signal and introduces harmonic frequencies.

Although this mode can be useful, it increases the intensity of the beam, which is another reason for using it only when necessary.

Figs 1.12 and 1.13 show the aliasing artefact. The high-velocity forward flow

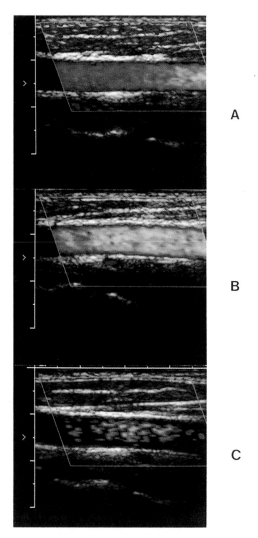

Fig. 1.11 Variation of gain in a Doppler image. The image content is very sensitive to gain setting: (a) shows too much gain, (b) too little.

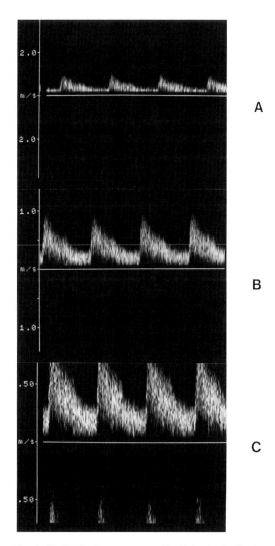

Fig. 1.12 Aliasing in a sonogram. The highest velocities in (c) appear in the reverse channel.

components, above the upper limit, appear as high-velocity reverse flow. Aliasing can be of value in colour Doppler imaging since it allows high-velocity jets to be identified. Power Doppler does not suffer from aliasing.

Effect of beam angle to flow direction

The quality of a Doppler signal depends on beam–vessel angle and, in particular, above 70° it degrades quite rapidly (Fig. 1.14). If the direc-

tion of an ultrasound beam is at 90° to the direction of the flowing blood, no Doppler signal is expected since, in the Doppler equation, $\cos 90° = 0$. However, a poor-quality Doppler signal is usually obtained for a number of reasons. First, the ultrasound beam may converge or diverge slightly from the beam axis, so all of it is never at 90° to the flow. Second, there may be some turbulence in the flow, in which case the blood cells are not all travelling in parallel paths at 90° to the beam. Third, as cells enter and leave the

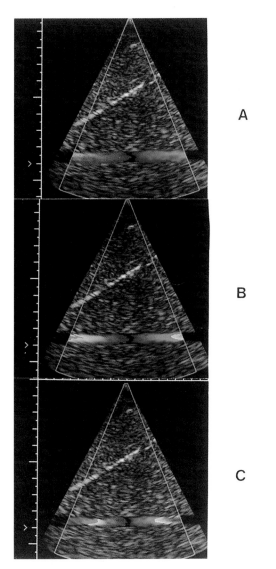

A

B

C

Fig. 1.13 Aliasing in a colour Doppler velocity image. Note that there is no black space between the red and blue pixels in the lateral colour displays, indicating that the pixel colour-coding has gone off the top of the red colours and wrapped round to the blue colours. However, there is a black space between the colour displays centrally, indicating reversal of flow direction in relation to the transducer.

beam they cause small fluctuations in the level of the reflected ultrasound. When this reflected signal is mixed with the reference signal in the instrument, fluctuations occur in the resultant processed signal which resembles a Doppler flow signal.

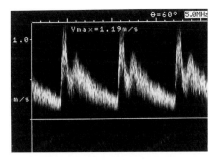

A

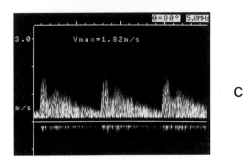

B

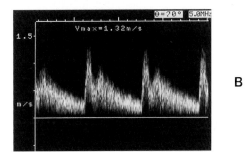

C

Fig. 1.14 Variation of quality of signal with beam–vessel angle: (a) at 60°; (b) at 70°; (c) at 80°.

Colour Doppler images obtained at 90° to the direction of flow appear dark or noisy, corresponding to absent or slow flow (Fig. 1.3). Power Doppler images are relatively insensitive to angle, except near 90°, where the low Doppler frequencies may fall below the clutter filter and no power signal is displayed (Fig. 1.3).

In a vessel in which the direction of flow alters with respect to the ultrasound beam, different regions of the vessel will be colour-coded differently. Note that this may be due to a genuine change in flow direction as seen in the normal carotid bulb, or merely due to the changing beam angle which is particularly common in sector scan imaging.

Effect of velocity scale

The choice of velocity scale can dramatically change the appearance of a colour flow image (Fig. 1.15). The scale should be chosen to accommodate the range of velocities thought to be present. Too low a scale will cause aliasing and too high a scale results in the flow being depicted as a few dark colours in colour Doppler imaging.

Unexpected machine artefacts

Doppler technology is developing rapidly and can still have gremlins in it. The operator must therefore check the performance and calibration of the instrument. This is most readily done in a situation where the flow pattern is considered to be well understood, such as in a clearly seen normal blood vessel or a flow test-object. Fig. 1.16 shows an unexpected artefact in which the maximum velocity measured varies with the beam position in the field of view. This has arisen because the transducer aperture used is a different size in the different positions, resulting in a different amount of spectral broadening.

Interference from neighbouring vessels

If part or all of a neighbouring vessel in addition to the vessel of interest is within the sample volume of a CW or PW instrument, the Doppler signal will contain a contribution from the extra vessel. Moving the sample volume or redirecting the ultrasound beam to try to interrogate only the vessel of interest may reduce this artefact.

Vessel compression

It is easy to compress superficial vessels by transducer pressure. Increased velocity of flow through the restriction in the compressed vessel results in a higher-pitched Doppler sound or a colour change in an image.

Factors affecting the patient

It is necessary to have as complete a knowledge as possible of the patient's physiological status

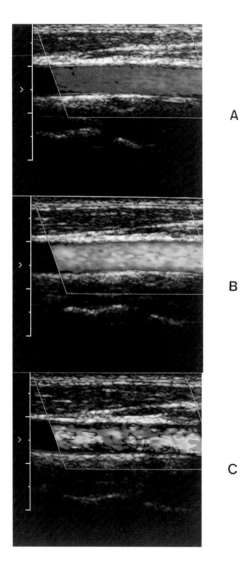

A

B

C

Fig. 1.15 Effect of changing velocity scale. (a) maximum velocity 77 cm s^{-1}, (b) maximum velocity 32 cm s^{-1}, (c) maximum velocity 8 cm s^{-1}.

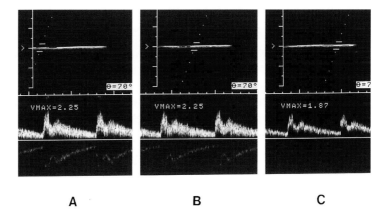

A   B   C

Fig. 1.16 Variation of sonogram for different beam positions in the field of view. A wider aperture is used near the centre of the array to increase focusing. This increases the range of angles of approach of ultrasound and hence increases spectral broadening.

when undertaking blood flow studies, since many factors affect the cardiovascular system. Examples of these factors are exercise, heart rate, temperature, anxiety, posture, food, smoking and other drugs.

Patient or vessel movement

If movement causes the sample volume of a CW or PW beam to interrogate a different region, the blood flow signal will obviously be altered. It can be difficult to eliminate this factor, especially in abdominal examinations, and it is not always clear whether respiration has actually affected the flow or just moved the vessel.

Flash artefact

Movement of the patient, an organ, or the transducer during Doppler imaging gives tissues a velocity relative to the transducer and hence scattered ultrasound is Doppler shifted; a large area of the image is therefore colour-coded for the duration of the movement. This artefact is more severe with power Doppler imaging due to its increased sensitivity.

Beam position within the vessel lumen

The Doppler signal obtained from a vessel depends on how the beam insonates the vessel.

The effect is less marked if the beam is wider than the vessel. A narrow beam through the centre of a vessel, however, overemphasizes the high velocities while a beam through the side of the vessel detects lower velocities.

One-dimensional scan

Blood flow often occurs in an unknown direction in space in relation to the transducer, for example in the heart or at a vessel bifurcation. Detecting the flow from one direction only measures the velocity component along that beam direction. Measurement of the actual velocity in these situations requires components to be measured in three directions not in the same plane. However, when laminar flow occurs in a vessel lying in an imaging scan plane, measurement of one velocity component and the beam–vessel angle permits measurement of the actual velocity.

SAFETY AND PRUDENT USE OF DOPPLER INSTRUMENTS

Ultrasound beams transmit energy into tissue so the possibility of hazard has to be considered. The most likely mechanisms for harmful effects are thought to be tissue heating as the ultrasound energy is absorbed, or cavitation in which microbubbles in the tissue react violently under the influence of the pressure fluctuations of the ultrasound field. The most sensitive structures are considered to be the developing fetus, the brain, the eye, the lung and bone–tissue interfaces.

There is a considerable amount of literature on bioeffects and safety of diagnostic ultrasound. The literature is scrutinized by several national and international bodies who produce statements on safety and the prudent use of ultrasound. Two active organizations are the European Federation of Societies for Ultrasound in Medicine and Biology (EFSUMB) and the American Institute of Ultrasound in Medicine (AIUM). It is still true to say that there are no confirmed harmful effects of diagnostic ultrasound. Often the possibility of an effect is reported but it is not confirmed by further work. There is a need for well-controlled studies but these are increasingly difficult to conduct since unscanned control populations are almost non-existent in the developed world. Although no harmful effects have been confirmed, there is some concern that the outputs of machines have been increasing by factors of as much as 3 or 5 since 1991, as manufacturers seek to produce better B-mode images and more sensitive Doppler units[15]. The situation is summed up in a commentary by ter Haar[16].

Until the early 1990s, attempts were made to specify the maximum intensities permissible for different clinical applications. This proved to be limiting and impractical, so the approach now is to use the ALARA principle (As Low As Reasonably Achievable) borrowed from the field of ionizing radiations. The user is now informed of the output of the machine and has the responsibility to keep the exposure to a low value which will still give a diagnosis. Some systems will display the output on the screen in terms of a thermal index (TI), related to tissue heating, and a mechanical index (MI), related to the possibility of producing cavitation. These indices are defined in the Output Display Standard (ODS)[17] developed in the USA.

EFSUMB puts out an annual statement on safety and in its most recent statement it says that the use of B-mode is not contraindicated in routine scanning during pregnancy[18]. However, it is more cautious with regard to pulsed Doppler, saying 'routine examination of the developing embryo during the particularly sensitive period of organogenesis using pulsed Doppler devices is considered to be inadvisable at present'.

Technical factors affecting prudent use and safety

1. Use the lowest transmit power which will give a diagnostic result. This involves keeping the MI and TI less than 1 if possible.
2. Use high receiver gain rather than high output power to achieve high sensitivity.
3. Use the minimum scan time possible.
4. Check that the transducer ceases to transmit when the imaging mode is frozen.
5. Take particular care when the fixed beam direction PW Doppler mode is being used near sensitive tissues.
6. Compare the maximum output values (intensity, power, pressure amplitudes) for your machine to those quoted in the published data of equipment surveys.
7. Safety considerations related to contrast agents need to be studied at frequent intervals during their developmental stage.

REFERENCES

1. White DN (1982) Johann Christian Doppler and his effect – a brief history. *Ultrasound Medicine and Biology* 8: 583–591
2. McDicken WN (1991) *Diagnostic Ultrasonics: Principles and Use of Instruments*. London: Churchill Livingstone
3. Evans DH, McDicken WN, Skidmore R, Woodcock JP (1989) *Doppler Ultrasound: Physics, Instrumentation and Clinical Applications*. Chichester: Wiley
4. Hoskins PR (1990) Measurement of arterial blood flow by Doppler ultrasound. *Clinical Physics and Physiological Measurement* 11: 1–26
5. Taylor KJW, Burns PN, Wells PNT (1988) Clinical applications of Doppler ultrasound. New York: Raven Press
6. Fish P (1990) *Physics and Instrumentation of Diagnostic Medical Ultrasound*. Chichester: Wiley
7. Wells PNT (1969) A range-gated ultrasonic Doppler system. *Medical and Biological Engineering* 7: 641–652
8. Kasai C, Namekawa K, Koyano A, Omoto R (1985) Real-time two-dimensional blood flow imaging using an autocorrelation technique. *Institute of Electrical and Electronics Engineers Transactions in Sonography and Ultrasonography* 32: 458–464
9. Rubin JM, Bude RO, Carson PL, Bree RL, Adler RS (1994) Power Doppler US: a potentially useful alternative to mean-frequency based colour Doppler US. Radiology 190: 853–856
10. Ophir J, Parker KJ (1989) Contrast agents in diagnostic ultrasound. *Ultrasound Medicine and Biology* 15: 319–333
11. Bommer WJ, Shah P, Allen H, Meltzer R, Kisslo J (1984) The safety of contrast echocardiography – report of the Committee on Contrast Echocardiography for the American Society of Echocardiography. *Journal of the American College of Cardiology* 3: 6–13
12. Williams AR, Kubowicz G, Cramer E, Schlief R (1991) The effects of the microbubble suspension SHU 454 (Echovist) on ultrasound-induced cell lysis in a rotating tube exposure system. *Echocardiography* 8: 423–433
13. Burns PN, Powers JE, Fritzsch T (1992) Harmonic imaging; new imaging and Doppler method for contrast-enhanced ultrasound. *Radiology* 182: 142
14. Porter TA, Xie F (1995) Transient myocardial contrast after initial exposure to diagnostic ultrasound pressures with minute doses of intravenously injected microbubbles. *Circulation* 92: 2391–2395
15. Henderson J, Willson K, Jago JR, Whittingham TA (1995) A survey of the acoustic outputs of diagnostic ultrasound equipment in current clinical use. *Ultrasound Medicine and Biology* 21: 669–705
16. ter Haar G (1996) Commentary: safety of diagnostic ultrasound. *British Journal of Radiology* 69: 1083–1085
17. American Institute of Ultrasound in Medicine/ National Electrical Manufacturers Association (1992) Standard for real-time display of thermal and mechanical acoustic output indices on diagnostic ultrasound equipment. American Institute of Ultrasound in Medicine. Rockville, MD
18. European Federation of Societies for Ultrasound in Medicine (1995) Clinical safety statement. *European Journal of Ultrasound* 2: 77

Haemodynamics and blood flow

2

PETER R. HOSKINS, W. NORMAN McDICKEN and PAUL L. ALLAN

PRINCIPLES OF BLOOD FLOW

This section describes the simple principles of blood flow which are of value in understanding the role of Doppler and for performing vascular ultrasound examinations. The underlying principles of fluid mechanics applied to the flow of blood are a complex subject, which is discussed in detail in a number of texts including those by McDonald[1], Caro *et al*[2], Strackee and Westerhof[3], and chapters in the Doppler ultrasound books by Evans *et al*[4] and Taylor *et al*[5].

The blood vessels carry blood from the heart through the pulmonary and systemic arterial circulations and back to the heart through the venous network. Atheroma develops in the arteries and impedes the flow of blood to a greater, or lesser, extent depending on the degree of obstruction that results from its presence.

Types of flow

The two essential flow states are laminar and turbulent. At low velocity, fluid flow is laminar (Fig. 2.1a). This is characterized by the motion of fluid along well-defined paths called streamlines. At very high velocities, fluid flow is turbulent (Fig. 2.1b); particular elements of the fluid no longer travel along well-defined paths, and there is a random component to the motion of the fluid.

Concepts of laminar and turbulent flow first arose from consideration of flow in long straight tubes. It was found that a dimensionless number called the Reynolds number (*Re*)

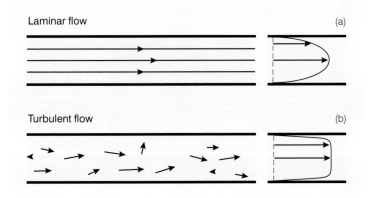

Fig. 2.1(a) Laminar flow consists of flow along well-defined streamlines; the velocity profile in a long straight tube under conditions of steady flow is parabolic. (b) The velocity vector magnitude and direction in turbulent flow have random components; the time-averaged profile is blunt.

Laminar flow (a)

Turbulent flow (b)

27

was useful in characterizing the fluid flow. The Reynolds number is defined as:

$$Re = \frac{\rho L V}{\mu}$$

where ρ is the fluid density, L is the vessel diameter, V is the mean velocity and μ is the fluid viscosity. For a wide variety of fluids the transition to turbulence takes place at a value of Re of about 2000. For flow in which Re is about 2000 the fluid flow will alternate between turbulent and laminar. When velocity is increased so that the Reynolds number is above the critical value, turbulence will take a small amount of time to develop. During pulsatile flow it is therefore possible for the flow to be laminar at values of Reynolds number higher than the critical value, because turbulence does not have time to develop before the blood velocity has decreased.

There is also a third flow state called disturbed flow, which refers to variations in velocity magnitude and direction which occur at low values of Reynolds number. The most important phenomenon is that of vortices, which are regions of circulating flow often produced when there is some obvious change in vessel geometry such as a stenosis, or the normal carotid bulb. The pattern of vortex production will change as the degree of stenosis and blood velocity increase. During steady flow at low Reynolds number the vortex will be stable and limited to the region immediately behind the stenosis. At low velocity the fluid flow within the vortex is actually laminar. At higher Reynolds number there will be vortex shedding at regular time intervals. Again this is not strictly turbulence, as the velocity magnitude and direction at any location is not random, but follows a regular pattern. At even higher Reynolds number the vortex shedding will be combined with the random flow patterns of true turbulence. Vortices which are shed travel a few diameters downstream and eventually die out as their energy is absorbed through viscous losses. During pulsatile flow, vortex shedding may occur for only a portion of the cardiac cycle.

The effect of the flow state on the Doppler waveform is illustrated in Fig. 2.2. Doppler spectra are shown from the normal femoral artery in Fig. 2.2a; in this case flow is laminar.

(a)

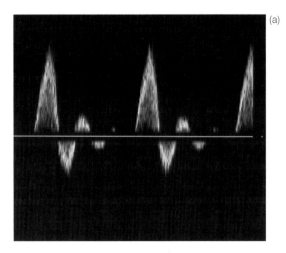

(b)

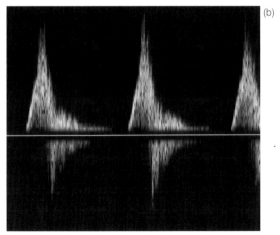

Fig. 2.2 Femoral artery Doppler waveforms. (a) From a normal segment; the waveform has a smooth outline and the spectral width is low. (b) From the poststenotic region; in the early systolic phase the waveform has a clearly defined outline associated with the passage of blood which was at rest in the poststenotic region during diastole through the insonation site. In the later part of the waveform, blood which has passed through the stenosis has developed turbulent, disturbed flow with increased velocity. This appears as a region in which there is spectral broadening and high-frequency spikes.

Within the sample volume the blood velocity magnitude and direction is similar for all of the red cells, hence the spectral width is low and the waveform outline is smooth. In the post-stenotic region of a diseased artery the Doppler waveform is more complex (Fig. 2.2b). The blood which was at rest in the poststenotic region during diastole is accelerated through the sample volume. For this blood, flow is laminar and the initial up-slope of the wave-form has a smooth outline with low spectral width, whereas blood which was in the prestenotic region during diastole has to pass through the stenosis, producing disturbed and turbulent flow within the sample volume. The variation in velocity magnitude and direction which this produces results in an increase in the spectral width (Fig. 2.2b), and the waveform outline is no longer smooth.

In the normal circulation, flow is mostly laminar; however, disturbed flow may occur in particular vessels such as the carotid arteries. Flow recirculation is commonly seen in the region of the bulb and there may be disturbed flow in the distal region. For the purposes of clinical Doppler ultrasound, very little prac-tical distinction is made between disturbed and turbulent flow. The presence of spectral broad-ening is often indicative of pathological change in the vessel. A summary of points concerning flow state is given below:

1. In the normal circulation, flow is mostly laminar.
2. Disturbed flow may occur in particular vessels, e.g. in the region of the carotid bulb.
3. Disturbed and turbulent flow occur in the poststenotic region.
4. Disturbed and turbulent flow both give rise to spectral broadening.

Pressure and energy

In the circulation the essential principle is that a pressure gradient must be created in order for blood to flow, this is produced by the contrac-tion of the heart and the resultant ejection of blood into the aorta and systemic vessels.

Energy is a useful concept in fluid mechanics. When there is steady flow of an incompressible frictionless fluid, the principles of conservation of energy can be used to give Bernoulli's equation.

Energy associated with blood pressure	+
Kinetic energy of moving blood	+
Potential energy associated with the height of the fluid above ground	= Constant

This is a simple expression which demonstrates that there will be an interchange between the different types of energy within the circulation. In the human body, however, the flow is non-steady and the above equation must be modi-fied slightly to account for the energy required to accelerate the fluid[4]. Energy is conserved in this simple ideal loss-less system. In the circula-tion, energy is lost in the form of heat through viscous effects, manifested through friction of the blood at the vessel wall and between adja-cent layers of blood. Energy losses are highest in the region of a stenosis, as there is consider-able friction during turbulent flow and vortex motion.

Within a stenosis there will be an increase in blood kinetic energy associated with increase in blood velocity, and according to the Bernoulli equation there is a corresponding fall in blood pressure. If there was no energy loss within the system then the decrease in velocity (and hence kinetic energy) in the poststenotic region would be compensated by a return of the pressure to the prestenotic level. In practice the loss of energy through turbulence and vortex shedding gives rise to a pressure drop across the stenosis whose magnitude is dependent on the degree of stenosis. These effects are explained in detail in Taylor et al[5].

The most common application of Bernoulli's equation is in the prediction of pressure drop across a stenosed cardiac valve[6]. The equation may be simplified to:

$$P = 4V^2$$

where V is the measured velocity in m s^{-1}, and P is the pressure drop in mmHg. Points concerning pressure and energy are summarized below:

1. The pressure drop across a stenosis is high as a result of energy loss in the poststenotic region.
2. For the estimation of the pressure drop across a cardiac valve stenosis, Bernoulli's equation may be simplified to $P = 4V^2$.

Velocity profiles

The Doppler ultrasound spectrum is critically related to the detailed variation of velocity within the vessel of interest. The velocity of the blood will vary as a function of its position within the vessel; this is called the velocity profile. The most commonly known velocity profile is called the parabolic velocity profile.

Strictly speaking, a parabolic velocity profile only applies to steady laminar flow in a long straight tube, when there is maximum velocity in the centre of the vessel and zero velocity at the edge of the vessel (Fig. 2.1a). The profile is radially symmetric, which means that it is the same regardless of which diameter is considered. The shape of the profile is an exact mathematical equation, that of a parabola.

Velocity profiles in vessels in the body are generally more complex, they may not be even

approximately radially symmetric and they vary with time during the cardiac cycle. It is worth exploring the various effects that will influence true velocity profiles in the circulation.

Entrance effect

The velocity profile in a vessel is strongly influenced by the distance of the region of interest from the entrance to the vessel. For a long straight vessel, when there is steady flow, the profile is initially flat at the entrance to the vessel. With increasing distance from the entrance the profile will change, becoming parabolic at a distance called the inlet length (Fig. 2.3).

Vessel narrowing

For steady flow, a gradual narrowing taper will tend to sharpen the velocity profile.

Vessel expansion

At regions where the cross-sectional area of the vessel increases, an adverse pressure gradient in the direction of flow is created; that is, there is a pressure decrease in the direction of flow, which tends to retard the flow. For the central high-velocity region, the high momentum opposes this, but at the edge of the vessel the velocities are low and the direction of motion near the wall will reverse if there is a sufficiently rapid increase in vessel cross-sectional

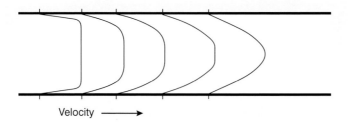

Velocity ⟶

Fig. 2.3 Velocity profiles during steady flow at different distances from the entrance to a long straight tube from a reservoir. The parabolic velocity profile is restored at a distance from the entrance, the 'inlet length'. Redrawn from Caro *et al*[2].

area with distance. The phrase 'flow separation' is often used to describe this phenomenon; that is, the high-velocity central jet is located next to a region in which the flow is of low velocity and recirculating. The production of vortices was noted above; both the central jet and vortices die out after a length equivalent to a few diameters and laminar flow is re-established. Fig. 2.4 shows the velocity profiles in the region of a small stenosis. When the expansion is less severe, such as a gradually widening taper, the velocity profile simply becomes more blunted.

Curved vessels

Fig. 2.5 shows that the velocity profile for steady flow in a curved vessel is skewed towards the outer wall when the entrance profile is parabolic, and skewed towards the inner wall when the entrance profile is flat.

Y-shaped junction

Fig. 2.6 shows the velocity profiles from a Y-shaped junction and it can be seen that the profiles are skewed within the two branches, so that the higher velocities occur on the inner aspects of the two branches.

Pulsatile flow

During pulsatile flow the velocity profile will vary throughout the cardiac cycle. Fig. 2.7 shows the profiles from a long straight tube

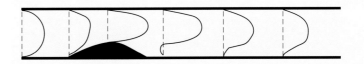

Fig. 2.4 Velocity profiles from a stenosis model; the region of recirculation in the poststenotic region can be seen on the lower aspect.

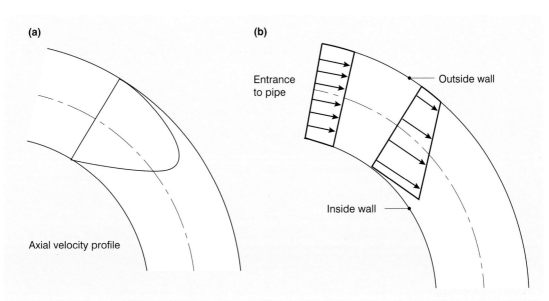

Fig. 2.5 Velocity profiles within a curved vessel during steady flow. (a) A parabolic velocity profile at the entrance results in higher velocities on the outer aspect of the curve. (b) A blunt velocity profile at the entrance results in the higher velocities occurring on the inner aspect. Reproduced from Caro *et al*[2].

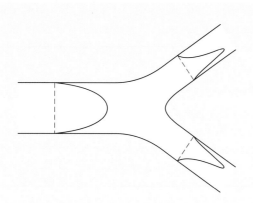

Fig. 2.6 Velocity profiles in a Y-shaped junction with skewing of the velocity profile and higher velocities on the inner aspects of the two branches.

with a velocity waveform similar to that found in the femoral artery.

Turbulence

As discussed above, the velocities during turbulence have a random component, so that it is necessary to take an average value over time. If this is done, then the averaged velocity profile during steady turbulent flow is found to be blunted, with high-velocity gradients near to the vessel wall (Fig. 2.1b).

Secondary flow motions

In many of the geometrical situations described above the components of flow are three-dimensional, which means that there will be some secondary flow motion in the plane perpendicular to the vessel axis. These motions may easily be demonstrated using flow models and dye-injection techniques, and there are a few *in vivo* studies which claim to have demonstrated this[7,8]. A summary of points concerning velocity profiles is given below:

1. Velocity profiles are influenced by a large number of factors, and it generally cannot be assumed that the profile is parabolic.
2. The displayed Doppler spectrum will be critically related to the velocity profile present within the sample volume of the Doppler system.
3. In the absence of arterial stenosis, it is best to align the beam axis with the vessel axis in order to obtain a waveform with a clearly defined outline.

A simple flow model

The creation of a pressure gradient within the arterial system is performed by ejection of

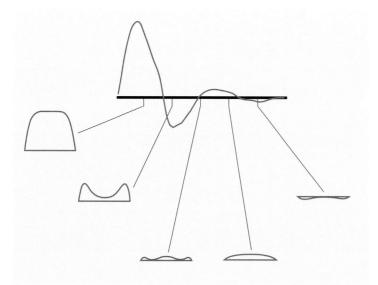

Fig. 2.7 Changes in the velocity profiles at various moments during pulsatile flow for a velocity waveform similar to that found in the femoral artery. Reproduced from Evans *et al*[4].

blood into the arterial tree by the heart. The resistance R to flow of a vessel segment may be defined as:

$$R = \frac{(P_1 - P_2)}{Q}$$

where Q is the flow through the vessel, and P_1 and P_2 are the pressures at the entrance and exit points of the vessel. One way of expressing this equation is to say that in order to maintain flow at a constant level, the pressure difference must be greater when the resistance to flow increases. Strictly speaking this formula only applies for steady flow conditions, it is therefore useful mainly as an aid in understanding general concepts of flow in arteries, and a more complex version of this equation must be used for pulsatile flow. For a long straight vessel the resistance to flow depends on the fourth power of the diameter. A segment of vessel 2 mm in diameter will therefore have a resistance 16 times that of a similar segment of 4 mm diameter.

A simple model of the flow to an organ is shown in Fig. 2.8. The net flow is controlled by a combination of the small vessel (arteriolar) resistance and the large vessel (arterial) resistance. In the non-diseased circulation, the main arteries have relatively large diameters and their resistance to flow is small; the main resistance vessels are the arterioles. The essential clinical manifestations of atherosclerosis may be understood with the aid of this model; an increase in resistance in a large distributing artery because of atheroma must be compensated by a decrease in the resistance of the small arteries and arterioles in order to preserve flow to the capillary bed. As the disease progresses, flow is maintained by

arteriolar dilatation until the point is reached where the arteriolar network is fully dilated. Further progression of the proximal disease results in a reduction in flow to the organ and the development of ischaemia because no further compensatory dilatation is achievable. In patients with lower limb claudication, the presence of severe proximal disease results in the distal arteriolar network being fully dilated at rest in order to maintain flow to the lower limb muscles. Whilst this is sufficient in the resting limb, the combination of the proximal stenosis and the maximum arteriolar dilatation means that no further increase in flow can be obtained to cope with the increased metabolic demands of limb exercise.

The concept of a critical stenosis follows from the above model. As the degree of narrowing at a single, isolated stenosis increases, a point is reached at which the distal arteriolar dilatation is maximum. Consequently, any increase in the degree of stenosis beyond this point leads to a reduction in flow. Experiments performed on animals suggest that this point of critical stenosis is reached with an area reduction of about 75%, which corresponds to a diameter reduction of approximately 50%. Two quantities of interest in Doppler ultrasound are the volume flow rate and the velocity of the blood; the relationship between these two parameters, according to the model developed above, is shown in Fig. 2.9[9]. As the calibre of the vessel is reduced, the volume of blood flowing along the vessel is maintained by increasing the velocity. However, above the point of critical stenosis (75% area stenosis), the volume of blood starts

Fig. 2.8 A simple model of flow from the heart to an organ through a large vessel (arterial) and small vessels (arterioles) to the capillary bed.

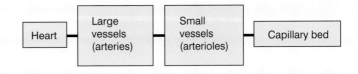

2

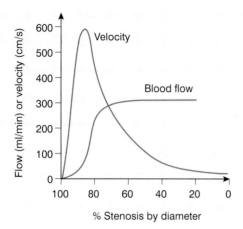

Fig. 2.9 Flow rate and velocity based upon a single arterial stenosis inserted into an otherwise normal artery. Redrawn from Spencer and Reid[9].

is an increase in the extraction efficiency of oxygen from blood. A summary for this section is given below:

1. The degree of constriction of the distal arteriolar bed is one factor used to control the flow rate to the organ.
2. As the resistance to flow of diseased arteries increases, flow rate is maintained within normal levels as a result of distal arteriolar dilatation.
3. Very high degrees of stenosis are accompanied by a low flow rate and low velocities.

Pulsatile flow and distal resistance

Doppler ultrasound is commonly used to assess distal resistance to flow. The origin of pulsatile waveforms and their relation to distal resistance are considered here.

For a particular element of blood it is the pressure gradient, not the actual pressure, which accelerates the blood. The pressure gradient is related to the difference between the pressures on either side of the element of blood (Fig. 2.10). When the pressure gradient is positive the blood will be accelerated along the vessel; when the gradient is negative the blood will be decelerated. The corresponding flow waveform is found by detailed calculation of the pressure gradient at the site of interest.

The blood ejected by the heart passes into the aorta. This causes local expansion of the aorta and distal arteries due to the local high pressure. The expanded region passes down the arterial tree in the form of a pressure wave (Fig. 2.11). If the artery were long and straight

to reduce. It should also be noted that the velocity peaks at about 85% diameter stenosis, subsequently tailing off, so that in very tight stenoses the velocity is relatively low.

Two stenoses in series have a larger overall resistance compared with either stenosis considered individually. In practice the combined resistance of stenoses in series is dominated by the one with the smallest luminal diameter.

The concept of a critical stenosis is useful but its application to atherosclerosis should not be taken too far. As atherosclerosis develops, various other compensatory mechanisms come into play in an attempt to preserve perfusion. These include the development of a collateral circulation and a degree of local dilatation of the affected arterial segment. In addition, there

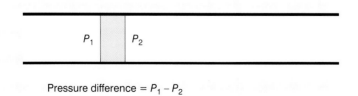

Fig. 2.10 The force acting on an element of blood is related to the difference in pressures on either side of that element.

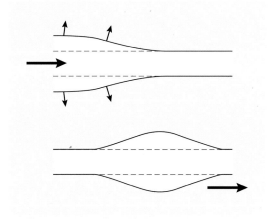

Fig. 2.11 The blood ejected by the heart causes expansion of the elastic arteries. This expansion passes down the arteries in the form of pressure and flow waves.

then, at a particular location along the vessel, the pressure would reach a maximum and then decline to the baseline value (Fig. 2.12a), resulting in a flow waveform with forward

flow only (Fig. 2.12b)[10]. In practice the pressure waves are reflected, primarily by the arteriolar network (Fig. 2.13), where there is an alteration, or mismatch, in the resistance to flow, with the arteriolar network having a higher resistance than the proximal arteries. The reflected pressure wave travels up the arterial tree and interacts with the forward-going pressure wave (Fig. 2.14). The resultant flow waveform has a period of negative flow (Fig. 2.15). The amplitude of the reflected pressure waves will depend on the extent of the mismatch in resistance; that is, the amplitude will depend on the state of constriction of the arteriolar bed. The consequence of this is that the degree of pulsatility of the velocity waveform will be related to the distal resistance to flow. This simple relation has been experimentally proven to work in some instances, such as the fetal placental circulation[11]. In this case, the normal placenta has a low resistance to flow and umbilical waveforms show flow throughout the cardiac cycle. Absent end-diastolic flow is associated with increased resistance to flow and abnormal placental development; there is an increased incidence of fetal compromise. A summary of this section is given below:

1. Reflected pressure waves from the distal arteriolar bed interact with the forward-

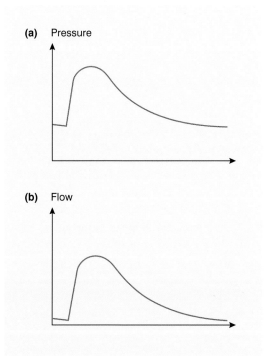

(a) Pressure

(b) Flow

Fig. 2.12 (a) and (b) Pressure and flow waves in the absence of distal reflection. Redrawn from Murgo et al[10].

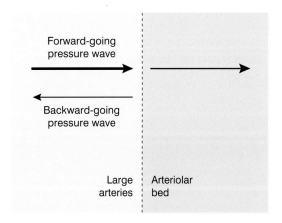

Forward-going pressure wave

Backward-going pressure wave

Large arteries   Arteriolar bed

Fig. 2.13 Reflected pressure and flow waves are produced from the distal arteriolar bed.

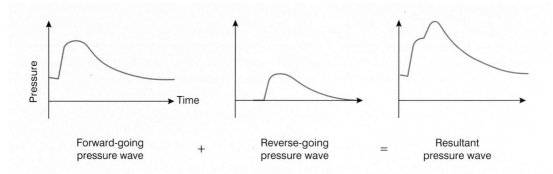

Fig. 2.14 The resultant pressure wave is a combination of the forward-going wave and the reverse-going wave.

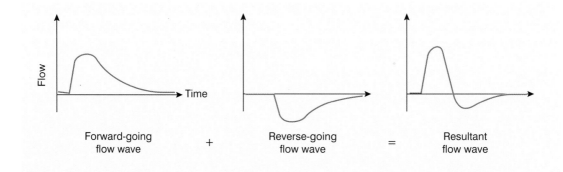

Fig. 2.15 The resultant flow wave can be considered to be a combination of a forward-going flow wave and a reverse-going flow wave.

going waves to produce the waveform causing increases in pulsatility of the flow waveform.

2. For some arteries the waveform pulsatility as measured using Doppler ultrasound may be a clinically useful indicator of disease.

QUANTITATIVE FLOW MEASUREMENT

Whilst it is possible to measure blood flow quantitatively, the error is usually rather large, probably between 20 and 100%[12, 13]. In some applications such errors may be tolerable, for instance when a large change in flow in the order of 300% from normal to abnormal flow exists. However, one factor which mitigates against blood flow being a sensitive indicator of disease affecting an organ or limb is that circulatory regulatory mechanisms can often

maintain the level of blood supply until the disease is quite advanced.

A variety of factors must be borne in mind when considering volume flow calculations in relation to the circulation of blood:

1. Flow is pulsatile, therefore the velocity varies over the cardiac cycle. The velocity also varies across the vessel lumen. In addition, turbulence and disturbed flow will result in vectors of flow off the central axis of the vessel, leading to inaccurate angle estimation and correction. Complex flow patterns can occur in curved vessels and near bifurcations, so that the assumption of laminar or plug flow should be carefully examined for each application. Turbulence observed in a sonogram or colour Doppler image makes accurate measurement of volume flow impossible.

2. In practice it is difficult to ensure uniform insonation of a blood vessel, and the resultant error in instantaneous average velocity can be very large, perhaps greater than 50%. Maximum velocity, for use in the calculation of instantaneous average velocity (see below), can be measured to around 5% by ensuring that the ultrasound beam passes through the centre of the vessel. It should always be borne in mind that spectral broadening errors can be large, up to 50%, when maximum velocity is measured by wide-aperture arrays[14].

3. The calibre of compliant arteries varies with the cardiac cycle. Pulsation of an artery can change its cross-section by up to 20%, hence an instantaneous diameter measurement (see below) should be used if possible.

4. The accuracy of the measurement of the vessel diameter, or cross-sectional area, is inversely related to the size of the vessel and measurement errors are usually quite large, up to 20% for a 10 mm diameter vessel, rendering the technique of doubtful value for small vessels. The cross-sectional area and the velocity should be measured at the same site; in addition, errors will occur if the scan plane is not exactly at right angles to the axis of the vessel. Special efforts should be made to reduce the error in diameter measurement, since diameter is squared in the formula for cross-section (area = πr^2) and this increases the error.

5. For laminar flow in a straight vessel the beam–vessel angle can be determined to within 2° or 3°. However, even with this accuracy, if the beam–vessel angle is made greater than 60°, the error in the calculated velocity rapidly rises above 10%, so that the calculated velocities will have significant errors associated with them in this situation.

Knowing the sources of error, steps may be taken to minimize them. A simple approach to measurement is based on the formula:

Instantaneous flow rate = instantaneous cross-section × instantaneous average velocity

'Instantaneous' means the value measured at the point in the cardiac cycle being considered.

The instantaneous average velocity may be calculated by taking the average of the velocities in the spectral display. Both the power level of each velocity in the spectrum and the velocity itself are used in this calculation. The power level for each velocity is a measure of the number of cells moving with that velocity. For this calculation to be accurate, the vessel must be uniformly insonated, which is not easy to achieve due to beam misalignment and distortion.

Another way to obtain the instantaneous average velocity is to measure the maximum velocity and assume a profile for the velocities across the vessel, for example a plug or a parabolic profile. With plug flow all of the blood cells are travelling with the same velocity, so the instantaneous average velocity equals the maximum. For parabolic flow the instantaneous average velocity equals half of the maximum velocity. The maximum velocity is readily measured from a spectral display, provided that part of the beam passes through the centre of the vessel.

The instantaneous cross-section is most easily calculated from the instantaneous diameter measured from an M-scan generated simultaneously with the sonogram; the assumption of a circular cross-section for a given diameter appears to be reasonable for arteries and introduces little error. The diameter can also be obtained from a B-scan provided that it is recorded at the same time and the same location as the spectrum being used from the sonogram.

Averaging the instantaneous flow rate over the cardiac cycle gives the average flow rate.

In practice, these measurements may not be easily achieved on some systems and the following is a more practical formula to use for volume flow rate, in ml min^{-1}.

Flow rate (ml min^{-1}) = TAV_{mean} (cm s^{-1}) × area (cm^2) × 60

In these cases the time-averaged maximum velocity (TAV_{max}) can be calculated over several cardiac cycles and, assuming parabolic flow, divided by two to give a calculated time-averaged mean velocity (TAV_{mean}). Some systems will calculate the time-averaged mean velocity directly from the spectral display. Similarly, only a few systems will provide a time-averaged diameter measurement and therefore an instantaneous diameter measurement must be used to calculate area, usually from an image frozen in systole. Alternatively, the area of the vessel can be measured directly from a transverse image of the vessel, providing care is taken to ensure that the section is a true cross-section of the vessel made at systole.

Measurement of volumetric flow is difficult and not generally attempted, as it is easy to produce errors of 100%[12], but there is little in the literature that gives accurate data on errors in practice. In general terms it should be considered as a research tool and the results treated with suitable caution with regard to the potential errors.

CONCLUSIONS

The study of haemodynamics involves the application of the principles of fluid mechanics to blood flow in the circulation and provides an insight into the events which occur in both normal and diseased vessels. It is essential to have an understanding of these haemodynamic principles in order to be able to carry out Doppler examinations and to understand the findings which are obtained during the procedures.

REFERENCES

1. McDonald DA (1974) *Blood Flow in Arteries*. London: Edward Arnold
2. Caro CG, Pedley TJ, Schroter RC, Seed WA (1978) *The Mechanics of the Circulation*. Oxford: Oxford University Press
3. Strackee J, Westerhof N (1993) *The Physics of Heart and Circulation*. Bristol: Institute of Physics
4. Evans DH, McDicken WN, Skidmore R, Woodcock JP (1989) *Doppler ultrasound: Physics, Instrumentation and Clinical Applications*. Chichester: Wiley
5. Taylor KJW, Burns PN, Wells PNT (1995) *Clinical Applications of Doppler Ultrasound*. New York: Raven Press
6. Holen J, Aaslid R, Landmark K, Simonsen S (1976) Determination of pressure gradient in mitral stenoses with a non-invasive ultrasound Doppler technique. *Acta Medica Scandinavica* 199: 455–460
7. Hoskins PR, Fleming A, Stonebridge P, Allan PL, Cameron DC (1994) Scan-plane vector maps and secondary flow motions. *European Journal of Ultrasound* 1: 159–169
8. Stonebridge PA, Hoskins PR, Allan PL, Belch JFF (1996) Spiral laminar flow in vivo. *Clinical Science* 91: 17–21
9. Spencer MP, Reid JM (1979) Quantitation of carotid stenosis with continuous wave (CW) Doppler ultrasound. *Stroke* 10: 326–330
10. Murgo JP, Col MC, Westerhof N, Giolma JP, Altobelli SA (1981) Manipulation of ascending aortic pressure and flow waveform reflections with the Valsalva manoeuvre: relationship to input impedance. *Circulation* 63: 122–132
11. Adamson SL, Morrow RJ, Langille BL, Bull SB, Ritchie JWK (1990) Site-dependent effects of increases in placental vascular resistance on the umbilical arterial velocity waveform in fetal sheep. *Ultrasound in Medicine and Biology* 16: 19–27
12. Evans DH (1986) Can ultrasonic duplex scanners really measure volumetric flow? In: Evans JA (ed.) *Physics in Medical Ultrasound*. York: Institute of Physical Sciences in Medicine
13. Gill RW (1985) Measurement of blood flow by ultrasound: accuracy and sources of error. Ultrasound in Medicine and Biology 11: 625–641
14. Hoskins PR (1996) Accuracy of maximum velocity estimates made using Doppler ultrasound systems. *British Journal of Radiology* 69: 172–177

The carotid and vertebral arteries; transcranial colour Doppler

PAUL L. ALLAN

THE CAROTID AND VERTEBRAL ARTERIES

Indications

Ultrasound of the extracranial cerebral circulation is used predominantly in the assessment of patients with symptoms which might arise from disease in the carotid arteries, such as amaurosis fugax and transient ischaemic attacks (TIA), in order to identify those patients with significant changes who will benefit from surgery. Two major trials have shown that endarterectomy for symptomatic patients with significant stenoses confers a significant advantage over medical management in terms of reducing morbidity and mortality[1,2]. The European Carotid Surgery Trial (ECST) data showed that, during the follow-up period, the percentage of subjects having ischaemic symptoms lasting more than 7 days was 16.8% for those on medical management, compared with 2.8% if surgery was performed. There was no significant advantage in having surgery with stenoses less than 30%. With regard to intermediate degrees of stenosis (30–69%), the initial analysis of the ECST data shows no advantage for surgery in these patients[3]. The main indications for ultrasound of the carotids are shown in Table 3.1.

Cerebral ischaemic symptoms

There are many causes of cerebral ischaemic symptoms apart from disease at the carotid bifurcation. These include cardiac arrhythmias, hypotensive episodes, emboli and atheromatous disease elsewhere in the circulation between the heart and the intracerebral arterioles. Many of these can be treated with medical therapy but it is only the extracranial section of the carotid artery which is amenable to surgery, and it is for this reason that so much effort is devoted to the assessment of this area. The main aim is to classify patients into five main groups.

1. Those without significant disease.
2. Those with mild disease (<50% diameter reduction), who will benefit from medical therapy if they are symptomatic.
3. Those with more severe disease (50–70% diameter stenosis), who will be treated medically and followed to assess progression of disease, particularly if they are symptomatic.

Table 3.1 Indications for carotid ultrasound.

- Transient ischaemic attacks (TIA)
- Reversible ischaemic neurological deficits (RIND)
- Mild resolving strokes in younger patients
- Atypical, non-focal symptoms which may have a vascular aetiology
- Arteriopaths/high-risk patients prior to surgery
- Post-endarterectomy
- Pulsatile neck masses
- Trauma, or dissection
- Screening for disease

39

4. Those patients with severe disease (>70% diameter reduction) who will benefit from surgery if they are symptomatic.

5. Those patients with a complete occlusion, who are therefore not candidates for surgery.

The relationship between the presence of carotid artery disease and the development of cerebral ischaemic symptoms is not straightforward and detailed discussion of this subject is beyond the scope of this book. However, patients who have suffered from temporary ischaemic symptoms, such as TIA, reversible ischaemic neurological deficits (RIND), or amaurosis fugax, are significantly more likely to suffer a stroke than asymptomatic subjects: 36% of patients who have a TIA will have an infarct within 5 years of the TIA, compared with an annual stroke rate of 1% for asymptomatic, elderly individuals[4]. Therefore it is reasonable to investigate patients with reversible ischaemic cerebral symptoms in order to identify those with a 70% or greater stenosis who will benefit from endarterectomy. Those with lesser degrees of stenosis can be treated medically and followed up; those who progress to more than 70% diameter stenosis can then be considered for surgery.

The situation regarding the examination of patients with asymptomatic carotid bruits is also complex. The authors, along with many people, would wish to know the status of their arteries if they were found to have an asymptomatic carotid bruit. Although the risk of ipsilateral stroke from an asymptomatic carotid stenosis is low, the Asymptomatic Carotid Atherosclerosis Study (ACAS) has reported that surgery is beneficial in reducing the risk of subsequent ipsilateral stroke by some 5% in asymptomatic patients with a stenosis of more than 60% diameter reduction, providing that the centre has a perioperative morbidity/mortality rate of less than 3%[5]. Ultrasound will therefore have a role in the identification of those patients who will be considered for

surgery. However, if there is a policy not to offer surgery to asymptomatic patients, then it might be argued that an ultrasound examination is unnecessary.

The policy for ultrasound in patients with strokes needs some consideration. Patients with a significant, persistent, established neurological deficit will not benefit from carotid surgery. Whereas individuals with a mild, resolving deficit, who are otherwise candidates for carotid endarterectomy, may be considered for surgery. It is therefore reasonable to suggest that an ultrasound examination is of benefit in younger patients with milder, resolving neurological deficits; whereas it is of little value in older patients with more permanent neurological signs.

Atypical symptoms

Some patients have unusual symptoms which may or may not be related to carotid disease. Atypical migraine, hyperventilation attacks and temporal lobe epilepsy may sometimes be difficult to diagnose and, in some patients, the possibility of carotid disease might be considered. Ultrasound is of value in excluding carotid disease as a cause of the symptoms in this group of patients, although some care must be given to patient selection to prevent large numbers of unnecessary examinations.

Patients at risk of perioperative stroke

Arterial disease is usually a generalized process, although it affects different arterial territories to varying degrees. Therefore, patients undergoing surgery for conditions such as coronary artery disease, peripheral arterial disease and aortic aneurysms may also have significant carotid disease; there is concern that perioperative morbidity from strokes can be increased in these patients as a result of emboli or inadequate perfusion. Diabetics can also have severe arterial disease and are at risk from perioperative strokes when undergoing major surgery.

Ivey *et al*[6] showed that there was no increase in risk associated with asymptomatic bruits in these patients, even if there was a haemodynamically significant stenosis; although they felt that patients with a bruit and a history of ischaemic symptoms should be considered for a staged, or simultaneous, endarterectomy if they were shown to have a stenosis of greater than 70% diameter reduction. However, this decision would depend on the relative urgency of the primary condition and many centres, whilst taking note of the carotid disease, will proceed with the main operation and consider subsequent endarterectomy in symptomatic patients.

Postendarterectomy patients

Complications following endarterectomy can be divided into three groups based on the timing of the events.

1. Early occlusion due to thrombosis, occurring within the first 24–48 hours after the operation.
2. Stenosis developing over 12–18 months due to neo-intimal hyperplasia.
3. Recurrence of atheroma over a period of several years resulting in restenosis.

Colour Doppler ultrasound provides a rapid and straightforward method for diagnosis of these complications.

Routine follow-up of asymptomatic patients is not justified by the pick-up rate for developing significant recurrent stenoses[7], but any patient suffering symptoms related to the operated side should be examined by colour Doppler in the first instance.

Pulsatile masses

Colour Doppler ultrasound provides a rapid technique for the assessment of pulsatile neck lumps. There are a variety of causes for these, the main ones are listed in Table 3.2.

Table 3.2 Causes of pulsatile neck masses.

- Normal but prominent carotid artery and bulb
- Ectatic carotid, innominate or subclavian artery
- Aneurysm of the carotid artery
- Carotid body tumour
- Enlarged lymph node adjacent to carotid sheath

Carotid dissection

Dissection of the carotid artery may develop from a variety of causes.

1. It may occur spontaneously consequent upon atheroma.
2. It may result from the extension of an aortic arch dissection.
3. It may develop following trauma to the neck such as occurs in whiplash injuries.
4. As a result of iatrogenic causes, such as carotid catheterization.

Colour Doppler can be used to identify different flow patterns on either side of the flap, or the presence of a thrombosed channel, and monitor subsequent progress.

Epidemiological studies and monitoring of therapy

The carotids provide a convenient window for the assessment of the whole arterial system. Patterns of development of atheroma vary for different arterial areas. Nevertheless it could be expected that changes in the carotids might be related to disease in other vessels, such as the coronary arteries, and that the changes in the carotids might allow some prediction of severity of this disease. In addition their examination could also provide a method for assessing the rate of progression, or regression of disease, if treatment regimens are being investigated, or epidemiological studies are being performed.

By far the largest group of patients will fall into the first group of indications relating to the diagnosis of carotid atheroma and stenosis as a cause of cerebral ischaemic symptoms. In the end the aim of the sonographer is to identify patients with carotid disease which may be the cause of their symptoms, and to assess the severity of the disease so that appropriate management decisions in relation to surgery or medical management can be taken.

Anatomy and scanning technique

The main steps in the examination are given in Table 3.3. The patient lies supine, with their neck a little extended by placing a pillow under their shoulders. The patient should be comfortable and excessive extension of the neck should be avoided. In addition, some patients with carotid or veretebral disease may find that neck extension compromises the flow of blood to the cerebral circulation, so if the patient appears to be asleep it is worth checking that they have not lost consciousness. Some patients may not be able to lie supine; if this is the case they can usually be examined adequately in a sitting position.

The examiner can sit beside the patient's thorax and scan the neck from this position, or sit at the patient's head and scan the neck from this location; this latter arrangement was favoured in the early days of carotid ultrasound as it was easier to obtain a standardized probe position, but it is no longer necessary with modern duplex or colour Doppler equipment. Furthermore, using this position at the head of the patient for carotid scanning during a general ultrasound list means that the couch and machine have to be moved around in the middle of the list, which is disruptive and time-consuming.

A high-frequency transducer (7–10 MHz) is used and the examination starts with a transverse scan of the carotid artery from as low in the neck as possible, to as high in the neck as possible behind the angle of the mandible. This approach will allow the depth and course of the vessels to be ascertained, together with the level of the bifurcation and the orientation of its branches (Fig. 3.1). In addition, areas of major disease will be identified and can be noted for further assessment.

Colour Doppler is then activated and the vessels are examined in the longitudinal plane, again from the lower neck upwards. Areas of abnormal flow are identified with colour Doppler, an initial assessment of their significance is made and the need to undertake a spectral examination can be considered. Just as

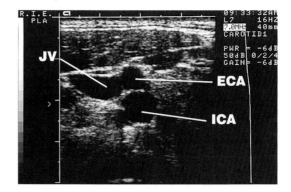

Fig. 3.1 The right carotid bifurcation on transverse scanning. The external carotid artery (ECA) lies anteriorly with the jugular vein lying adjacent to it (JV), the internal carotid artery (ICA) lies behind the ECA.

Table 3.3 Basic steps in the examination.

1. Transverse scan from low in the neck up to behind the angle of the mandible to locate bifurcation
2. Longitudinal colour scan to identify areas of abnormal flow and disease
3. Positive identification of the external carotid artery and internal carotid artery
4. Spectral Doppler
    (a) in normal vessels take readings from common carotid artery, internal carotid artery, external carotid artery
    (b) in abnormal vessels take readings from areas of disease in addition to standard readings from common carotid artery, internal carotid artery, external carotid artery
5. Examine the vertebral arteries

importantly, areas of normal flow are seen so that the normal segments of the vessel can be identified rapidly and excluded from further investigation (Fig. 3.2). It may be necessary to try a variety of scan planes in order to see the bifurcation in some subjects; the normal approach is from an anterolateral or lateral direction but more posterior planes may be required and, in a few individuals, the approach may be from under the mastoid process and behind the sternomastoid muscle. In patients who have undergone recent carotid surgery, access can be problematical due to the skin incision and oedema of the soft tissues, so that a variety of approaches may need to be tried; sufficient information can usually be obtained to confirm flow in the vessel, or the absence of flow. Beards are not usually a problem but if they are particularly extensive and luxuriant they may interfere with access; liberal application of gel usually allows access to the carotids, although there is some impairment of resolution.

Identification of the internal and external carotid arteries

The common carotid artery on the right arises from the innominate artery behind the right sternoclavicular joint (Fig. 3.3), where the origin can usually be seen on ultrasound. On the left it usually arises directly from the aorta, so that its origin on the left cannot be seen on scanning from the neck. The level of the carotid bifurcation is usually at about the

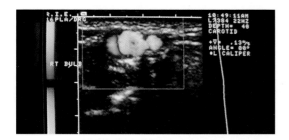

Fig. 3.2 Transverse colour Doppler image of the carotid bifurcation. The normal area of reversed flow is seen in the bulb of the internal carotid artery, represented in blue.

level of the upper border of the laryngeal cartilage but it may vary considerably. The two branches of the common carotid artery are the internal carotid artery and the external carotid artery. It is essential that they are identified positively, otherwise there is the possibility that disease in one vessel will be mistakenly attributed to the other, which may lead to further inappropriate investigations. The external carotid artery is usually the easier of the two branches at the bifurcation to recognize positively and the criteria to look for are listed in Table 3.4.

The external carotid artery has branches just above the bifurcation (Fig. 3.4); the superior thyroid, ascending pharyngeal and lingual arteries may all arise from the external carotid artery below, or around, the level of the angle of the mandible.

The external carotid artery is nearly always the more anterior of the two branches. In one study it lay anteromedial to the internal carotid artery in 48.5% of bifurcations studied, anterior in 34.5% and anterolateral in 13%; other positions accounted for only 4% of vessels[8].

The external carotid artery supplies the relatively high-resistance vascular bed of the facial muscles, pharynx, tongue and scalp. Therefore the external carotid artery has relatively less diastolic flow, which makes it appear more pulsatile on colour Doppler and to have a characteristic waveform on spectral Doppler with relatively low diastolic flow (Fig. 3.5a). In addition the dichrotic notch of the pulse wave is usually more prominent in the external carotid artery spectrum than in the internal carotid artery spectrum.

The superficial temporal artery is one of the terminal branches of the external carotid artery, and if this is tapped by a finger as it passes over the zygoma it will produce rapid, clear fluctuations in the waveform in the external carotid artery, whereas there is little or no effect in the ipsilateral common carotid artery or internal carotid artery.

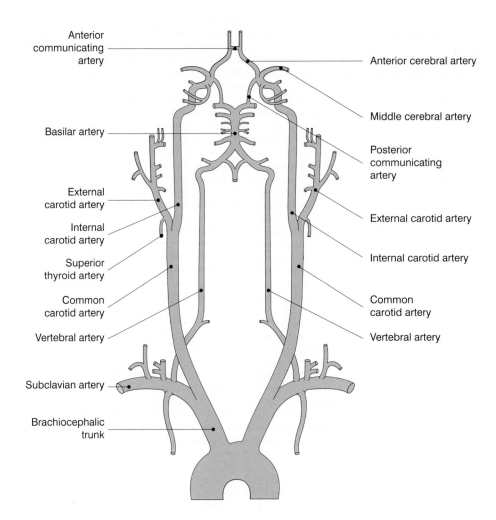

Fig. 3.3 Carotid and vertebral arteries.

Once the external carotid artery has been identified positively then it can be assumed that the other large vessel arising from the carotid bifurcation is the internal carotid artery. This vessel is nearly always the more posterior of the two branches and tends to run deeply and more posteriorly. It does not have visible branches at this level but the bulge of the carotid bulb is usually apparent in subjects without severe disease. The spectrum is less pulsatile and more sustained than that of the external carotid artery, with relatively high diastolic flow (Fig. 3.5b).

Diseased vessels may be more difficult to distinguish as plaques can obscure visual details; local and remote disease can lead to alterations in the normal patterns of flow, so that distinction on the basis of the appearance of the waveform may be impossible. In addition some high bifurcations are very difficult to see well enough to allow reliable assessment.

Standard velocity measurements

Once the bifurcation and its branches have been identified and assuming that no areas of significant disease are present, it is good practice to

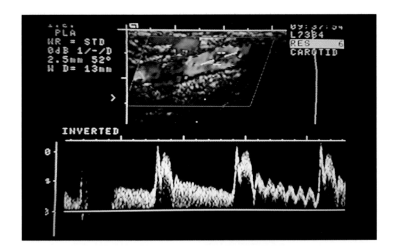

Fig. 3.4 The external carotid artery showing a branch arising just above the bifurcation and fluctuations induced in the spectrum by tapping the superficial temporal artery at the level of the zygoma.

Table 3.4 Identification of the external and internal carotid arteries.

The external carotid artery
Branches present
Anterior position
Waveform characteristics:
High resistance pattern with relatively little diastolic flow
Appears more pulsatile on colour Doppler
Dichrotic notch is more prominent
Positive 'temporal tap'

The internal carotid artery
The other branch of the bifurcation
Bulb at origin
Posterior position and course angled posteriorly
Less pulsatile waveform on colour Doppler with relatively high diastolic flow

take peak systolic velocity measurements from the common carotid artery, the internal carotid artery and the external carotid artery in order to have a record of the examination. These are obtained using spectral Doppler from the upper common carotid artery 2–3 cm below the bifurcation; the internal carotid artery from 1–2 cm above the bulb, or as high as possible, in order to allow the normal bulbar turbulence to settle; and from the lower external carotid artery. For routine measurements the sample volume is set at about half the total diameter and placed in the centre of the vessel in order to avoid the natural turbulence at the edge of the lumen and 'wall

thump' from inclusion of the vessel wall in the sample volume. The Doppler angle is kept as low as possible, ideally less than 60°, certainly less than 70°; it is good practice to try and keep to a specific angle, such as 55° or 60°, in order to improve the reproducibility of results between examinations. For tight stenoses it is better to reduce the size of the sample volume, as this allows the area of the peak systolic flow signal to be better defined. The precise final location of the sample volume is chosen using a combination of the audible Doppler signal and the spectrum so that the clearest, highest-frequency audible signal and the best spectral trace are obtained.

Measuring the intima-medial thickness (IMT)

This is not always required but should it need to be measured, for instance as part of a population survey, then it can be measured on an image of the distal common carotid wall where the echoes from the intima–media complex are most easily distinguished. The machine settings should be set to give a clear, uncluttered image of the vessel wall and the position of the transducer adjusted to show the characteristic double-line appearance of the vessel wall (Fig. 3.6). The image should be magnified as much as possible to make the measurement easier to perform. The IMT is best demonstrated in the

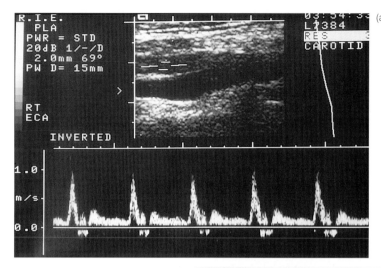

(a)

Fig. 3.5 (a) The external carotid artery and the characteristic spectrum seen in normal vessels. There is relatively low diastolic flow and a prominent dichrotic notch compared with the spectrum from the internal carotid artery. (b) The internal carotid artery and its characteristic spectrum with more flow throughout diastole.

(b)

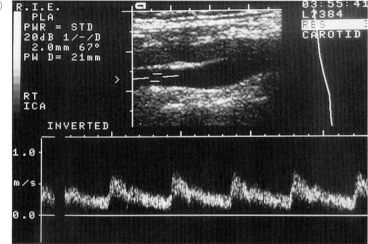

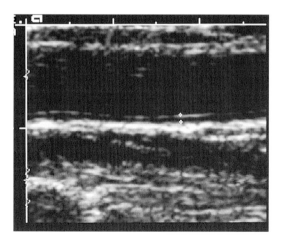

Fig. 3.6 A normal IMT of 0.6 mm measured in the upper common carotid artery.

upper common carotid artery where the vessel is usually at right angles to the ultrasound beam. The internal carotid artery is more difficult to assess as the vessel slopes obliquely away from the transducer face in many cases. With careful attention to detail it is possible to measure the IMT with satisfactory, reproducible accuracy. The precise upper limit of the normal range is a matter of some discussion. It does increase with age but values of less than 0.8 mm correlate well with lack of coronary artery disease, whereas an increasing thickness above this level (Fig. 3.7) is associated with increasingly severe coronary artery disease[9] and an increased risk of myocardial infarction[10].

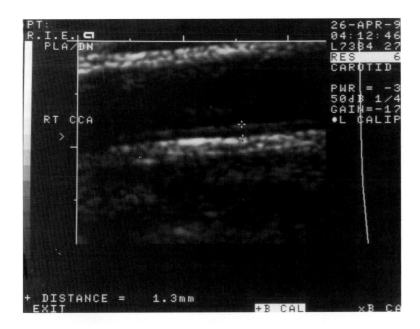

Fig. 3.7 Thickening of the IMT which has been shown to correlate with an increased incidence of coronary artery disease.

The vertebral arteries

Once both carotids have been examined the vertebral arteries are assessed. The vertebral artery on each side is the first branch of the subclavian artery (Fig. 3.3). It passes posteriorly and upwards to the vertebral foramen in the transverse process of the sixth cervical vertebra, and from there it passes upwards in the vertebral canal to the level of the axis (C2). It emerges from the vertebral canal at C2, passing behind the lateral mass of the atlas (C1) to enter the skull through the foramen magnum and join with the vessel from the other side in front of the brain stem to form the basilar artery.

The vertebral arteries are most easily located by placing the transducer longitudinally over the common carotid artery and angling it medially so that the vertebral bodies are identified; the transducer is then moved laterally so that the transverse processes of the vertebrae and the spaces between them are visualized, the vertebral artery and vein may then be seen in these gaps (Fig. 3.8). If the vertebral artery cannot be identified in the vertebral canal, it may be looked for in the lower neck as it passes backwards from the subclavian artery towards C6; or in the upper neck behind the mastoid process as it passes around the atlas (C1) and into the foramen magnum.

There may be marked variation in the size of the vertebral arteries and their relative contribution to basilar artery flow; when there is disparity of size, the left artery is usually the larger of the two and in 7–10% of individuals there are significant segments of hypoplasia, which result in the artery not being visible[11]. Clear visualization of the vein but not the artery suggests that the artery may be either thrombosed or congenitally absent.

Colour Doppler makes assessment of flow direction in the vertebral arteries straightforward (Fig. 3.9). They should have the same colour as the common carotid artery in front of them. Care needs to be taken in the diagnosis of reversed flow, particularly if the spectral Doppler trace has been inverted during the examination: if subclavian steal is suspected it is worth confirming that the machine is set up appropriately in order to avoid making an error. In some patients reversed flow may only occur with the arm in certain positions, or after a period of exercise;

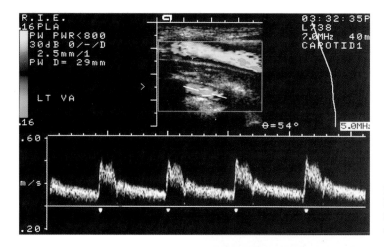

Fig. 3.8 The vertebral artery seen between the transverse processes of the cervical vertebrae. The vertebral artery is the same colour as the CCA.

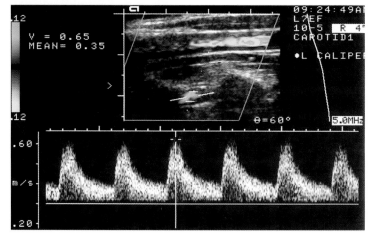

Fig. 3.9 Reversed flow in the vertebral artery in a patient with a proximal left subclavian artery stenosis. The vertebral artery is the opposite colour (blue) from the CCA.

therefore scanning after a period of arm exercise, such as elbow flexions holding a book, or some other relatively heavy object, should be considered if the history is suggestive of a steal syndrome. Alternatively a pressure cuff can be inflated to occlude blood flow to the arm and then released after 2–3 min. The resulting reactive hyperaemia produces an increased demand for blood and reversal of flow in the relevant vertebral artery.

Assessment of disease

Measurement of the degree of stenosis

Two types of information can be used to assess the degree of stenosis: direct measurement

using the callipers on the machine; and velocity criteria derived from spectral Doppler.

Direct visualization and measurement

If the stenosis and plaque can be seen clearly then it is possible to measure the calibre of the residual lumen and the original calibre of the vessel. Diameter reduction ratios, or area reduction ratios, are the usual methods for describing the reduction in vessel calibre; percentage residual lumen can also be used. Diameter measurements are generally a little quicker to perform but are slightly less representative of the stenosis, as they do not take account of variations in plaque thickness around the circumference of the vessel and there is the potential to underestimate, or overestimate, the degree of

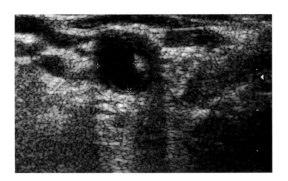

Fig. 3.10 Transverse view of a plaque in the common carotid artery with the diameter reduction calculated from the diameter measurements. Note that an inappropriate longitudinal scan plane (x–x) could result in a significant underestimation of the degree of stenosis.

stenosis (Fig. 3.10). Care must be taken to examine a diseased segment of vessel in both transverse and longitudinal views so that the distribution of plaque can be clearly assessed and the most appropriate diameter measurement can be made; this is usually the shortest diameter. Measuring stenoses by area reduction, although more time-consuming, overcomes this problem with the eccentricity of the plaque being taken into account as the luminal and vessel areas are measured.

It is important that the type of measurement used is clearly defined as either a diameter reduction or an area reduction, because significant misunderstandings may occur in the interpretation of the results. For a given stenosis, a 50% diameter reduction corresponds to a 70% area reduction, so that misinterpretation of a 70% area stenosis as a diameter reduction will result in a significant overestimation in the assessment of calibre reduction, possibly leading to unwarranted surgery (Fig. 3.11). It is good practice always to define the value of a stenosis as either an area or a diameter reduction and this is essential if the measurement is in a different form from that normally used.

Most stenoses are relatively short in longitudinal extent, usually no more than a centimetre for the maximum degree of narrowing. Some patients, however, have longer segments of varying calibre reduction and it is important to remember that, although the degree of pressure drop across a stenosis is related primarily to the reduction in radius, it is also related to the length of the stenosis. However, length has a much smaller effect, as the resistance is related to the first power of the length, rather than the fourth power of the radius (Poiseuille's Law):

$$R = \frac{8l\eta}{\pi r^4}$$

Doppler criteria

In many cases the region of the stenosis is not seen clearly due to complex plaque structure and calcification. In these cases direct measurement cannot be used to quantify the degree of stenosis and Doppler criteria must be used. Over the years, much work has been done correlating

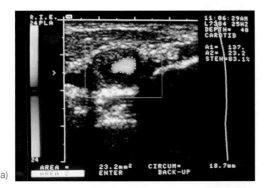

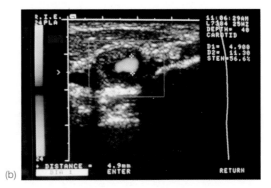

Fig. 3.11 A stenosis measured with (a) an area-reduction calculation and (b) a diameter-reduction calculation. Note that the same calibre reduction gives an area reduction of 83%, and a diameter reduction of 56%.

Doppler findings with degrees of stenosis found on arteriography, or at surgery. It has been shown that carefully obtained Doppler criteria correspond well with the degree of stenosis, and values which allow the severity of internal carotid artery stenoses to be predicted have been developed. However, the literature can be confusing, with apparently widely varying velocities being quoted for specific levels of stenosis. One of the first studies suggested that a peak systolic velocity of >1.3 m s^{-1} was appropriate for diagnosis of a diameter stenosis of 60% or greater[12]. However, other workers have reported velocities of 1.7 m s^{-1} for a 60% stenosis[13], 2.25 m s^{-1} for a 70% stenosis[14] and 1.3 m s^{-1} for 70% diameter stenosis[15]. This apparent lack of consensus emphasizes the fact that there is some variation from one department to another depending on the equipment and technique used. Each department must therefore develop and audit criteria which they find work in their environment and complement the clinical criteria and practices used in their institution.

The peak systolic velocity (PSV), end-diastolic velocity (EDV) and the ratio of peak systolic velocities in the internal and common carotid arteries (IC/CC systolic ratio) are the most useful measurements in general practice[14]

(Fig. 3.12). Spectral broadening and filling in of the window under the spectrum are subjective, difficult to quantify and can be affected significantly by gain control settings; however, they do indicate abnormal flow if they are present. The IC/CC diastolic ratio can also be measured but this does not usually add to the information obtained from the three main criteria. The main levels which need to be distinguished are 50% diameter reduction, where blood flow starts to decline, and 70% diameter reduction, which is the level strongly associated with clinical symptoms and for which surgery will be considered. The values for the criteria which the authors have found to be useful in their practice to predict these levels of stenosis in the internal carotid artery are shown in Table 3.5 and are based on those reported by Robinson et al[14]. It is important to remember that the peak systolic and diastolic values refer only to the internal carotid artery, not to the common carotid artery or external carotid artery. Furthermore, it should be borne in mind that physiological variations due to heart rate, cardiac output and contralateral occlusion may affect the velocities in a vessel, potentially leading to a false diagnosis of a pathologically high velocity, although these cases should be clarified by the use of the

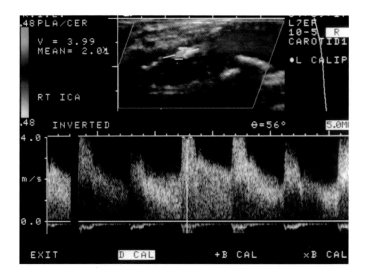

Fig. 3.12 A stenosis of the internal carotid artery showing a peak systolic velocity of nearly 4 m s^{-1} and an end-diastolic velocity of over 2 m s^{-1}.

Table 3.5 Diagnostic criteria for Doppler diagnosis of stenoses of 50% and 70%. Based on Robinson et al[14].

Diameter stenosis %	Peak systolic velocity ICA[a] m s^{-1}	End diastolic velocity ICA[a] m s^{-1}	IC/CC systolic ratio
50	>1.5	>0.5	>2
70	>2.3	>0.75	>3

[a]ICA = internal carotid artery.

velocity ratios. It should also be remembered that peak velocities decline with very high degrees of stenosis (>90% diameter stenosis).

Attempts have been made to use colour Doppler criteria to assess the severity of stenoses[16]. In addition to the direct measurement of the residual lumen demonstrated by the colour map, a cursor with angle correction can be placed over the colour map and used to provide an estimate of the mean velocity in the underlying pixel. This allows the mean velocities in a stenotic segment to be estimated. However, these correlate less well with the degree of stenosis than peak systolic or diastolic velocities. Although experienced operators can often get a good idea of the severity of a stenosis from the colour map changes, it is better to use the colour map to identify areas of abnormal flow and to position the sample volume for spectral Doppler analysis.

Effects of disease elsewhere

The velocities and flow characteristics seen in any given section of a vessel depend not only on local conditions but also on conditions elsewhere along the vessel, in other vessels connected to that vascular territory and to other factors, such as heart rate, cardiac output and blood pressure (Table 3.6). The best example of this is vertebral or subclavian steal, where a proximal occlusion of the subclavian artery results in reversed flow in the ipsilateral vertebral artery. Carotid occlusion can lead to an increase in the volume of blood flow in the contralateral carotid. This is achieved by the blood flowing more quickly, therefore there is the potential to mistakenly suggest that an increased velocity

measurement is compatible with a degree of stenosis. The use of ratios, mainly the IC/CC peak systolic ratio, helps identify such a situation as the velocity in both the common carotid artery and the internal carotid artery is increased and the ratio does not alter; whereas if there is local disease affecting the internal carotid artery, velocities in this vessel are increased but the common carotid artery velocities are unchanged, so that the ratio is also increased.

Carotid occlusion

Occlusion can affect the internal carotid artery or common carotid artery separately, or together. Occlusion of the common carotid artery does not always result in occlusion of the internal carotid artery, as sufficient blood flow may be provided by retrograde flow down the ipsilateral external carotid artery to maintain patency of the internal carotid artery. This pattern of abnormal flow may be quite confusing if it is not recognized but it is of clinical importance, as these patients can still suffer ischaemic events in the relevant internal carotid artery territory. If an occlusion is suspected it is essential that care is taken to ensure that the Doppler settings on the

Table 3.6 Factors affecting the waveform.

Local	Atheroma and plaques Tortuosity
Proximal	Common carotid artery origin disease Aortic valve disease
Distal	Carotid siphon disease Intracranial vessel disease
Remote	Contralateral carotid occlusion
Physiological	High cardiac output states

machine are appropriate for locating any low-velocity, small-volume flow that may be present in a narrow residual lumen in the segment under investigation. Spectral Doppler must be carefully performed and colour Doppler can help in the diagnosis of occlusion, as it allows a better appreciation of adjacent vessels or collateral channels which might be confused with an occluded carotid[17], giving a mistaken impression of flow. Conversely, colour Doppler or power Doppler may show the location of a residual channel in a vessel that was otherwise thought to be occluded; echo-enhancing agents are of value if there is any persisting uncertainty.

Occlusion of the internal carotid artery results in the reduction of diastolic flow in the ipsilateral common carotid artery, so that the common carotid artery waveform becomes more like that seen in the external carotid artery. Reduction of common carotid artery diastolic flow may therefore be an initial clue to the presence of an internal carotid artery occlusion, or a very severe stenosis. Care should be taken, however, as the development of collateral channels between the external carotid artery and internal carotid artery circulations in the orbit and meninges can result in 'internalization' of the external carotid artery flow with relatively high diastolic flow in the external carotid artery; this results in a mistaken impression of a patent internal carotid artery, if it is not recognized. The 'temporal tap' manoeuvre can usually clarify the situation.

If there is occlusion of both the internal carotid artery and external carotid artery then the ipsilateral common carotid artery also usually occludes. Before thrombosis occurs, however, a to-and-fro pattern of flow may be seen in the common carotid artery, which signifies that there is no net forward flow of blood up the vessel (Fig. 3.13).

Plaque characterization

Much effort has been expended in attempting to classify atheroma and plaques on ultrasound, particularly in the carotids, where high-resolution ultrasound gives good images of many plaques. Steffen *et al* proposed a classification of plaque which takes account of the different types of plaque and its components (Fig. 3.14)[18]. Types 1 and 2 were predominant in symptomatic arteries, whereas types 3 and 4 were more common in asymptomatic patients. This supports the suggestion that the more friable, lipid-containing, soft plaques are more

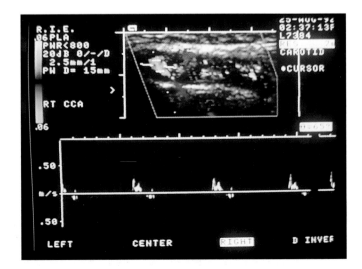

Fig. 3.13 Blood flow in the common carotid artery of a patient with distal occlusion showing alternating forward and reverse flow, the result of which is no forward flow up the vessel.

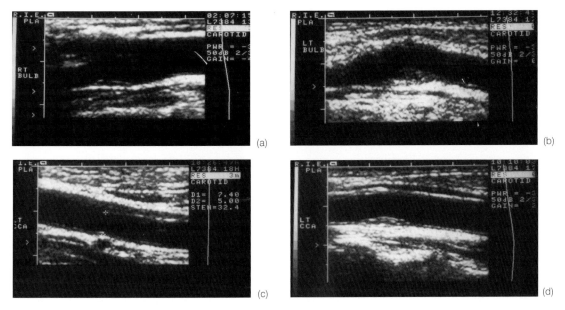

Fig. 3.14 Different types of plaque seen on ultrasound. (a) Type 1, dominantly echolucent with a thin echogenic cap. (b) Type 2, substantially echolucent lesions with small areas of echogenicity. (c) Type 3, dominantly echogenic lesions with small areas of echolucency of <25%. (d) Type 4, uniformly echogenic lesions.

likely to result in plaque disruption and produce symptoms than firmer, more fibrous and coherent plaques.

The value of ultrasound in predicting the complications associated with plaques is more difficult to define. These complications include intraplaque haemorrhage, surface ulceration and adherent thrombus. The presence of intraplaque haemorrhage has been inferred from the presence of hypoechoic areas within the plaque. However, it is also possible that many of these areas are aggregates of lipid rather than areas of haemorrhage. Sometimes an ulcer in the plaque can be clearly seen, but many plaques are irregular without being ulcerated and, conversely, an ulcerated plaque may not be identified on ultrasound. Thrombus adherent to the surface is suggested by an anechoic or hypoechoic area adjacent to the plaque surface on colour or power Doppler. It is important that the system is set up appropriately, otherwise the lack of colour on the image may be due to technical factors, rather than the presence of thrombus.

Some studies have shown a good correlation between the ultrasound appearances and those found at operation[19, 20], but the results from others have been less satisfactory, with poor prediction of ulceration or haemorrhage[21, 22]. However, if there is a good view of the diseased segment, the plaque can be described in terms of its type (1–4), extent (focal, diffuse, circumferential) and any obvious associated complications (ulceration, thrombus, haemorrhage) (Fig. 3.15). If visualization is moderate or poor then discretion is necessary and only those features which are clearly seen should be noted. For example, it may be difficult to distinguish between a plaque ulcer and a gap between two adjacent plaques, or to decide if a colour void associated with the plaque surface is really due to adherent thrombus or to technical factors.

An attempt has been made to standardize these descriptions for carotid disease in relation to ultrasound and other non-invasive modalities[23]. This proposes that lesions can be described in terms of the degree of

3

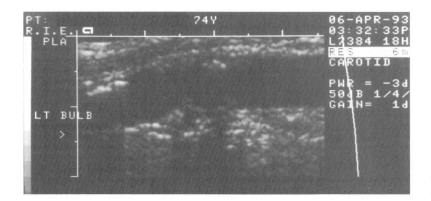

Fig. 3.15 An ulcerated plaque.

stenosis, the morphologic plaque components and the surface characteristics, where these can be clearly visualized. The suggested classification is given in Table 3.7. A lesion listed as H4, S2, P2 therefore represents a lesion which is producing a stenosis of more than 80% diameter reduction (H4), which has an irregular surface (S2) and is heterogeneous (P2).

In practical terms, a smooth, homogeneous, predominantly echogenic plaque is less likely to be associated with symptoms, whereas an irregular, heterogeneous or hypoechoic lesion is of greater concern. Ulceration should only be diagnosed if the plaque and the ulcer are clearly seen, otherwise plaques should be described as smooth or irregular. It should be remembered that

many diseased segments are not clearly seen due to the presence of calcification, which makes attempts at plaque characterization very difficult, or impossible.

Pulsatile masses

The main causes of pulsatile neck masses are given in Table 3.2. Normal but prominent carotids and ectatic carotid or subclavian arteries are easily identified with colour Doppler and do not usually require any further investigation.

Aneurysms of the carotid arteries can also be identified as they are in continuity with the artery (Fig. 3.16). The majority arise following surgery but they may also occur following trauma. The flow in the aneurysm may be seen with colour Doppler, unless there is thrombosis of the lumen of the dilated segment. In some cases of aneurysm of the common carotid artery, it may be difficult to identify the internal carotid artery above the dilatation and care must be taken to establish whether it is patent or not; flow in the ipsilateral ophthalmic artery is not necessarily evidence of patency, as this may come from collateral filling via the circle of Willis.

Lymph nodes and other masses adjacent to the carotids will transmit pulsations and require distinction from intrinsic vascular lesions. This

Table 3.7 Classification of carotid plaques. From Thiele et al[23].

Haemodynamic classification

H1	0–20% Diam. reduction	Normal to mild
H2	20–60% Diam. reduction	Moderate
H3	60–80% Diam. reduction	Severe
H4	80–99% Diam. reduction	Critical
H5	Occluded	

Morphological components

P1	Homogeneous
P2	Heterogeneous

Surface characteristics

S1	Smooth
S2	Irregular (defect <2 mm)
S3	Ulcerated (defect >2 mm)

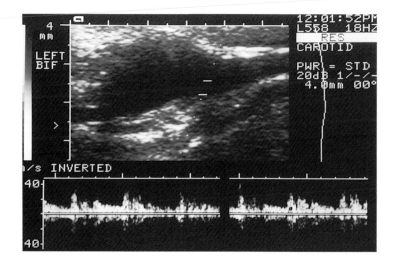

Fig. 3.16 An aneurysm of the origin of the internal carotid artery in a young patient who sustained a whiplash injury in a car accident.

is not usually a problem, but occasionally a deposit will surround the carotid artery (Fig. 3.17) and, unless there is a previous history of malignancy, diagnosis can be difficult. Adherence to the carotid sheath can be assessed by gentle palpation and getting the patient to swallow so that relative movement between the mass and the carotid can be assessed[24].

Carotid body tumours are rare tumours but can be diagnosed easily with ultrasound. Characteristically there is a hypoechoic mass between the two branches at the bifurcation, spreading them apart in a 'wine glass' deformity (Fig. 3.18). Colour Doppler shows a highly vascular lesion and the external carotid usually shows a low resistance pattern of flow on spectral Doppler[25].

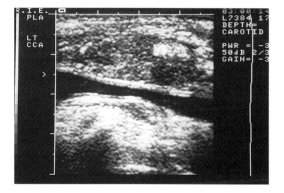

Fig. 3.17 Tumour recurrence from an oropharyngeal malignancy closely applied to the carotid sheath.

Dissection of the carotid arteries

The ultrasound findings in this condition can vary considerably. The vessel may be occluded completely; show a smooth tapering stenosis, with or without a recognizable haematoma/thrombosed false lumen being visible (Fig. 3.19); or a membrane with a double lumen may be seen with variable flow patterns in the two channels on either side[26]. Recanalization of the occluded vessel is a recognized occurrence and occurs in up to 60% of cases[27].

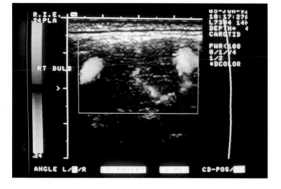

Fig. 3.18 A carotid body tumour splaying apart the internal carotid artery and external carotid artery. Colour Doppler shows the abnormal tumour circulation.

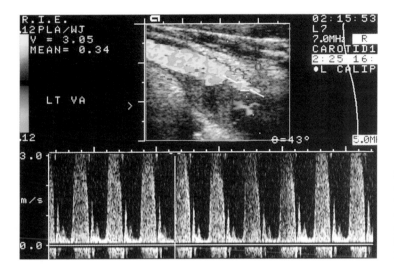

Fig. 3.19 Dissection of the common carotid artery extending up from a dissection of the aortic arch. One channel has thrombosed, producing a haematoma in the wall of the vessel posteriorly which is narrowing the residual lumen.

Problems and pitfalls in carotid ultrasound

Problems and pitfalls can arise from a variety of sources. These can be divided into those resulting from poor or faulty technique and those arising from pathological or physiological causes (Table 3.8). Technical aspects of setting up the system are discussed elsewhere (see Appendix 1) but other aspects which can lead to problems should be considered.

Long and eccentric lesions

The amount of pressure reduction across a stenosis is related primarily to the fourth power of the radius; however, as noted previously, it is also related to the length of the stenosis. This is not relevant for many stenoses, as they are relatively short, but some stenoses, particularly in the common carotid artery, may be longer. Therefore, whilst a 40% diameter stenosis extending over 5–8 mm length is not haemodynamically significant, a 40% diameter stenosis extending over 5–8 cm may well result in some reduction in pressure and a decrease in flow, resulting in cerebral perfusion problems in some circumstances, and this should be taken into account in the assessment of the patient.

Eccentric lesions may cause problems if the exact disposition of plaque around the circumference of the vessel is not appreciated (Fig. 3.10). Care should be taken to examine areas of disease transversely, as well as longitudinally, as discussed earlier. Another problem with eccentric lesions is that the high-velocity jet may emerge from the stenosis at an unusual angle that is not parallel to the vessel wall, as many people would assume. Colour Doppler is useful in identifying these oblique jets and allows for a more accurate angle correction to be achieved.

Tortuous vessels

Sharp twists in the course of a vessel result in changes to the pattern of blood flow in the lumen: blood on the outer margin flows faster

Table 3.8 Problems and pitfalls.

Technique related
Incorrect Doppler sample volume position or size
Doppler angle too large (>60–65°)
Doppler settings too high for low-velocity, low-volume flow
Good Doppler angles give poor images and vice versa

Disease related
Long lesions
Eccentric lesions
Tortuous vessels
High-grade stenosis
Lesions at the bifurcation
Disease elsewhere in the vascular tree

than blood on the inside of the bend (Fig. 2.5); in addition, turbulence is generated, even if plaques are not present. Furthermore, assessing the angle of flow for calculation of velocity can be difficult, so that accurate, representative velocities are hard to define, especially if there is associated disease. Whenever possible, flow characteristics should be assessed as far as possible from the curved segment.

High-grade stenoses

In critical stenoses (>90%) velocity decreases; in addition, there is only a small volume of blood flowing through the narrow residual lumen. The signal strength is therefore poor and the Doppler shift is lower than might be expected. It is important to ensure that the machine is set up appropriately to detect these weaker, lower Doppler shifts, if they are not to be missed and a false diagnosis of occlusion reached (Fig. 3.20). The higher sensitivity of power Doppler and the increase in signal strength obtained with echo-enhancing agents are two developments which both individually and together improve the success of ultrasound in discriminating between an occlusion and a small residual lumen[28].

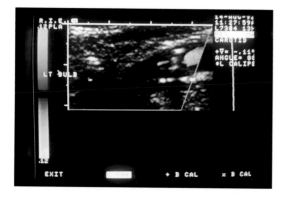

Fig. 3.20 A very severe/critical stenosis showing a small residual lumen and relatively low velocity in a patient with a stenosis in the region of 95% diameter reduction.

Lesions at the bifurcation

These can cause problems as a significant amount of plaque may be present in the bulb but, because of the relative dilatation of the lumen which is normally present here, this does not result in any narrowing of the flow channel between the common carotid artery and the internal carotid artery. Although this will not have any effect on the overall flow in the vessel, this disease may provide a source of emboli and may not be recognized if spectral criteria alone are used to identify stenotic segments, as there will not be a significant increase in velocity.

Disease elsewhere in the vascular tree

Vascular ultrasound allows direct assessment of much of the extracranial cerebral circulation from the clavicular region into the upper cervical area and disease in these segments can be measured directly. However, changes in vessels remote from those under examination may affect the findings at any given point. As discussed previously, contralateral occlusion results in increased flow through the patent carotid with higher than normal velocities as a result of this. Aortic valve stenosis or common carotid artery origin stenosis on the left will not be visualized directly on carotid examination; the presence of disease in these areas can only be inferred from damping of the waveform with, or without, turbulence. Similarly disease more distal in the carotid siphon region will not be detected by cervical carotid examination.

Accuracy in relation to other techniques

Arteriography

Many studies have shown that spectral Doppler and, more recently, colour Doppler have satisfactory accuracy in the diagnosis and assessment of disease when compared with arteriography. Some care must be taken when considering studies comparing the two techniques, as different types of angiography are used as the gold standard: direct carotid injection, arch injection, digital subtraction arteriography (DSA) and venous DSA have all been used. Different methods of measuring the degree of stenosis are also used (Fig. 3.21)[29–31]. These will result in different degrees of stenosis for a bifurcation lesion depending on whether the diameter of the residual lumen is compared with the diameter of the common carotid artery, the diameter of the internal carotid artery, the estimated diameter at the bulb as calculated from calcification in the wall, or from the alignment of the vessels. Indeed, the North American Symptomatic Carotid Endarterectomy Trial (NASCET) and ECST[1, 2] used different techniques for measuring the degree of angiographic stenosis, so that the results of the two studies are not directly comparable; an 80% ECST diameter stenosis for a given lesion corresponds to a stenosis of 50% in the NASCET study for the same lesion. There is also a degree of variation between different observers in the estimation of stenosis on arteriography, which may be up to 20%[32]. However, even allowing for these reservations, the overall performance of Doppler ultrasound compared with arteriography is good. Cardullo *et al*[33] reviewed 16 spectral Doppler studies with 2146 Doppler–arteriogram comparisons; non-colour duplex Doppler had an overall sensitivity of 96%, specificity of 86%, positive predictive value of 89%, negative predictive value of 94% and accuracy of 91% for the diagnosis of a diameter stenosis greater than 50%. Subsequently, further studies have confirmed the value of colour Doppler with similar or better levels of accuracy and also its value in improving diagnostic confidence, clarifying difficult situations and reducing exam-

1. ECST method

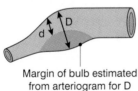

$$\frac{D - d}{D} = \% \text{ diameter stenosis}$$

Margin of bulb estimated from arteriogram for D

Example

$$\frac{10 - 2}{10} = 80\% \text{ diameter stenosis}$$

2. NASCET method

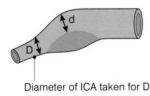

Diameter of ICA taken for D

Example

$$\frac{4 - 2}{4} = 50\% \text{ diameter stenosis}$$

3. Common carotid diameter method

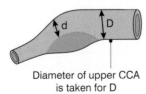

Diameter of upper CCA is taken for D

Example

$$\frac{8 - 2}{8} = 75\% \text{ diameter stenosis}$$

Fig. 3.21 Methods for estimating % diameter stenosis in arteriography.

ination times[34]. In particular the difficult distinction between a critical stenosis and a complete occlusion can be achieved in nearly all cases with the use of colour Doppler[17].

Magnetic resonance angiography and computed tomography angiography

Developments in computed tomography (CT) technology and techniques have made the use of CT for the assessment of larger vessels a realistic proposition. Magnetic resonance angiography (MRA) is also developing at a rapid pace. These two techniques have an advantage over ultrasound as they provide information on disease at the origins of the carotids and also in the intracranial circulation. However, they also have significant drawbacks: they both 'image' the blood and infer the wall characteristics from the shape of the blood flowing in the vessel, whereas colour Doppler provides information on the wall of the vessel as well as the flowing blood. MRA is still limited to some extent by signal voids at relatively high velocities, as well as problems from signals arising in plaque haemorrhage and lipid deposits[35]. Although advances in the technique over the coming years will reduce this problem, magnetic resonance imaging (MRI) has not yet reached a sufficient degree of refinement to replace ultrasound or arteriography[36, 37]. Spiral CT protocols need to limit scanning to a 5–8 cm length of vessel at a time in order to obtain the resolution required. They also need to be reconstructed carefully in order to distinguish between contrast in the blood and calcification in the wall of the vessel and adjacent vertebrae. In addition the technique requires relatively high radiation and intravascular contrast dosage and it remains to be seen whether it will find a role in relation to Doppler and MRA[29].

Compared with these two techniques, Doppler ultrasound is relatively cheap, rapid, non-invasive and accurate for extracranial carotid disease. Whilst it will not provide information on siphon disease this is not usually a significant problem in most patients in relation to the decision to perform an endarterectomy. However, if a policy to operate without arteriography is to be implemented then the scanning protocols and results must be continuously reviewed and care taken to identify patients who will benefit from further imaging.

TRANSCRANIAL DOPPLER OF THE CEREBRAL CIRCULATION

The use of ultrasound to assess intracranial structures is not a new phenomenon. One of the first clinical applications of ultrasound as a diagnostic technique was in the assessment of midline intracranial structures with A-scan equipment. More recently, high-quality imaging and Doppler studies have been obtained in neonates through the patent fontanelles, or through the relatively thin bone of the neonatal skull. Transcranial Doppler was first described by Aaslid in 1982[38] and the technique of pulsed transcranial Doppler has subsequently been developed in many centres. This technique provides useful information on the direction and velocity of blood flow and the changes which may occur in these with various physiological, pharmacological or pathological conditions. However, it is a difficult technique to learn and to perform reliably as the vessels must be located without any imaging information.

Modern ultrasound equipment can now be configured to get some imaging detail and colour Doppler information from within the adult skull in many cases; best results are obtained with dedicated transducers and software. This allows localization and positive identification of the major arteries and specific segments of these. The main problem is the bone of the skull vault, where it has been estimated that the attenuation can vary from 15–25 dB to 40–60 dB depending on the type and thickness of the bone for a single passage across the skull vault[39]. As the sound pulse has to penetrate the skull on both the inward and outward segments of its passage, there is therefore considerable loss of energy. Power Doppler is of value in locating the vessels and the advent of intravascular ultrasound contrast agents has improved the signal-to-noise ratio significantly; it also makes the location of intracranial vessels more straightforward[40].

Technique

There are three potential sites of access for transcranial examinations in the adult: the transtemporal window, the suboccipital approach and the transorbital approach. The transtemporal window is used for assessment of the internal carotid arteries, the middle, anterior and posterior cerebral arteries. The window is located by applying liberal amounts of acoustic coupling gel to the hair and skin of the temporal region in front and above the external auditory meatus. Slowly moving the transducer around will allow the point of best transmission to be identified. In some 10% of subjects it may not be possible to get worthwhile images and Doppler signals[41]; there tends to be greater attenuation in older patients, females and black patients[42].

The pituitary fossa and suprasellar cistern are the most recognizable structures in the transverse plane. Once these have been identified, colour Doppler can be used to locate the main arteries and the direction of flow in these vessels (Fig. 3.22). The ipsilateral middle cerebral artery is seen passing peripherally from the end of the internal carotid artery. It cannot often be seen in its entirety in a single scan plane and the transducer position must be varied to follow it out to the Sylvian fissure, where it turns posteriorly. The origin of the contralateral middle cerebral artery can also usually be identified. The proximal segments of the anterior cerebral arteries are also seen from the transtemporal approach. The direction of flow in the ipsilateral anterior cerebral

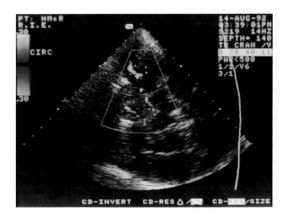

Fig. 3.22 The anterior and middle cerebral arteries on transcranial colour Doppler ultrasound through the transtemporal window.

artery is normally away from the transducer and towards the transducer in the contralateral vessel. This arrangement will be altered if there is occlusion of an internal carotid artery and collateral flow through the anterior communicating artery is present. In this situation, flow in the anterior cerebral artery on the side away from the occluded carotid will be reversed. The posterior cerebral arteries can be seen arising from the vertebral artery and passing around the cerebral peduncles.

The suboccipital window is located by scanning transversely in the midline under the occipital bone. It is often better to position the transducer slightly to one side or the other of the midline as the nuchal ligament can interfere with the clarity of the image. The vertebral arteries can be seen passing around the atlas and into the foramen magnum. The point where they join to form the vertebral artery may be seen if it lies low enough in relation to the foramen magnum.

The major cerebral veins and venous sinuses are more difficult to demonstrate due to their anatomical locations and slow flow within them, but contrast agents have been reported to improve this situation[40].

The transorbital approach is used in pulsed transcranial Doppler to assess the anterior cerebral arteries, but it is not very convenient for colour Doppler examinations as the transducers are relatively larger. Care must be taken, if this approach is used, to ensure that the transmit power is low in order to reduce the risk to the retina.

Indications

Transcranial colour Doppler has several advantages when compared with conventional transcranial Doppler. Visualization of the intracranial anatomy allows rapid localization and identification of specific vessels and specific segments of particular vessels. The colour Doppler signal allows rapid identification of flow patterns and direction, so compression studies are less necessary in order to assess collateral flow. The ability to perform angle-corrected velocity measurements produces more accurate readings and the ability to measure at specific sites allows better consistency for serial measurements.

Although still largely a research tool, the technique does have several potential applications. These were reviewed in 1989 by the American Academy of Neurology (Table 3.9)[43]. In particular the ability to bring the ultrasound machine to the patient allows the technique to be used to monitor cerebral blood flow in a variety of cerebrovascular disorders, such as subarachnoid haemorrhage and stroke.

Table 3.9 Application of transcranial Doppler. From American Academy of Neurology[43].

- Detection of significant (>65%) stenosis of major intracranial vessels
- Assessment of collateral pathways
- Evaluation of vasospasm, especially after subarachnoid haemorrhage
- Detection of arteriovenous malformations and assessment of their blood supply
- Assessment of possible brain death
- Assessment of patients with migraine
- Monitoring during surgical procedures
- Evaluation of patients with dilated vasculopathies
- Research into physiological and pharmacological aspects of cerebral blood flow
- Evaluation of children with sickle cell disease, moya moya, etc.

CONCLUSIONS

Colour Doppler ultrasound provides a useful technique for the assessment of the carotid and vertebral arteries in the neck. Careful attention must be paid to the standard techniques which are used for the examinations and each centre should use the Doppler criteria for stenosis that provide the most accurate and reproducible results in their experience. The availability of the technique should reduce the necessity for carotid arteriography in most departments. Magnetic resonance angiography and CT angiography continue to improve but ultrasound provides information on the nature of the plaque which is not available from these techniques.

REFERENCES

1. European Carotid Surgery Trialists' (ECST) Collaborative Group (1991) MRC European Carotid Surgery Trial: interim results for symptomatic patients with severe (70–99%) or with mild (0–29%) carotid stenosis. *Lancet* **337**: 1235–1243
2. North American Symptomatic Carotid Endarterectomy Trial (NASCET) Collaborators (1991) Beneficial effect of carotid endarterectomy in symptomatic patients with high-grade carotid stenosis. *New England Journal of Medicine* **325**: 445–453
3. ECST Collaborative Group (1996) Endarterectomy for moderate symptomatic carotid stenosis: interim results from the MRC European Carotid Surgery Trial. *Lancet* **347**: 1591–1593
4. Zwiebel WJ (1992) Duplex sonography of the cerebral arteries: efficacy, limitations and indications. *American Journal of Roentgenology* **158**: 29–36
5. National Institute of Neurological Disorders and Stroke (1994) Clinical advisory: carotid endarterectomy for patients with asymptomatic internal carotid artery stenosis. *Stroke* **25**: 2523–2524

6. Ivey TD, Strandness DE, Williams DB, Langlois Y, Misbach GA, Kruse AP (1984) Management of patients with carotid bruit undergoing cardiopulmonary bypass. *Journal of Thoracic and Cardiovascular Surgery* 87: 183–189

7. Naylor AR, Merrick MV, Sandercock PAG *et al* (1993) Serial imaging of the carotid bifurcation and cerebrovascular reserve after carotid endarterectomy. *British Journal of Surgery* 80: 1278–1282

8. Trigaux JP, Delchambre F, Van Beers B (1990) Anatomical variations of the carotid bifurcation: implications for digital subtraction angiography and ultrasound. *British Journal of Radiology* 63: 181–185

9. Salonen JT, Salonen R (1991) Ultrasonically assessed carotid morphology and the risk of coronary heart disease. *Arteriosclerosis and Thrombosis.* 11: 1245–1249

10. Geroulakos G, O'Gorman DJ, Kalodiki E, Sheridan DJ, Nicolaides AN (1994) The carotid intima-media thickness as a marker of severe symptomatic coronary artery disease. *European Heart Journal* 15: 781–785

11. Berguer R, Kiefer E (1992) The aortic arch and its branches: anatomy and blood flow (1992) In: *Surgery of the Arteries to the Head*, pp 5–31. New York: Springer Verlag

12. Bluth EI, Stavros AT, Marich KW, Wetzner SM, Aufrichtig D, Baker JD (1988) Carotid duplex sonography: a multicentre recommendation for standardized imaging and Doppler criteria. *RadioGraphics* 8: 487–506

13. Carpenter JP, Lexa FJ, Davies JT (1995) Determination of 60% or greater carotid artery stenosis by duplex Doppler ultrasonography. Journal of Vascular Surgery 22: 697–705

14. Robinson ML, Sacks D, Perlmutter GS, Marinelli DL (1988) Diagnostic criteria for carotid duplex sonography. *American Journal of Roentgenology* 151: 1045–1049

15. Hood DB, Mattos MA, Mansour A *et al* (1996) Prospective evaluation of new duplex criteria to identify 70% internal carotid artery stenosis. *Journal of Vascular Surgery* 23: 254–262

16. Erickson SJ, Mewisson MW, Foley WD (1989) Stenosis of the internal carotid artery: assessment using colour Doppler imaging compared with angiography. *American Journal of Roentgenology* 152: 1299–1305

17. Mattos MA, Hodgson KJ, Ramsey DE, Barkmeier LD, Sumner DS (1992) Identifying total carotid occlusion with colour flow duplex scanning. *European Journal of Vascular Surgery* 6: 204–210

18. Steffen CM, Gray-Weale AC, Byrne KE, Lusby RJ (1989) Carotid artery atheroma: ultrasound appearances in symptomatic and asymptomatic vessels. *Australia and New Zealand Journal of Surgery* 59: 529–534

19. O'Donnell TF, Erdoes L, Mackey WC *et al* (1985) Correlation of B-mode ultrasound imaging and arteriography with pathologic findings at carotid endarterectomy. *Archives of Surgery* 120: 443–449

20. Bluth EI, Kay D, Merritt CRB *et al* (1986) Sonographic characterization of carotid plaque: detection of haemorrhage. *American Journal of Roentgenology* 146: 1061–1065

21. Ratliff DA, Gallagher PJ, Hames TK, Humphries KN, Webster JHH, Chant ADB (1985) Characterisation of carotid artery disease: comparison of duplex scanning with histology. *Ultrasound in Medicine and Biology* 11: 835–840

22. O'Leary DH, Holen J, Ricotta JJ, Roe S, Schenk EA (1987) Carotid bifurcation disease: prediction of ulceration with B-mode US. *Radiology* 162: 523–525

23. Thiele BL, Jones AM, Hobson RW *et al* (1992) Standards in non-invasive cerebrovascular testing. *Journal of Vascular Surgery* 15: 495–503

24. Mann WJ, Beck A, Schreiber J, Maurer J, Amedee RG, Gluckmann JL (1994) Ultrasonography for evaluation of the carotid artery in head and neck cancers. *Laryngoscope* 104: 885–888

25. Barry R, Pienaar A, Pienaar C (1993) Duplex Doppler evaluation of suspected lesions at the carotid bifurcation. *Annals of Vascular Surgery* 7: 140–144

26. de Bray JM, Lhoste P, Dubaz F, Emile J, Saumet JL (1994) Ultrasonic features of extracranial carotid dissections: 47 cases studied by angiography. *Journal of Ultrasound in Medicine* 13: 659–664

27. Steinke W, Rautenberg W, Schwartz A, Hennerici M (1994) Non-invasive monitoring of internal carotid artery dissection. *Stroke* 25: 998–1005

28. Sitzer M, Fürst G, Siebler M *et al* (1994) Usefulness of an intravenous contrast medium in the characterization of high-grade internal carotid stenosis with colour Doppler-assisted duplex imaging. *Stroke* 25: 385–389

29. Alexandrov AV, Bladin CF, Magisano R, Norris JW (1993) Measuring carotid stenosis. Time for a reappraisal. *Stroke* 24: 1292–1296

30. Rothwell PM, Gibson RJ, Slattery J, Warlow CP (1994) Prognostic value and reproducibility of measurements of carotid stenosis: a comparison of three methods on 1001 angiograms. *Stroke* 25: 2440–2444

31. Phillips DJ (1990) Recent advances in carotid artery evaluation. In: Taylor KJW, Strandness DE (eds) *Clinics in Diagnostic Ultrasound 26: Duplex Doppler Ultrasound*, pp 25–44. Edinburgh: Churchill Livingstone

32. Chikos PM, Fisher LD, Hirsch JH, Harley JD, Thiele BL, Strandness DE (1983) Observer variability in evaluating extracranial carotid stenoses. *Stroke* 14: 885–892

33. Cardullo PA, Cutler BS, Brownell Wheeler H (1986) Detection of carotid disease by duplex ultrasound. *Journal of Diagnostic and Medical Sonography* 2: 63–73

34. Carroll BA (1991) Carotid sonography. *Radiology* **178**: 303–313

35. Sellar RJ. Imaging blood vessels of the head and neck. *Journal of Neurology, Neurosurgery and Psychiatry* **59**: 225–237

36. Masaryk TJ, Obuchowski NA (1993) Non-invasive carotid imaging: *caveat emptor. Radiology* **186**: 325–328

37. Polak JF (1993) Non-invasive carotid evaluation: *carpe diem. Radiology* **186**: 329–331

38. Aaslid R, Markwalder TM, Nornes H (1982) Non-invasive transcranial Doppler ultrasound recording of flow velocity in basal cerebral arteries. *Journal of Neurosurgery* **57**: 769–774

39. White DN, Curry GR, Stevenson RJ (1978) The acoustic characteristics of the skull. *Ultrasound in Medicine and Biology* **4**: 225–252

40. Bauer A, Becker G, Krone A, Fröhlich T, Bogdahn U (1996) Transcranial duplex sonography using ultrasound contrast enhancers. *Clinical Radiology* **51**(Suppl 1): 19–23

41. Ringelstein EB, Kahlscheuer E, Niggemeyer E, Otis SM (1990) Transcranial Doppler sonography: anatomical landmarks and normal velocity values. *Ultrasound in Medicine and Biology* **16**: 745–761

42. Halsey JH (1990) Effect of emitted power on waveform intensity in transcranial Doppler. *Stroke* **21**: 1573–1578

43. American Academy of Neurology (1990) Assessment: transcranial Doppler. Report of the American Academy of Neurology, Therapeutics and Technology Assessment Subcommittee. *Neurology* **40**: 680–681

THE CAROTID AND VERTEBRAL ARTERIES; TRANSCRANIAL COLOUR DOPPLER

The peripheral arteries

PAUL L. ALLAN

Atheroma occurs to different degrees in different parts of an individual's cardiovascular system and the lower limb arteries are particularly prone to the development of atherosclerosis. Approximately 2% of adults in late middle age in Western countries have intermittent claudication[1] and each year in England and Wales around 50 000 patients are admitted to hospital with a diagnosis of peripheral arterial disease; 15 000 of these will require amputation[2]. There are many factors which may influence the development of disease and, in general terms, the prevalence of peripheral vascular disease detected by non-invasive procedures is about three times greater than the prevalence of intermittent claudication[3]. This chapter concentrates on the use of ultrasound in the assessment of disease in the lower limb arteries, as this is the area where most work is generated, but the value of ultrasound in the investigation of a variety of upper limb arterial disorders is also discussed.

INDICATIONS

Peripheral vascular disease

The main indications for performing Doppler ultrasound of the arteries of the upper and lower limbs are given in Table 4.1. The most common indication is the assessment of

Table 4.1 Indications for Doppler ultrasound of the peripheral arteries.

- Assessment of disease in patients with ischaemic symptoms of the upper or lower limb
- Follow-up of bypass graft procedures
- Follow-up of angioplasty procedures
- Diagnosis and follow-up of aneurysms of the peripheral arteries
- Diagnosis and treatment of false aneurysms
- Diagnosis of pulsatile lumps
- Assessment of dialysis shunts

patients with ischaemic symptoms of the lower limb in order to determine if they are likely to benefit from angioplasty or a bypass graft. The ultrasound findings provide information on the extent and severity of disease, allowing any subsequent arteriogram to be scheduled as either a straightforward mapping examination prior to bypass grafting, or as a more time-consuming angioplasty procedure[4]. Patients with severe, limb-threatening ischaemia will normally proceed straight to arteriography prior to surgery, but patients who are not surgical candidates may have an ultrasound scan to see if there is any lesion appropriate for angioplasty, which may improve circulation and reduce the likelihood of amputation. At the other end of the spectrum, patients with atypical symptoms that might be due to ischaemia can be examined to exclude the presence of significant arterial disease.

Bypass grafts and angioplasty

A variety of problems can occur with surgically inserted bypass grafts, especially in the first 2 years after the operation. A graft surveillance programme using ultrasound allows the identification of grafts at risk of failure and early remedial action to be taken. Similarly patients in whom angioplasty has been undertaken can be followed with ultrasound to confirm residual patency, identify restenosis and assess improvements to flow following the procedure.

False aneurysms and other pulsatile masses

The assessment of pulsatile masses in relation to the arteries of the upper and lower limbs can be performed rapidly and easily using ultrasound. Aneurysms can be distinguished from non-vascular masses which lie adjacent to the artery. The complications of catheterization procedures, including haematomas, arteriovenous fistulae and false or pseudoaneurysms, can be assessed and differentiated; in many cases, pseudoaneurysms can be treated under ultrasound control, thereby removing the need for a surgical procedure.

Haemodialysis fistulae

Arteriovenous fistulae created for haemodialysis can be examined using ultrasound, allowing identification of complications associated with stenosis or occlusion, as well as estimation of blood flow through the shunt, particularly if this is thought to be inadequate or excessive.

ANATOMY AND SCANNING TECHNIQUE

Anatomy – lower limb

The arteries of the lower limb arise at the bifurcation of the abdominal aorta (Fig. 4.1), the *common iliac arteries* run down the poste-

rior wall of the pelvis and divide into the internal and external iliac arteries in front of the sacroiliac joint. The *internal iliac artery* continues down into the pelvis and is difficult to demonstrate with transabdominal ultrasound, although transvaginal or transrectal scanning will show some of its branches. The *external iliac artery* continues around the side of the pelvis to the level of the inguinal ligament, it lies anteromedial to the psoas muscle and is normally superficial to the external iliac vein.

The *common femoral artery* runs from the inguinal ligament to its division into superficial and deep femoral arteries in the upper thigh; this division is usually 3–6 cm distal to the inguinal ligament. The deep femoral artery, or *profunda femoris artery*, passes posterolaterally to supply the major thigh muscles. The importance of the profunda femoris lies in its role as a major collateral pathway in patients with significant superficial femoral artery disease. Several other branches arise from the external iliac, common femoral and profunda femoris arteries and occasionally one of these may be mistaken for the profunda femoris artery, especially if it is enlarged as a collateral supply.

The *superficial femoral artery* passes downwards along the anteromedial aspect of the thigh lying anterior to the vein; in the lower third of the thigh it passes into the adductor canal, deep to sartorius and the medial component of quadriceps femoris. Passing posteriorly behind the lower femur it enters the popliteal fossa and becomes the *popliteal artery*, which lies anterior to the popliteal vein and gives off several branches, the largest of which are the superior and inferior geniculate arteries. Below the knee joint the popliteal artery divides into the anterior tibial artery and the tibioperoneal trunk, although the exact level of the division may vary; after 2–4 cm the latter divides into the posterior tibial artery and the peroneal artery.

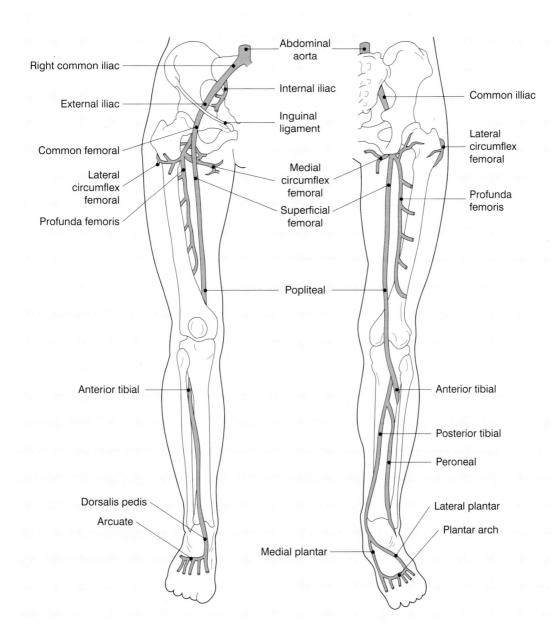

Fig. 4.1 The lower limb arteries.

The *anterior tibial artery* passes forwards through the interosseous membrane between the fibula and tibia. It then descends on the anterior margin of the membrane, deep to the extensor muscles on the anterolateral aspect of the calf (Fig. 4.2). At the ankle it passes across the front of the joint to become the dorsalis pedis artery of the foot.

The *posterior tibial artery* passes down the deep medial aspect of the calf to pass behind the medial malleolus, after which it divides into the medial and lateral plantar arteries of

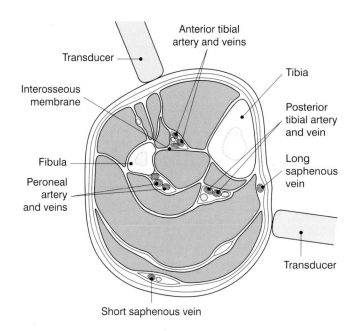

Fig. 4.2 Cross-section of calf, showing major relations of calf arteries and the two main access points for demonstrating these vessels.

the foot. The *peroneal artery* passes down the calf behind the tibia and interosseous membrane and divides into several periarticular branches behind the ankle joint. The size of the calf arteries can be quite variable, the posterior tibial artery is the least variable in calibre but the anterior tibial and peroneal arteries may vary considerably in calibre and overall length in the calf.

Scanning technique – lower limb

Common femoral, profunda femoris and superficial femoral arteries

The examination begins with the patient lying supine on the couch. The main steps in the examination are given in Table 4.2. A linear array transducer is used; this may be 5–10 MHz depending on the performance of the ultrasound system and the build of the patient. The distal external iliac/common femoral artery is located using colour Doppler as it leaves the pelvis under the inguinal ligament lateral to the femoral vein. Even if flow

appears normal on colour Doppler and there is no evidence of local disease, a spectral Doppler trace should be recorded, as changes in this may indicate the presence of significant disease proximally, necessitating a careful direct examination of the iliac vessels. The bifurcation of the common femoral artery into the profunda femoris and superficial femoral arteries is then examined using colour and spectral Doppler. The profunda femoris artery should be examined over its proximal 5–10 cm, especially in patients with severe superficial femoral disease, in order to assess the amount of collateral flow, or its potential value as a graft origin.

The superficial femoral artery is then followed along the length of the thigh using colour Doppler. It is often better to move the transducer in sequential steps, rather than sliding it down the thigh, as most machines require a few frames of sampling at each position to provide a steady image. In addition, the moving transducer generates colour Doppler noise over the image, obscuring vascular details. Doppler spectra are obtained

Table 4.2 Basic steps in the examination of the lower limb.

1. Patient supine: scan common femoral, proximal profunda and superficial femoral artery down to adductor canal

2. Patient decubitus: scan adductor canal, popliteal artery to bifurcation, scan posterior tibial and peroneal arteries

3. Patient supine: scan anterior tibial arteries. Scan iliac arteries and lower aorta if waveform in common femoral artery suggests significant iliac disease

as necessary at points of possible disease. Even in the absence of colour Doppler abnormalities, it is good practice to obtain routine spectral assessments from the superficial femoral artery in the upper, middle and lower thigh, in order to confirm that there is no alteration in the waveform that might suggest disease. Sometimes the artery is difficult to see on colour or power Doppler as the signals are weak or absent. In these cases the artery may be visible by virtue of calcified plaques in the wall of the vessel. Alternatively, the superficial femoral vein, lying behind the artery, can be used as a guide to the position of the artery and spectral Doppler used to demonstrate the presence or absence of arterial flow. Echo-enhancing agents can be used if there is any continuing uncertainty concerning the patency of the artery.

There are three indirect signs of significant disease which might be apparent during the examination and which should prompt a careful review if a cause for these changes has not been identified.

1. Colour Doppler may show the presence of collateral vessels in the muscles of the thigh (Fig. 4.3a).
2. Collateral vessels may be seen leaving the main artery (Fig. 4.3b).
3. The character of the spectral waveform may show a change between two levels, indicating a segment of disease somewhere between the two points of measurement.

The adductor canal and popliteal fossa

The patient is then turned into a lateral decubitus position so that the medial aspect of the leg being examined is uppermost (Fig. 4.4).

This position is better than the prone position as it allows access in continuity to the lower superficial femoral artery, the adductor canal area, the popliteal region and the medial calf. The region of the adductor canal must be examined with great care as it is a site where a short-segment stenosis or occlusion may be present, and this section of the vessel can be difficult to visualize as it passes deep to the thigh muscles. In some cases the use of a lower-frequency transducer may help in visualization. The superficial femoral artery is examined as far down as it can be followed on the medial aspect of the thigh; the popliteal artery is then located in the popliteal fossa and followed superiorly. In difficult cases a mark can be put on the skin of the medial thigh to show the lowest segment of vessel visualized in the supine position; the popliteal artery is then followed superiorly in the decubitus position until the transducer reaches the level of the skin mark, ensuring that the vessel has been examined in continuity. The popliteal artery is then examined and followed down to the point of division into the tibioperoneal trunk and anterior tibial artery.

Calf arteries

The complexity of the assessment of the calf arteries depends on the clinical situation. If the examination is to exclude significant proximal disease that would benefit from angioplasty or bypass grafts, then it is usually sufficient to assess the three calf arteries at the upper and mid-calf level, recording whether they are patent or not, in order to provide some assessment of the state of the distal run-off. Occasionally a more detailed examination is

(a)

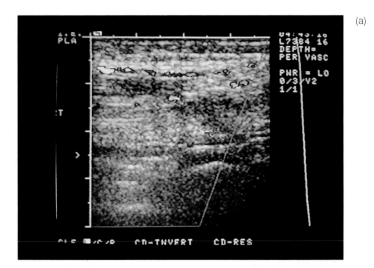

(b)

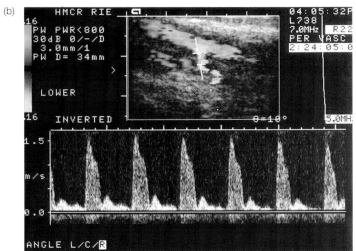

Fig. 4.3 (a) Collateral vessels in the muscles of the thigh. (b) A larger collateral vessel leaving the lower superficial femoral artery.

required to clarify changes seen on arteriography, or if a distal insertion point for a bypass graft is being sought. The increased sensitivity of power Doppler is useful in detecting weak signals from small or diseased but patent vessels.

The posterior tibial artery is usually the easier of the two branches of the tibioperoneal trunk to locate. Often it can be located by placing the transducer in a longitudinal position on the medial aspect of the mid-calf area behind the tibia, using colour or power Doppler to show the course of the vessel, which can then be followed up and down the calf (Fig. 4.2). In obese or oedematous legs, or

if blood flow is impaired by disease, the posterior tibial artery and the other calf arteries may be difficult to locate. Scanning with colour Doppler in the transverse plane using some angulation towards the head or feet may show the relative positions of the posterior tibial and peroneal arteries. Alternatively, the associated veins can be used to identify the region of the relevant artery: squeezing the foot or lower calf will augment flow in the deep veins, allowing these to be identified in either a longitudinal or transverse scan plane. The posterior tibial artery can also be located as it passes behind the medial malleolus, where its position is constant, and then followed back up the leg.

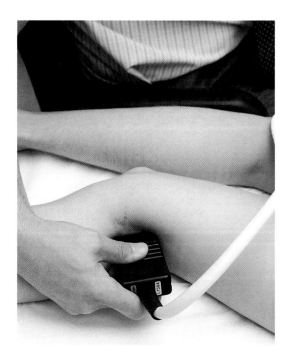

Fig. 4.4 The position of the patient for examination of the adductor canal and popliteal fossa; the line on the lower thigh shows the lowest extent at which the artery was visible on scanning down the thigh.

The peroneal artery runs more deeply down the calf than the posterior tibial artery, lying closer to the posterior aspect of the tibia and the interosseous membrane. It can be examined from two approaches: firstly from a posteromedial approach similar to that used for the posterior tibial artery; alternatively, it can often also be seen from the anterolateral approach used for the anterior tibial artery as it runs behind the interosseous membrane (Fig. 4.2).

The anterior tibial artery is examined from an anterolateral approach through the extensor muscles lying between the tibia and fibula. The two bones can be identified on transverse scanning and the interosseous membrane located passing between them. The anterior tibial artery lies on the membrane and can be located using colour Doppler in either the longitudinal or transverse plane. It usually lies nearer the fibula than the tibia (Fig. 4.2).

The foot vessels are not usually examined but the dorsalis pedis artery may be examined in front of the ankle joint before it passes deep to the metatarsals.

The advent of power Doppler and echo-enhancing agents has extended the role of ultrasound in the assessment of vascular disease. In the proximal lower limb and iliac vessels, the location of the vessel and confirmation of occluded segments has been made easier and, in the distal part of the leg, they make assessment of the smaller vessels of the calf and foot easier. However, more work is required to evaluate further their role[5].

Iliac arteries

Examination of the iliac vessels is carried out if the clinical picture suggests disease affecting these vessels, or if the Doppler findings at the groin suggest the likelihood of significant proximal disease. The ease with which they can be visualized depends on the build of the patient and the amount of bowel gas present. It is usually necessary to use a 3–4 MHz transducer for satisfactory visualization. Some examiners will prepare patients for iliac Doppler examinations with laxatives and low-residue diets if it is considered likely that these vessels will be examined, although most centres do not do this routinely. However, it is important not to make a false diagnosis of occlusion because the vessel is obscured by bowel gas.

The external iliac artery can be followed up from the groin for a variable distance; the vein, lying behind the artery, can be used to identify the probable location of the artery if this is not apparent. Colour or power Doppler may also help locate the vessel, even if it is not visible on the real-time scan image. Superiorly the common iliac artery can be identified arising from the aortic bifurcation and then followed distally. Firm pressure with the transducer will displace intervening amounts of bowel gas to a large extent, although care must be taken not to compress the artery and produce a false impression of a stenosis. The internal iliac artery may be seen arising from the common iliac artery and passing deeply into the pelvis. This is a useful landmark as visualization of the internal iliac artery origin, on tracking both the external iliac artery upwards and the common iliac artery downwards, means that the iliac vessels have been examined in their entirety.

The orientation of the iliac vessels as they pass round the pelvis and the use of sector or curved–array transducers can lead to problems with beam–vessel geometry and obtaining satisfactory angles of insonation. However, careful attention to positioning the transducer will usually allow an appropriate angle to be obtained.

Anatomy – upper limb

The *subclavian arteries* arise from the brachio-cephalic trunk on the right and directly from the arch of the aorta on the left (Fig. 4.5); however, there is considerable normal variation in the patterns of their origination. The origin of the right subclavian artery can be examined behind the right sternoclavicular joint, where the brachiocephalic trunk divides into the right common carotid artery and the subclavian artery. The origin of the left subclavian artery from the aortic arch cannot be demonstrated, although the more distal segments can be seen as on the right side. The subclavian artery on each side runs from its point of origin to the outer border of the first rib where it becomes the axillary artery, the subclavian vein lies in front of the artery. The main branches of the subclavian artery are the vertebral arteries, the thyrocervical trunk, the internal thoracic (mammary) artery and the subscapular artery.

The *axillary artery* runs from the lateral border of the first rib to the outer, inferior margin of the pectoralis major muscle. It gives

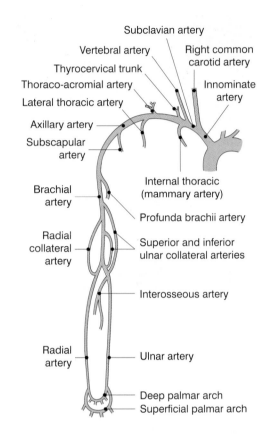

Fig. 4.5 The upper limb arteries.

rise to several branches which supply the muscles around the shoulder, the largest of these are the thoracoacromial trunk, the lateral thoracic artery and the subscapular artery.

The *brachial artery* passes down the medial aspect of the upper arm to the cubital fossa below which it divides into the radial and ulnar arteries; the point of division sometimes lies higher in the upper arm. Apart from muscular branches, the main branches of the brachial artery are the profunda brachii artery, which is given off in the upper arm and passes behind the humerus; the superior and inferior ulnar collateral arteries arise from the lower part of the brachial artery.

The *radial artery* runs down the radial (lateral) aspect of the forearm to the wrist, where it passes over the radial styloid process, and over the lateral aspect of the carpus. It then passes down through the first interosseous space to form the lateral aspect of the deep palmar arch. It also has a superficial branch which anastomoses with the equivalent branch of the ulnar artery to form the superficial palmar arch. In the upper forearm the radial artery gives off the radial recurrent artery, which anastomoses with the profunda brachii artery, and several muscular branches in the forearm and at the wrist.

The *ulnar artery* passes down the anterior ulnar (medial) aspect of the forearm to the medial aspect of the wrist, where it runs over the flexor retinaculum and then divides into superficial and deep branches which anastomose with the equivalent branches of the radial artery to form the superficial and deep palmar arches. It gives off recurrent ulnar arteries below the elbow and the common interosseous artery, which forms anterior and posterior divisions, running on either side of the interosseous membrane.

Scanning technique – upper limb

A 7–10 MHz transducer may be used in most cases for examining the arteries in the upper limb, as there is less tissue to penetrate than in the leg. The patient lies in a supine position with their head turned away from the side being examined, the arm is abducted with the elbow flexed and the back of the hand resting on the pillow by the patient's head, so that the axilla and medial aspect of the upper arm can be examined. Alternatively, the arm can be abducted and supported on a suitable shelf, or by asking the patient to hold onto a suitable part of the ultrasound machine. The distal innominate artery on the right and the mid-subclavian artery on the left can be visualized from a supraclavicular approach by angling the transducer down towards the mediastinum from above the medial clavicle and sterno-clavicular joint. The subclavian arteries on

both sides are seen behind the subclavian vein as they run up to cross the first rib. In patients with possible arterial compression syndromes, the artery is examined with the arm in various positions so that any narrowing or occlusion may be demonstrated.

The artery beyond the first rib is best examined from below the clavicle and followed distally. It can be followed in continuity as it runs deep to the pectoralis muscles through the axilla and into the medial aspect of the upper arm; from here it can be tracked down to the cubital fossa. The division of the artery into the two main forearm branches usually occurs below the cubital fossa and each branch can be followed to the wrist; if either the radial or the ulnar artery is difficult to trace down from the elbow, then the vessel should be sought at the wrist and followed back up the forearm.

ASSESSMENT OF DISEASE

The assessment of lower limb atheroma is more complex than for the carotids as the potential for collateral supply around stenoses or occlusions is very much greater. The distinction must be made between haemodynamically significant disease and clinically significant disease. Two individuals may have the same degree of stenosis in their superficial femoral artery, but an 80% diameter reduction which develops acutely will be significantly symptomatic, whereas the same degree of stenosis developing over a period of time, allowing collateral channels to open, may be much less disabling. The findings on Doppler must therefore not be considered in isolation but in the light of the full clinical picture.

Colour Doppler allows the rapid identification of normal and abnormal segments of vessel. In addition, some stenoses may show a colour Doppler tissue 'bruit' due to the tissue vibrations set up by the blood passing through the stenosis. It is valuable to relate the level of any diseased segments demonstrated on ultrasound to bony landmarks which can be seen on angiography; this allows the appearances on the two examinations to be compared and confirm that the abnormality on the arteriogram is at the level of the lesion seen on ultrasound or vice-versa. The groin skin crease corresponds to the superior pubic ramus and can be used for lesions in the upper part of the thigh; the upper border of the patella can be used for lesions in the lower part of the thigh; and the tibiofemoral joint space for popliteal lesions.

Some patients will show extensive diffuse disease along much, or all, of the superficial femoral artery but do not show any specific, localized stenoses. It is important to note this appearance, as the overall haemodynamic effect may be severe enough to produce a significant pressure drop along the vessel, thereby reducing limb perfusion, although this pattern of disease is not suitable for angioplasty. Other patients may have several stenoses along the length of the vessel, each of which is not haemodynamically significant but the effects of these are additive, so that there is still a significant drop in perfusion pressure distal to the affected segment[6]. In addition, the presence of serial stenoses can affect the estimation of the degree of stenosis, if it is not recognized[7].

The same principles apply to the assessment of disease in the upper limb, but the type and distribution of disease in the arm is different from that seen in the leg. Ischaemic symptoms in the arm may be the result of compression, embolic occlusion, or vasospasm and are less frequently due to localized atheroma.

The main diagnostic criteria which are of value in the assessment of lower limb atheroma are direct measurement of the stenosis, peak systolic velocity ratios and waveform changes.

Direct measurement

Direct measurement of a stenosis is often quite difficult in the lower limb arteries as these are relatively small, and it may be difficult to see the lumen clearly in the deeper parts of the thigh, particularly if there is disease present. However, direct measurement of a stenosis may be possible in the lower external iliac, common femoral, profunda femoris and upper superficial femoral arteries. Measurement of the diameter reduction is performed after assessment of plaque distribution in both longitudinal and transverse planes, so that the most appropriate diameter is selected. When a segment of stenosis or occlusion is detected the length of the affected segment should be measured, as this will be relevant to the suitability of the lesion for angioplasty; segments of disease, particularly occlusions, longer than 10 cm will not normally be considered for percutaneous treatment[8].

Peak velocity ratios

Direct measurement of a stenosis is often not possible in the lower limb and the severity of the stenosis must then be estimated from the change in peak systolic velocity produced by the stenosis. Normal velocities in the lower limb arteries at rest are approximately 1.2 m s^{-1} in the iliac segments, 0.9 m s^{-1} in the superficial femoral segments and 0.7 m s^{-1} in the popliteal segment[9]. Various criteria have been put forward for the quantification of lower limb arterial stenosis. Those of Cossman et al[10] have produced satisfactory results in the author's department and have the advantage of being easy to remember (Table 4.3). These criteria are based on the peak systolic velocity at the stenosis and the ratio of the peak systolic velocity at the

Table 4.3 Velocity criteria for the assessment of lower limb stenoses. Reproduced from Cossman et al[10].

% Stenosis	Peak systolic velocity (m s^{-1})	Velocity ratio
Normal	<1.5	<1.5:1
0–49	1.5–2.0	1.5–2:1
50–75	2.0–4.0	2–4:1
>75	>4.0	>4:1
Occlusion	—	—

stenosis compared with the velocity 1–2 cm upstream. Colour Doppler allows the position and direction of peak velocity flow in the stenosis to be identified and the sample volume can be placed appropriately, final adjustments of position being performed by listening to the pitch of the frequency shift. A further velocity measurement is then made in a 'normal' segment of artery 1–2 cm upstream from the stenosis and the ratio calculated (Fig. 4.6).

Waveform changes

The normal waveform in the main arteries of the resting lower limb has three components;

four, or occasionally five, may be seen in fit young individuals. These represent the pressure changes which occur in the lower limb arteries during the cardiac cycle. First there is the rise in pressure and acceleration of blood flow at the onset of systole. There is then a short period of reversed flow as the pressure wave is reflected from the constricted distal arterioles. This is followed by a further period of forward flow produced by the elastic compliance of the main arteries in diastole (Fig. 4.7a). These changes are discussed in more detail in Chapter 2.

Exercise modifies this pattern by reducing the peripheral resistance. This results in the

(a)

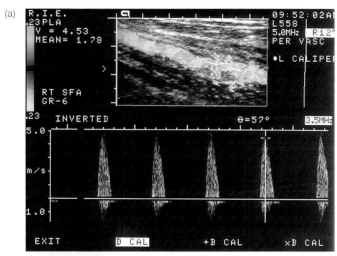

(b)

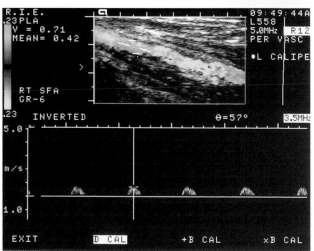

Fig. 4.6 Measurement of the peak systolic velocity ratio at a stenosis. (a) Velocity at the stenosis is 4.5 m s⁻¹; a visible tissue bruit is present at the stenosis. (b) Velocity above the stenosis is 0.7 m s⁻¹, giving a ratio of >6.

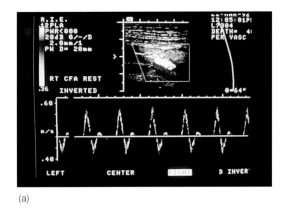

(a)

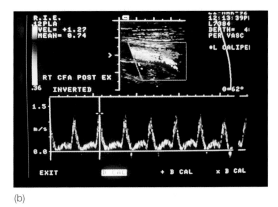

(b)

Fig. 4.7 The normal femoral artery waveform. (a) In a limb at rest the three components are visible. (b) Following exercise there is increased diastolic flow.

reversed component being lost and increased diastolic flow throughout the cardiac cycle (Fig. 4.7b). It is for this reason that ultrasound examination of the lower limb arteries should be performed in patients who have not had significant exercise of the leg muscles for about 15 min. Conversely, examination after exercise, or reactive hyperaemia, may be used in order to 'stress' the lower limb circulation and reveal stenoses which are not significant at rest, when blood flow is relatively low, but which become apparent with the higher volumes flowing when the distal circulation to the muscles opens up[11].

Disease in the vessel at the point of measurement, above it or below it, can affect the waveform, and if the vessel cannot be visualized in continuity then a change in the waveform between two points is indicative of disease. The two main features which may be altered are the overall shape of the waveform and the degree of spectral broadening as a result of flow disturbance[9]; the major changes are shown in Table 4.4 and illustrated in Fig. 4.8. Proximal disease above the point of measurement results in loss firstly of the third and then of the second components of the waveform, as the normal passage of the pressure wave along the artery is impaired. This interference with the passage of the pulse wave along the vessel is also manifest

by the slowing of the systolic acceleration time. The width of the first, systolic complex is increased and the overall height is decreased. These changes result in 'damping' of the waveform, which is most marked when there is a proximal occlusion. The turbulence generated beyond a stenosis shows in the spectrum as spectral broadening and its presence therefore also indicates proximal disease, although not its severity, as mild turbulence may be due to a minor stenosis close by, or a more severe stenosis further away. The spectral broadening may be seen throughout the spectrum if the stenosis is close to the point of measurement; as the distance from the stenosis increases, the spectral broadening is seen in the postsystolic deceleration phase only. The disturbance of flow created by a stenosis may take several centimetres to resolve. The spectral broadening is lost and the systolic forward flow component is regained, but the reverse component and third component are much less likely to reappear distal to disease. In addition, if the distal limb is ischaemic, this will result in dilatation of the capillaries and increased flow throughout diastole. The presence of some, or all, of these changes requires that the vessel be carefully examined proximally to identify their source.

The presence of distal disease will also affect the waveform, resulting in increased pulsatility,

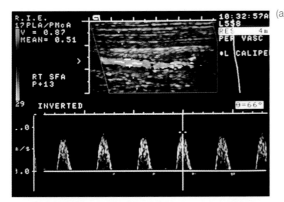
(a)

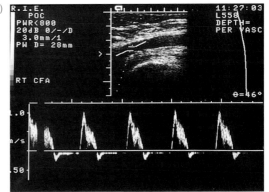
(b)

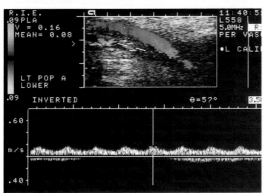

(c) **Fig. 4.8** Abnormal lower limb artery waveforms. (a) Loss of reverse component. (b) Broadening of the waveform and turbulence secondary to a proximal stenosis. (c) Damped waveform in the popliteal artery secondary to a proximal occluded segment.

with reduced diastolic flow, evident from the loss of the third component; in addition, the peak systolic velocity is reduced. This situation is most often seen at the origin of a superficial femoral artery with significant distal disease, although the precise changes are variable, depending on the degree of obstruction and the capacity of any collateral channels[12].

Assessment of aortoiliac disease

The clinical findings, or the appearances of the waveform at the groin, may suggest the presence of significant disease in the aortoiliac segments. The best method for assessment of these segments is by direct visualization with colour Doppler and measurement of velocities as for the leg vessels. Satisfactory examinations have been reported in up to 90% of cases with careful scanning and preparation[13]. However, even if adequate direct visualization is not achieved, the likeli-

hood of significant proximal disease should be noted and, depending on the clinical severity, assessed by arteriography, if necessary. The main indirect indicators of significant iliac artery disease are spectral broadening, due to the turbulence set up by the stenosis, and widening of the systolic complex as a result of the stenosis slowing the systolic acceleration. As noted earlier, power Doppler and echo-enhancing agents show promise in improving visualization and assessment using ultrasound[5].

ARTERIAL BYPASS GRAFTS

A variety of bypass grafts may be employed to alleviate ischaemic symptoms (Table 4.5). Autologous vein is the preferred material and usually the long saphenous vein is used,

---

Table 4.4 Waveform changes associated with disease in the lower limb.

- Loss of third and then second phase of the waveform
- Increased acceleration time
- Widening of the systolic complex
- Damping of the waveform
- Spectral broadening
- Absent flow in occlusion

Table 4.5 Types of bypass graft.

Types of graft

Femoropopliteal – may arise from external iliac artery
   rather than common femoral artery
Femorodistal – to calf vessels or dorsalis pedis
Femorofemoral crossover
Iliofemoral
Axillofemoral

Materials used for graft

Vein
   In situ vein
   Reversed vein
Synthetic
   Polytetrafluoroethylene (PTFE)
   Goretex

although other veins may occasionally be employed. Synthetic material is used if the long saphenous veins are unsuitable or unavailable. Several problems may occur which result in graft failure (Table 4.6) and it has been shown that a programme of graft surveillance in the postoperative period can reduce the number of failed grafts[14].

The timing of graft failure is related to the cause of the problem. Failures occurring within 6–8 weeks of surgery are usually due to technical problems arising from the surgery; 3–5% of grafts fail at this stage, approximately 25% of all graft failures. Failures developing in the period beginning 3 months and extending to 2 years after surgery are usually due to

Table 4.6 Causes of graft failure.

Intrinsic	Extrinsic
Stenosis	Inflow disease progression
Proximal or distal	Outflow disease progression
anastomosis	Entrapment or kinking
Mid-graft	
Diffuse myointimal	Clamp injury
hyperplasia	Thromboembolism
Aneurysm	Hypercoagulation states
Anastomotic	Sepsis
Mid-graft	

Haemodynamic failure occurs when the graft is patent but the limb remains ischaemic

myointimal hyperplasia; 12–37% of grafts fail during this period, approximately 70–80% of all graft failures; most of these will occur in the first 12 months. Beyond 2 years after surgery the usual cause of failure is progression of atherosclerosis, either in the native vessels or in the graft itself[15]. In addition to graft stenosis or occlusions other problems may occur, including dehiscence at the origin or insertion and false aneurysm formation, arteriovenous fistulae, infected collections and compression or kinking.

The timing of the surveillance scans is based on this time scale for problems. An early scan 4–6 weeks after the operation is performed, subsequently a scan is done at 3 months and then at 3-monthly intervals until the end of the first year. It is not usually necessary to continue beyond this if no cause for concern exists, as the majority of failures will occur in the first year. However, if there are particular reasons for concern, such as mild or moderate stenosis (velocity ratio <2), then surveillance can be extended as appropriate. Surveillance programmes have been shown to be beneficial for both autologous vein and synthetic grafts[14, 16], although the latter have a slightly increased tendency to fail without warning. Symptomatic grafts should always be examined, as a treatable lesion may be demonstrated prior to complete graft thrombosis and failure.

Technique of examination

It is of value if the request for a graft assessment gives details of the surgery and the type of graft inserted; ideally, a diagram of the course of the graft should be provided. The examination should begin at the groin and the graft located; transverse scanning is helpful with identification of the graft origin. Once located the graft should be followed up to its point of origin from the native artery. The majority of grafts are femoropopliteal and run from the common femoral artery, or lower external iliac artery, to the upper or lower popliteal artery; occasionally the graft may originate from deeper in the pelvis, lower down the superficial femoral artery, or from the profunda femoris artery. The native artery above the graft is assessed and the velocity of blood flow measured with spectral Doppler. The origin of the graft is then examined carefully and any increase in velocity, or disturbance of flow, noted (Fig. 4.9).

The graft is followed down the length of the thigh. Most grafts run along the medial aspect of the thigh; however some grafts, particularly repeat grafts, may follow unusual courses, even crossing the thigh to run down the lateral aspect of the leg. Velocity measurements are obtained at any point of disturbed flow; if no disturbance is present, two to three velocity measurements are taken along the length of the graft to ensure that there is satisfactory flow.

At the graft insertion, the flow above, at and below the anastomosis is examined and any significant changes in the velocities assessed as possible signs of stenosis. Some care must be taken in the interpretation of velocity increases at both the origin and insertion of grafts, as moderate changes may be the result of disparity in size between the graft and the

native vessel and therefore not pathological in origin, particularly at the distal insertion, if this is into a relatively small calf artery or the dorsalis pedis artery.

Synthetic grafts are relatively straightforward to assess, as any problems usually occur at the origin or insertion, rather than along the length of the graft. Vein grafts, however, can develop problems at any point along their length, particularly at sites of avulsed valves or tied perforating veins. Stenoses can occur secondary to surgery, or as a result of intimal hyperplasia, which can be stimulated by the turbulence at an irregularity in the vein wall. *In situ* vein grafts may also have persistent arteriovenous communications if a perforating or superficial communicating vein has been overlooked during the operation. These may be quite small but their presence should be suspected if there is a rapid, unexplained drop in velocity along the graft, or if pulsatile venous flow is seen in the common or superficial femoral veins. Scanning transversely along the line of the *in situ* graft makes it easier to identify these communicating vessels and demonstrate their course.

A note should also be made of any collections seen along the track of the graft. In the postoperative period these are usually small collections of serous fluid, haematomas, or

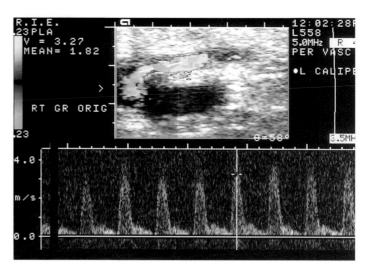

Fig. 4.9 Origin of a femoropopliteal bypass graft with a high velocity of 3.27 m s⁻¹.

small lymphocoeles; normally these resorb over a few weeks (Fig. 4.10). If infection is suspected then a fine needle (20–22G) can be used to perform a diagnostic aspiration, although care should be taken not to introduce infection into a sterile collection.

If an occluded graft is demonstrated but the leg is asymptomatic then it is worth checking if the patient has had more than one bypass procedure, as a second, patent graft may be present elsewhere in the leg.

Features of a graft at risk

The main features which suggest that a graft is at risk of failing are shown in Table 4.7. There is good correlation between these criteria and the incidence of subsequent graft failure. The finding of a fall in the ankle/brachial pressure index (ABPI) of more than 0.15 in addition to the presence of a stenosis of more than 70%, or low velocity, is a strong indicator of a graft at risk[14].

Other abnormalities which may be seen in relation to a bypass graft are a false aneurysm at the origin or insertion due to dehiscence of the anastomosis (Fig. 4.11), or an arteriovenous fistula.

DIALYSIS SHUNTS

Various types of arteriovenous communication may be fashioned to allow for haemodialysis. Colour Doppler can be used to examine the supplying artery, the anastomosis and the draining veins. In grafts which are not functioning well it should be remembered that problems can occur with the artery anywhere along its length, at the anastomosis, in the vein immediately distal to the anastomosis where dialysis needles are inserted, or in the veins proximally around the groin or clavicle.

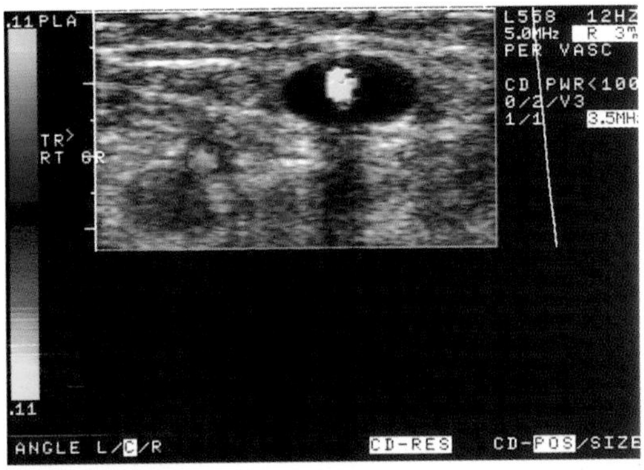

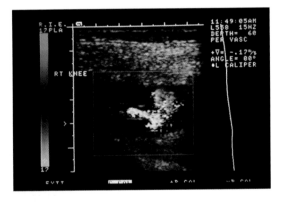

Fig. 4.10 Small lymphocoele around a femoropopliteal bypass graft.

Fig. 4.11 Dehiscence at the insertion of a graft into the lower popliteal artery.

Table 4.7 Doppler criteria for graft stenosis and grafts at risk.

Direct measurement of stenosis	Moderate >50% diameter stenosis
	Severe >70% diameter stenosis
Peak systolic velocity changes	>1.5 m s^{-1} = 50–70% diameter stenosis
	>2.5 m s^{-1} ≥ 70% diameter stenosis
End diastolic velocity	>0.2 m s^{-1} ≥ 70% diameter stenosis
Velocity ratio	>2.5 ≥ 50% diameter stenosis
	>3.5 ≥ 70% diameter stenosis
Peak systolic velocity	<45 cm s^{-1} at narrowest segment

Technique

The examination of upper limb arteriovenous dialysis fistulae begins with the axillary or upper brachial artery, which is then followed with colour Doppler distally until the anastomosis with the vein or graft is identified. The region of the anastomosis is then examined carefully for any evidence of stenosis. The amount of flow through such a fistula is normally sufficiently high and turbulent to produce tissue vibrations, which may obscure the lumen; however, making sure that transducer pressure is minimal, and therefore not producing any venous compression, may reduce this visible tissue vibration. Alternatively, gentle compression of the brachial artery with a pressure cuff or manual pressure may reduce flow sufficiently for the tissue vibrations to be reduced and allow visualization of the vessel and anastomosis. The venous drainage is then followed back up the arm to the subclavian vein; several veins may contribute to the drainage of the fistula, and each needs to be followed proximally. If a stenosis is suspected on the venous side, then the veins should be examined carefully, making sure that transducer pressure is as light as possible to ensure that inadvertent compression is not responsible for any narrowing which may be demonstrated. The cephalic vein may be narrowed as it passes through the clavipectoral fascia, and careful assessment of this region should be carried out if venous problems are suspected.

Stenosis and other abnormalities

A stenotic lesion may affect a dialysis fistula on the arterial side, at the anastomosis, or on the venous side. The criteria used for lower limb arterial lesions do not apply in these circumstances, as flow velocities are generally high with inherent turbulence in the presence of a fistula and visible tissue 'bruits' can occur in the absence of a stenosis. However, a sudden significant increase in velocity should be assessed carefully. In addition, a significant stenosis in the artery or at the anastomosis may result in a fall in the velocity and volume of blood flowing along the venous side of the fistula.

Apart from stenosis affecting the inflow, outflow, or anastomosis, other problems which may be identified in relation to dialysis fistulae are true or false aneurysms at the sites of needle insertion, haematomas and abscesses; these result from the repeated trauma of cannulation. Segmental thrombosis may occur on the venous side and complete thrombosis of the fistula may occur, usually affecting the venous rather than the arterial side.

Fistula steal syndrome

The low resistance of the fistula means that flow to the distal parts of the limb may be impaired if too much blood is diverted through the fistula. This is not normally a problem but coexistent arterial disease in the distal limb can result in significantly impaired perfusion pressure. Steal syndromes can be assessed by examining the distal arteries whilst compressing the venous side of the fistula; if this results in a significant increase in distal flow then it is likely that flow reduction surgery to the fistula will be beneficial, and an estimate of the fistula flow volume should be obtained in order to allow the degree of reduction to be calculated.

Volume flow in the fistula

The assessment of volume blood flow using Doppler ultrasound is beset by various inherent problems which result in a wide standard deviation for most flow measurements, as discussed in Chapter 1. However it is possible to measure dialysis fistula flow sufficiently accurately to divide it into three broad groups: <200 ml min^{-1}, which is inadequate for dialysis; 200–800 ml min^{-1}, which is satisfactory; and >800 ml min^{-1}, which is excessive and may be associated with high cardiac output problems at rates over 1400–1600 ml min⁻¹ depending on the cardiac reserve of the patient. A fistula flow rate of at least 200 ml min⁻¹ is required for adequate dialysis, ideally rates of 300–400 ml min⁻¹ are desirable. Some patients may tolerate flow rates in excess of 1000 ml min⁻¹ but others will start to show signs of cardiac decompensation at and above this level of flow[17].

The venous side of the fistula may show branching into two or more venous channels; one of these is usually dominant and used for dialysis needle puncture. However, the multiplicity of venous channels, together with the turbulence of flow, can make assessment of fistula flow volume difficult to estimate on the venous side. On the arterial side it is reasonable to assume that the greatest proportion of blood in the supplying brachial or radial artery will go through the fistula when the arm is in the resting state, and therefore to estimate the blood flow volume in the fistula from the supplying artery. If necessary the distal arterial supply can be occluded with a pressure cuff.

Techniques for measuring volume flow have been discussed in Chapter 1. The most straightforward method for estimating volume flow is by multiplying the time-averaged mean velocity in the vessel by the cross-sectional area at the point of measurement (Fig. 4.12). Three aspects of technique should be remembered: the time-averaged mean velocity must be measured, not the time-averaged maximum velocity; the sample volume for the velocity measurement should encompass the complete cross-section of the vessel; and the cross-sectional area should be measured at right angles to the long axis of the vessel in order to obtain the best estimate of volume flow.

FALSE ANEURYSMS

These are usually straightforward to diagnose on colour Doppler ultrasound, although occasionally there may be some difficulty if there is also a large haematoma present. The characteristic appearance is a hypoechoic space which shows swirling blood flow on colour Doppler (Fig. 4.13). It is important that the track between the aneurysm and the native artery is identified, as this is the point which needs to be obliterated by compression, or by surgery, if the aneurysm is to be treated adequately; in cases of a multiloculated false aneurysm, it is essential to identify the point of arterial leakage if successful compression therapy is to be applied. Spectral Doppler of the track, or aneurysm neck, shows a characteristic 'to and fro' flow signal as blood flows in during systole and out during diastole. Rarely, a

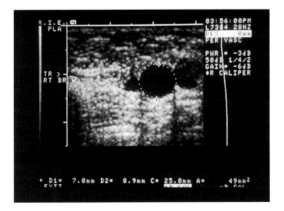

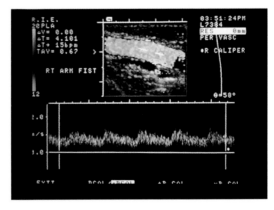

Fig. 4.12 Estimation of dialysis fistula flow volume. (a) Arterial cross sectional area is 0.49 cm². (b) Time average mean velocity is 0.67 cm s⁻¹. Calculated flow rate is therefore 0.49 cm² × 67 cm s⁻¹ × 60 = 1970 ml min⁻¹ (an excessively high flow).

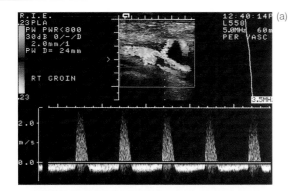

(a)

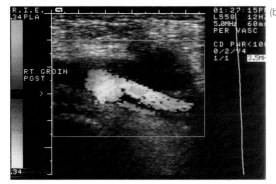

(b)

Fig. 4.13 (a) A false aneurysm showing a patent lumen on colour Doppler and the characteristic 'to and fro' flow on spectral Doppler. (b) The same false aneurysm after successful compression.

false aneurysm is associated with an arterio-venous fistula passing from the cavity to an adjacent vein. The clue to the presence of the fistula is the loss of the 'to and fro' flow in the track from the artery, with only forward flow being shown which increases towards end-diastole.

Ultrasound-guided compression therapy of false aneurysms

The ability of colour Doppler to demonstrate flowing blood in the aneurysm and track allows the operator to apply graded compression to these using pressure from the transducer, so that flow into the aneurysm is stopped, whilst allowing flow to continue down the native artery. This allows the aneurysm and track to thrombose and therefore remove the need for surgery[18]. Although some false aneurysms will

thrombose spontaneously, particularly during the first week after development, it is worth considering compression in most cases. There are, however, some circumstances where it is recognized that compression is unlikely to succeed and direct referral for surgery should be considered; these are shown in Table 4.8. The most common contraindications for compression are the age of the aneurysm and warfarin therapy; if it has been present for more than 7–10 days then the track will have started to develop an endothelium and the surrounding tissues are less compliant, so that adequate compression becomes difficult.

The procedure is quite time-consuming for the operator and uncomfortable for the patient, so it is better to give some analgesia to the patient prior to the commencement of prolonged compression. The aneurysm and its track are identified and compression is applied by pressing the transducer increasingly firmly down on these until flow in them has ceased but flow is still present in the native artery. This degree of pressure is then maintained for 10–15 min before being released slowly. If flow is then seen in the lumen, compression is reinstated for a further period of 10 min before again gently relaxing the pressure. These cycles of compression and relaxation are repeated until all flow in the aneurysm lumen has stopped. Usually the lumen of the aneurysm thromboses in an irregular fashion from the outside inwards, until complete obliteration is achieved. In one large series[18], the average time for successful treatment of a simple unilocular aneurysm was 43 min (SD ± 40 min) and 69 min (SD ± 54 min) for complex multiloculated

Table 4.8 Circumstances when compression of a false aneurysm is less likely to succeed.

- Aneurysms more than 7–10 days old
- Associated infection
- Severe pain/discomfort
- Large haematoma
- Aneurysms above the inguinal ligament

83

lesions. Following successful obliteration the patient is scanned after 24 hours to confirm that the aneurysm remains occluded (Fig. 4.3b). Some operators prefer to dispense with transducer compression and use manual compression with their fingers or a fist pressing over the site of the false aneurysm and its neck; ultrasound is used intermittently to assess the development of thrombosis. A variety of mechanical compression devices have also been proposed but results with these are variable.

Other pulsatile masses

Aneurysms

Aneurysms of the lower limb arteries may occur in isolation, or as multiple lesions. As with aortic aneurysms they can enlarge over a period of time; their size and rate of enlargement can be followed with ultrasound. Their main clinical significance is that they can act as a source of emboli to the distal lower limb, or may thrombose leading to acute ischaemia.

Cystic adventitial disease

This is a rare condition in which fluid-filled cysts are found in the wall of the artery, usually the popliteal artery, or superficial femoral artery in the adductor canal (Fig. 4.14). The aetiology of these cysts is unclear and various theories, including repeated trauma, ectopic synovial tissue, or a congenital abnormality linking the cyst to the adjacent knee joint space or to adjacent tendons, have been proposed[19].

BRACHIAL COMPRESSION SYNDROMES

Thoracic outlet syndrome, or compression of the subclavian artery as it crosses the first rib, may be due to congenital fibrotic bands at the insertions of the anterior and middle scalene muscles, or to compression associated with a cervical rib. The accompanying vein is also usually affected. Some degree of compression may be seen in up to 20% of normal subjects[20]. The compression is often positional, typically occurring when the arm is elevated above the head, so various positions of the arm and shoulder may need to be assessed. Sometimes the symptoms only occur with the patient in a particular position such as standing or lying down. Usually the diagnosis is straightforward on clinical grounds, with the pulse in the affected arm disappearing when the arm is in the appropriate position. However, in some cases the diagnosis, or the cause, is less clear cut

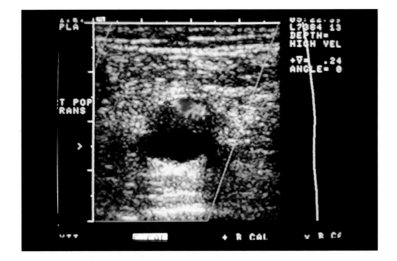

Fig. 4.14 Cystic adventitial disease of the popliteal artery. The cystic component is seen behind the patent lumen.

and colour Doppler can be used to image the subclavian artery as the arm is moved into various positions with the patient supine or erect. The transducer is usually placed in the supraclavicular position but scanning under the clavicle may be useful, particularly when the arm is fully elevated. Careful examination of the artery as it passes over the first rib may show changes in the waveform as the vessel is compressed (Fig. 4.15).

Popliteal artery compression

In cases of suspected entrapment of an artery or graft in the adductor canal or popliteal fossa, direct examination of the vessel is often restricted by the limited access to the popliteal fossa with the knee flexed. However, careful examination of the lower popliteal artery or posterior tibial artery with the knee in different positions of flexion will demonstrate changes in the arterial wave-form resulting from compression. Athletes may get compression of the popliteal artery between the lateral femoral condyle or upper tibia and the hypertrophied soleus and plan-taris muscles. This can be demonstrated on Doppler ultrasound by scanning with the foot in a neutral position and then in a posi-tion of forced plantar flexion[21].

ACCURACY IN RELATION TO OTHER TECHNIQUES

The gold standard for the assessment of the accuracy of Doppler ultrasound is usually arte-riography. The reservations on the accuracy of arteriography, which are discussed in Chapter 3 on carotids, are also applicable to peripheral arterial disease. Cossman *et al* compared colour Doppler with arteriography in 84 limbs[10], from the iliac to lower popliteal segments, using the criteria discussed earlier. For the detection of stenoses greater than 50%, they found an overall sensitivity of 87% (156/180 segments), specificity of 99% (444/449), accuracy of 95% (600/629), posi-tive predictive value of 96% (156/162) and negative predictive value of 95% (444/467). For the diagnosis of arterial occlusion the overall sensitivity was 81% (76/94), with speci-ficity of 99% (463/466), accuracy of 96% (539/560), positive predictive value of 95% (76/80) and negative predictive value of 96% (463/481).

Polak reviewed five studies performed between 1989 and 1992[22], including the study by Cossman *et al*. Colour Doppler was compared to arteriography and the overall sensitivity for the detection of a stenosis greater than 50% was 87.5% (316/361 seg-ments), for an occluded segment the sensitivity

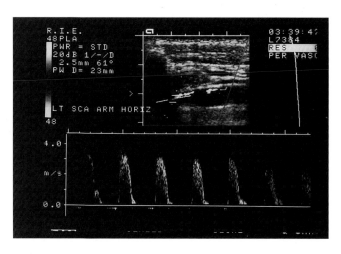

Fig. 4.15 Compression of the subclavian artery as the arm is elevated/abducted, showing narrowing of the artery as it emerges from behind the clavicle on the left of the picture.

was 92.6% (403/435), and the overall specificity for the identification of normal segments was 97% (1247/1282).

Magnetic resonance arteriography is now being applied to the peripheral arteries with some promising results, particularly with contrast enhancement, but availability and complexity, together with poor resolution in the smaller calf vessels, mean that this is still being developed, rather than a generally available technique. Computed tomography (CT) arteriography can be used for the assessment of brachial artery compression and is useful in demonstrating the relation of the artery to adjacent bone and other musculoskeletal structures.

CONCLUSIONS

Providing that the examination is performed carefully, Doppler ultrasound provides a relatively cheap and an accurate technique for the assessment of many patients with disease or previous surgery to the peripheral arteries, particularly in the lower limbs. In symptomatic patients it can be used as a first-line test to identify those patients without significant disease, those patients who may benefit from angioplasty and patients who are likely to require surgical bypass. It has been suggested that ultrasound can be used alone prior to surgery, but many vascular surgeons will still prefer an arteriogram in order to assess the distal run-off and to obtain a visual appreciation of the disease. Power Doppler and echo-enhancing agents will increase the diagnostic sensitivity of Doppler ultrasound and need for arteriography in many cases should be substantially reduced.

REFERENCES

1. Fowkes FGR (1988) Epidemiology of atherosclerotic disease in the lower limbs. *European Journal of Vascular Surgery* 2: 283–291
2. Department of Health and Social Security, Office of Population Censuses and Surveys (1988). *Hospital Inpatient Enquiry.* London: HMSO
3. Leng GC, Evans CJ, Fowkes FGR (1995) Epidemiology of peripheral vascular diseases. *Imaging* 7: 85–96
4. Edwards JM, Coldwell DM, Goldman ML, Strandness DE Jr (1991) The role of duplex scanning in the selection of patients for transluminal angioplasty. *Journal of Vascular Surgery* 13: 69–74
5. Langholz J, Schlief R, Schürmann R, Wanke M, Heidrich H (1996) Contrast enhancement in leg vessels. *Clinical Radiology* 51 (Suppl 1): 31–34
6. Flanigan DP, Tullis JP, Streeter VL, Whitehouse WM, Fry WJ, Stanley JC (1977) Multiple subcritical arterial stenoses: effect on poststenotic pressure and flow. *Annals of Surgery* 186: 663–668
7. Allard L, Cloutier G, Durand LG, Roederer GO, Langlois YE (1994) Limitations of ultrasonic duplex scanning for diagnosing lower limb arterial stenoses in the presence of adjacent segment disease. *Journal of Vascular Surgery* 19: 650–657
8. Whyman MR, Allan PL, Gillespie IN, Fowkes FG, Ruckley CV (1992) Screening patients with claudication from femoropopliteal disease before angioplasty using Doppler colour flow imaging. *British Journal of Surgery* 79: 907–909
9. Jager KA, Ricketts HJ, Strandness DE Jr (1985) Duplex scanning for evaluation of lower limb arterial disease. In: Bernstein EF (ed.) *Noninvasive Diagnostic Techniques in Vascular Disease* pp 619–631. St. Louis: CV Mosby
10. Cossman DV, Ellison JE, Wagner WH et al (1989) Comparison of contrast arteriography to arterial mapping with color-flow duplex imaging in the lower extremities. *Journal of Vascular Surgery* 10: 522–529
11. van Asten WN, van Lier HJ, Beijnevald WJ, Wijn PF, Pieters BF, Skotnicki SH (1991) Assessment of aortoiliac obstructive disease by Doppler spectrum analysis of blood flow velocities in the common femoral artery at rest and during reactive hyperaemia. *Surgery* 109: 633–639
12. Zierler RE (1990) Duplex and color-flow imaging of the lower extremity arterial circulation. *Seminars in Ultrasonography, Computed Tomography and Magnetic Resonance* 11: 168–179
13. Rosfors S, Hoglund N, Eriksson M, Johansson G (1993) Duplex ultrasound in patients with suspected aortoiliac occlusive disease. *European Journal of Vascular Surgery* 7: 513
14. Bandyk DF (1993) Essentials of graft surveillance. *Seminars in Vascular Surgery* 6: 92–102
15. Mills JL (1993) Mechanisms of graft failure: the location, distribution and characteristics of lesions that predispose to graft failure. *Seminars in Vascular Surgery* 6: 78–91

16. Sanchez LA, Suggs WD, Veith FJ *et al* (1993) Is surveillance to detect failing polytetrafluoroethylene bypasses worthwhile: 12-year experience with 91 grafts. *Journal of Vascular Surgery* **18**: 981–990

17. Landwehr P (1995) Haemodialysis shunts. In: Wolf K-J, Fobbe F (eds) *Colour Duplex Sonography*, pp 92–109. New York: Thieme Medical Publishers

18. Coley BD, Roberts AC, Fellmeth BD, Valji K, Bookstein JJ, Hye RJ (1995) Postangiographic femoral artery pseudoaneurysms: further experience with US-guided compression repair. *Radiology* **194**: 307–311

19. Flanigan DP, Burnham SJ, Goodreau JJ, Bergan JJ (1979) Summary of cases of adventitial disease of the popliteal artery. *Annals of Surgery* **189**: 165–175

20. Longley DG, Schwabacher S, Yedlicka JW, Hunter DW, Molina EJ, Letourneau JG (1992) Thoracic outlet syndrome: evaluation of the subclavian vessels by colour duplex sonography. *American Journal of Radiology* **158**: 623–630

21. Turnipseed WD, Pozniak M (1992) Popliteal entrapment as a result of neurovascular compression by the soleus and plantaris muscles. *Journal of Vascular Surgery* **15**: 285–294

22. Polak JF (1995) Peripheral arterial disease. Evaluation with color flow and duplex sonography. *Radiology Clinics of North America* **33**: 71–90

The peripheral veins

5

PAUL L. ALLAN

The peripheral veins may be affected by a variety of disorders, which can be assessed by ultrasound. Deep vein thrombosis and thrombo-embolic disease are the most common indications for investigation of the peripheral veins but venous insufficiency and vein mapping are also reasons for examining the veins. Anderson *et al* found an average annual incidence of 48 initial cases, 36 recurrent cases of deep vein thrombosis and 23 cases of pulmonary embolus per 100 000 population in the Worcester DVT study[1]. The prevalence of varicose veins and chronic venous insufficiency is more difficult to quantify, but it has been estimated that 10–15% of males and 20–25% of females in an unselected Western population over 15 years of age have visible tortuous varicose veins; 2–5% of adult males and 3–7% of females have evidence of moderate or severe chronic venous insufficiency, with a point prevalence for active ulceration of 0.1–0.2%[2].

INDICATIONS

The indications for ultrasound of the venous system are shown in Table 5.1. The most frequent indication for ultrasound of the veins is for the investigation of possible deep vein thrombosis in the lower limb and, occasionally, in the upper limb – especially if there have been central venous catheters inserted for intensive

care monitoring, chemotherapy, dialysis or parenteral feeding. Similarly, indwelling femoral catheters are prone to induce thrombosis and patients should be examined early if this is suspected. Ultrasound provides a non-invasive, reliable method for examining the venous system, particularly with respect to the diagnosis, or exclusion, of dangerous proximal thrombus in symptomatic patients[3]. The results for asymptomatic thrombus in the lower limbs are less encouraging and this should be recognized when using ultrasound to screen for deep vein thrombosis in asymptomatic patients[4].

Recurrence of varicose veins following surgery can pose many problems for the clinician trying to clarify the venous anatomy. Colour Doppler can be used instead of venography and varicography in many cases and may be the only examination required to define the anatomy and function in patients with recurrent varicose veins[5].

Table 5.1 Indications for venous ultrasound.

- Diagnosis or exclusion of deep vein thrombosis in the upper or lower limb, spontaneous or related to indwelling catheters
- Assessment of secondary/recurrent varicose veins
- Investigation of chronic venous insufficiency and postphlebitis syndrome
- Vein mapping prior to bypass grafts
- Localization of veins for cannulation

The impact of postphlebitis syndromes and chronic venous insufficiency is a rather larger problem than is apparent from its relatively low clinical profile. In one large epidemiological study of 4376 subjects, 62% had some evidence of varicose veins; signs of chronic insufficiency were present in 22%[6]. Varicography shows perforator veins which are obviously incompetent and some incompetent superficial and deep venous segments, but ultrasound has the advantage that the segments of the deep and superficial systems can be examined and the direction of blood flow within each segment can be demonstrated. In addition, it is less unpleasant for the patient and allows multiple assessments to be performed without discomfort. The main disadvantage is that it is fairly time-consuming, particularly in complex cases, and requires a significant degree of expertise in order to perform examinations efficiently.

The superficial veins of the legs and, occasionally, the arms may be used for bypass grafts for the coronary or lower limb arteries. If there is any doubt about their suitability as a conduit following previous varicose vein surgery, or in terms of their calibre, ultrasound can be used to assess the diameter and length of vein available. In addition, the sonographer can map out the course of the vein to allow easier harvesting.

It may be difficult occasionally to locate a suitable vein for central venous cannulation, particularly in patients who have had multiple previous central venous lines, such as intensive care or chemotherapy patients. Ultrasound can be used to clarify the location and patency of potentially suitable veins and, in difficult cases, the puncture may be made under direct ultrasound visualization.

ANATOMY AND SCANNING TECHNIQUE

The anatomy of the venous system in the limbs is more complex and variable than that of the arteries. The meanings of the terms 'proximal' and 'distal' may cause confusion as the veins start at the periphery and blood flows centrally towards the heart so that 'upstream' is peripheral and 'downstream' is central, which is the opposite from the situation in the arteries. The convention is that proximal describes locations nearer the heart and distal refers to points further from the heart; these terms are used in this way in this chapter.

Anatomy – lower limb

The veins of the lower limb are divided into deep and superficial systems. These are linked by a variable number of perforator veins which carry blood from the superficial to the deep systems (Figs 5.1 and 5.2).

The deep veins

The anatomy of the lower limb veins is rather variable. Generally the veins accompany the arteries but their number may vary and the communications with other veins along the way can show a variety of patterns; however, a general arrangement is usually apparent. In the calf there are veins running with the main arteries: the *posterior tibial, peroneal* and *anterior tibial veins*; there are usually two, occasionally three veins with each artery (Fig. 5.3). In addition there are venous channels, or sinuses, which drain the major muscle groups in the posterior calf. These are seen in the upper calf as they pass upwards to join the other deep veins in the lower popliteal region; the *gastrocnemius* and *soleal veins* are the largest of these. The gastrocnemius vein is the more superficial and may be mistaken for the short saphenous vein; clues to its true identity are that it is usually accompanied by the artery to the muscle and it can be followed distally down into the muscle rather than outwards to lie subcutaneously on the fascia around the calf, which is the position of the short saphenous vein.

The calf veins join to form the *popliteal vein*, or veins – there may be two, or sometimes

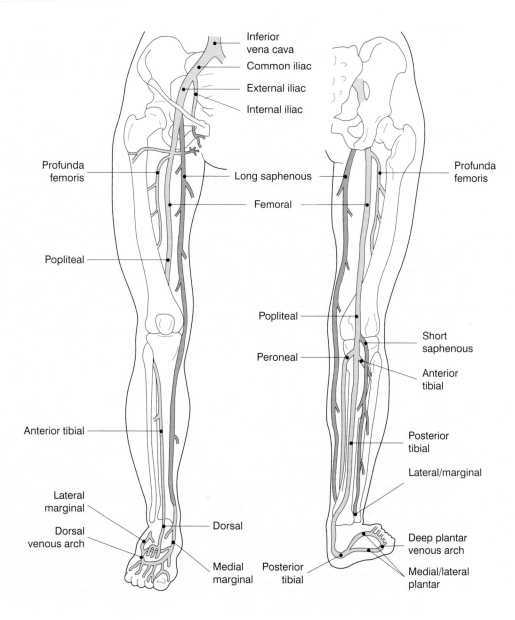

Fig. 5.1 The veins of the lower limb, showing the superficial and deep systems.

three channels, especially if there is a dual superficial femoral vein. The popliteal vein runs up through the popliteal fossa, lying more posterior and usually medial to the artery. As well as the veins from the calf and calf muscles, it is joined by the *short saphenous vein* at the saphenopopliteal junction.

The popliteal vein becomes the *superficial femoral vein* at the upper border of the popliteal fossa; rarely, the popliteal vein runs more deeply to join with the profunda femoris vein. The superficial femoral vein runs up the medial aspect of the thigh, posterior to the superficial femoral artery to join with the

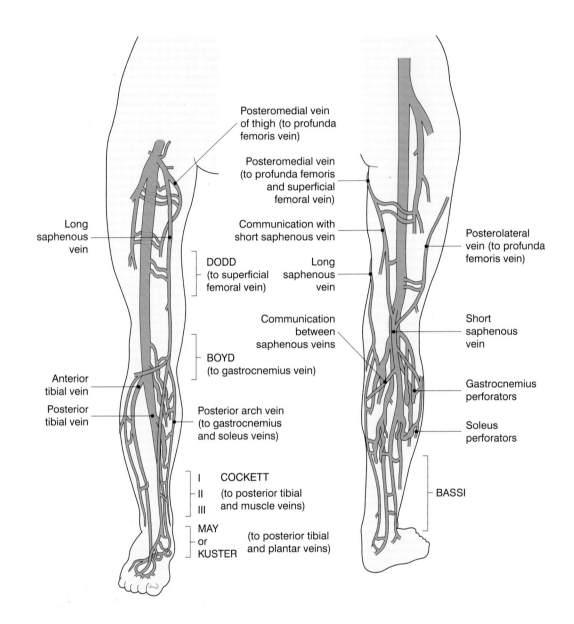

Fig. 5.2 The major perforating veins in the lower limb.

profunda femoris vein in the femoral triangle below the groin; the profunda femoris vein drains the thigh muscles. The confluence of the superficial femoral and profunda femoris veins to form the common femoral vein is normally a little more caudal than the bifurcation of the common femoral artery into the superficial femoral and profunda femoris arteries. The superficial femoral vein may have significant segments of duplication along its length in up to 25% of subjects[7], these dual segments may have a variable relation to the artery, so that they may be overlooked unless care is taken in the examination of the thigh veins.

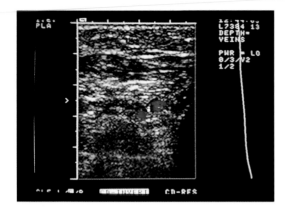

Fig. 5.3 Paired deep calf veins running with the artery.

In the pelvis and groin, the anatomy is generally consistent. The superficial femoral vein and profunda femoris vein join to form the *common femoral vein*, which lies medial to the common femoral artery. The common femoral vein is joined by the *long saphenous vein* at the saphenofemoral junction (Fig. 5.4a); the appearance of the common femoral vein, long saphenous vein and artery in transverse section is sometimes referred to as the 'Mickey Mouse' view (Fig. 5.4b). The common femoral vein is also joined by veins from the muscles around the hip. These veins are variable in size and number, and occasionally one of these is large enough to be confused with the long saphenous vein or profunda femoris vein but careful attention to the anatomy should clarify the situation. The common femoral vein becomes the *external iliac vein* after it has passed under the inguinal ligament, then it passes posteriorly along the posterior pelvis, running alongside the external iliac artery. The *internal iliac vein*, which drains the pelvic structures, joins with the external iliac vein deep in the pelvis to form the *common iliac vein* (Fig. 5.5). The two common iliac veins then join at the level of the aortic bifurcation to form the *inferior vena cava*, which normally passes cranially on the right side of the aorta. The left common iliac vein passes behind the right common iliac artery just distal to this confluence. In a small number of individuals this confluence does not occur and the two common iliac veins continue cranially as dual inferior venae cavae; this reflects the arrangement of paired cardinal veins in the embryo.

The deep veins have a series of valves along their course. These are somewhat variable in their number and location. They are most numerous in the veins below the knee; in the thigh, the superficial femoral vein usually has one just below the confluence with the profunda femoris vein and at several levels below this. The iliac veins, in contrast, have relatively few valves[8]; rarely a valve may be seen in the inferior vena cava.

The superficial veins

The two main superficial venous channels in the lower limb are the long and short

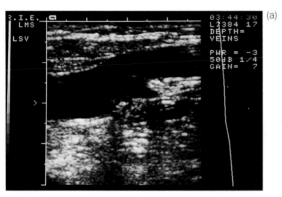

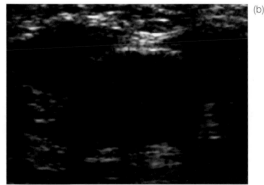

Fig. 5.4 The saphenofemoral junction in longitudinal section (a) and the transverse 'Mickey Mouse' view (b).

5

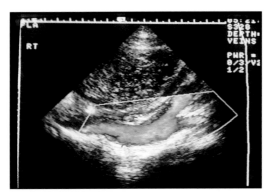

Fig. 5.5 The confluence of the internal and external iliac veins forming the common iliac vein.

saphenous veins. The *long saphenous vein* arises from the medial aspect of the dorsal venous arch of the foot and passes in front of the medial malleolus to run up the medial aspect of the calf and knee into the thigh. In the upper thigh, the long saphenous vein curves laterally and deeply to join the common femoral vein just below the inguinal ligament. The long saphenous vein receives many superficial tributaries and is connected to the deep veins by perforating veins. The standard sites for the perforators are at the level of the junction between the middle and lower thirds of the thigh and in the calf, although many other communicating veins have been recorded and described (Fig. 5.2)[9]. In the region of the saphenofemoral junction the long saphenous vein receives several tributaries draining the groin, lower abdominal wall and perineum. These veins are of significance in the recurrence of varicose veins following high ligation, as they provide a network of collateral channels which may bypass the resected segment.

The *short saphenous vein* arises from the lateral aspect of the dorsal venous arch of the foot, passing below and behind the lateral malleolus to run up the posterolateral aspect of the calf to the popliteal fossa, where it passes through the deep fascia to join the popliteal vein. It usually enters the lateral aspect of the popliteal vein at the level of the popliteal skin crease or within a few centimetres above this. Occasionally it passes upwards to join the profunda femoris vein in the lower thigh (Giacomini vein), and very rarely may join its superficial venous companion, the long saphenous vein.

Scanning technique – lower limb

The technique varies depending on the clinical indication. The most common indication is the diagnosis or exclusion of deep vein thrombosis in the lower limb. This section therefore concentrates on this aspect and variations in technique for other indications will be dealt with in subsequent sections (Table 5.2). A 5 MHz linear transducer is the most suitable frequency as it provides sufficient penetration, particularly in large or oedematous thighs. A higher-frequency transducer may be used for superficial veins. It is important to ensure that the system is set up for the slower velocities found in veins, rather than the significantly higher arterial velocities.

It is advantageous if there is a tilting couch available so that the patient can be moved from the horizontal to various degrees of head-up elevation as necessary. In the absence of a tilting couch it is better if the patient can be

Table 5.2 Basic steps in the examination for thrombosis.

1. Patient sitting on couch/trolley: compression of common femoral vein, superficial femoral vein from groin to adductor canal
2. Colour Doppler with augmentation, examine common and superficial femoral veins
3. Patient decubitus, or with leg elevated: compression and Doppler examination of popliteal vein(s)
4. Patient sitting, if possible, with legs dependent: examine the calf veins with compression and colour Doppler
5. Patient supine: examine iliac veins if thrombus suspected in these

examined with the thorax higher than the legs, as this produces some distension of the lower limb veins, which makes them easier to identify and the assessment of compression more straightforward.

There are three components to the ultrasound examination of the veins for deep vein thrombosis: imaging, Doppler and compression. Thrombus may be seen in the vein, Doppler may show abnormal, or absent, flow signals and compression refers to the fact that a normal vein is easily compressible – light pressure with the transducer will obliterate the lumen of the vein. Two points should be noted in relation to compression: first, compression should be performed in the transverse plane (Fig. 5.6) for the reason that if it is done in the longitudinal plane a thrombosed vein may disappear as it is no longer in the scan plane, rather than because it has been compressed. Second, fresh thrombus is soft and gelatinous, so that firm pressure can produce a degree of compression, which may give a false impression of patency. The use of colour Doppler should clarify this situation but care must be taken if this is not available. A further reason for scanning in the transverse plane is that dual segments of the superficial femoral vein will be identified more reliably.

The examination begins at the groin, where the common femoral vein is located on a transverse scan and compressed. Compression is then repeated at intervals of 3–5 cm down the length of the thigh to the adductor canal. At this point the superficial femoral vein is difficult to compress from an anterior approach as it is well supported by the bulk of the anterior

thigh muscles. Compression is better achieved in this region by placing a hand behind the medial thigh and pushing up with the fingers against the transducer. The scan plane is then changed to longitudinal and the vein examined with colour Doppler, or power Doppler, as the transducer is moved up the thigh. Squeezing the calf gently will augment flow and allow easier detection of areas of flow or thrombosis; alternatively, the patient can be asked to plantar-flex their toes, which results in calf muscle contraction and emptying of the calf veins.

Colour Doppler signals are often sufficient, in conjunction with the findings on compression, to confirm or exclude a diagnosis of deep vein thrombosis (Fig. 5.7). If there is any doubt then a spectral assessment will allow a better appreciation of damped flow, absent respiratory variation and impaired augmentation.

Once the thigh veins have been examined the patient is turned into a lateral position, with the medial aspect of the leg being examined uppermost, so that the popliteal veins can be examined. Again, compression and colour Doppler are used to assess the veins. Some patients, particularly postoperative patients, may not be able to move into a decubitus position. In these cases the popliteal veins are examined with the knee partially flexed up off the couch, with external rotation, if possible,

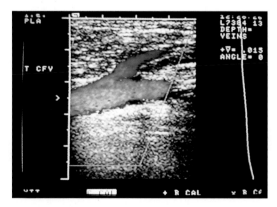

Fig. 5.7 The normal saphenofemoral junction showing complete colour fill-in across the vein lumen.

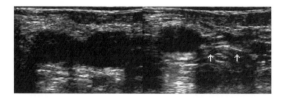

Fig. 5.6 Normal compression: the lumen of the vein is completely obliterated by pressure from the transducer.

95

so that the transducer can be positioned in the popliteal fossa; a curved array can be of benefit in gaining access in this situation. Alternatively, the leg can be elevated and supported off the couch by an assistant.

The calf veins can be examined after the popliteal vein with the patient in the decubitus position on a tilted couch, or in the supine position with the knee flexed up off the mattress, if the patient is relatively immobile. Alternatively, the patient can sit on the couch with their legs over the side so that the dependent calf veins are well distended. The posterior tibial and deeper peroneal vessels are most easily located by scanning in the transverse plane from the medial side of the calf and identifying the arterial signals on colour Doppler (Fig. 4.2). These veins may also be located on a longitudinal scan; again the arterial signal provides a useful guide to the position of the veins. If there are difficulties identifying the posterior tibial veins at the mid-calf level then scanning the lower calf just above the medial malleolus, where the vessels are superficial and constant in location, may be of value; the posterior tibial vessels can then be followed back up the calf with augmentation of flow as necessary in order to assess patency. In the mid- and lower calf, squeezing the calf can produce motion artefacts from movement of the calf muscles which obscure the flow signals from the veins; in these cases, squeezing the foot will produce adequate augmentation of flow. The anterior tibial veins are examined from an anterolateral approach: scanning transversely, the tibia, fibula and interosseous membrane are identified. The anterior tibial vessels are found on the superficial aspect of the interosseous membrane, although it should be noted that these veins are rarely involved in deep vein thrombosis in isolation from the other calf veins. The peroneal veins may also be visualized deep to the interosseous membrane in many patients from this anterolateral aspect, allowing their examination if

they have not been identified from a postero-medial approach.

The iliac veins are examined by following the external iliac vein upwards from the common femoral vein into the pelvis. A 3 or 4 MHz transducer is usually necessary for adequate penetration. Firm pressure may be required to displace bowel gas. This may produce narrowing or effacement of the more superficial segments of vein, resulting in an absence of signal and a possible false diagnosis of occlusion. If the pelvic veins are difficult to trace superiorly then the common iliac vein can usually be identified just distal to the inferior vena cava and aortic bifurcation; this can then be followed peripherally. In some patients it is impossible to identify the deeper pelvic portion of the iliac veins; however, if there is a patent external iliac vein which shows respiratory variation with good augmentation and a patent upper common iliac vein, then it is highly unlikely that there is significant thrombus in the invisible segment. Trans-vaginal scanning will show the deeper pelvic veins and may be considered if there is a need to visualize these vessels directly. In thinner patients, or patients with good pelvic access, the proximal internal iliac vein may be seen joining the external iliac vein in the pelvis (Fig. 5.5). The inferior vena cava is examined if thrombus is seen extending into this vessel. It is important, whenever thrombus is diagnosed in a leg vein, that the proximal extent of the clot is identified, as this may have a significant impact on management decisions in relation to anticoagulation therapy, or the placing of a filter.

In pregnant women in the later part of pregnancy, the uterus will lie on the iliac veins in the supine position and compress them, thus reducing flow and impairing augmentation in the lower limb veins. This can be alleviated by asking the patient to turn into a semi-decubitus position, with the side being examined uppermost, so that the uterus falls away, allowing better flow in the pelvic veins. An alternative is to examine the patient standing, as the uterus moves forward away from the iliac veins in this position.

Anatomy – upper limb

The veins of the upper limb are also divided into deep and superficial groups (Fig. 5.8). The *deep veins* are paired and accompany the arteries: the *radial, ulnar* and *brachial* veins. There is a variable pattern of communicating veins between the deep venous channels and between the deep venous channels and the superficial veins. The superficial system is more variable than in the leg but there are usually two main channels: the *cephalic vein* on the radial aspect of the arm and the *basilic vein* on the ulnar side. These communicate at the

cubital fossa by way of the *median cubital vein* and they also communicate with the deep brachial veins at this level. The basilic vein pierces the deep fascia on the medial aspect of the mid-upper arm to join the brachial veins and this combined venous channel becomes the *axillary vein* when it enters the axilla. The cephalic vein passes more cranially along the lateral aspect of the biceps. At the level of pectoralis major it turns medially and deeply to pierce the clavipectoral fascia below the clavicle and joins the upper axillary vein. The axillary vein also receives other tributaries from the region of the shoulder joint and the lateral chest wall.

The axillary vein becomes the *subclavian vein* as it crosses the first rib, where it lies in front of the artery; the main tributary of the subclavian vein is the external jugular vein. The subclavian vein joins with the internal jugular vein behind the medial end of the clavicle to form the innominate vein, which is also known as the *brachiocephalic vein*.

Scanning technique – upper limb

Examination of the upper limb veins is normally performed with the patient supine and the arm abducted to about 90°; the patient may require some support for the arm, or they can be asked to hold onto some suitable part of the ultrasound machine beside them. A transducer frequency of 5–10 MHz can be used. The examination begins at the sternoclavicular joint, where the distal innominate vein can be assessed and the confluence with the internal jugular vein examined, particularly if central lines have been inserted. The subclavian vein is examined from above and then below the clavicle; it is seen lying in front of the subclavian artery as it runs over the first rib. The axillary vein is then followed across the axilla into the upper arm, from where the brachial veins can be examined down to the elbow. The veins below this are not usually examined unless

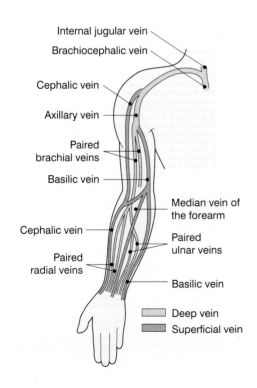

Internal jugular vein
Brachiocephalic vein
Cephalic vein
Axillary vein
Paired brachial veins
Basilic vein
Median vein of the forearm
Cephalic vein
Paired ulnar veins
Paired radial veins
Basilic vein

☐ Deep vein
▨ Superficial vein

Fig. 5.8 The veins of the upper limb, showing the main superficial and deep veins.

there is some specific reason, such as the presence of a dialysis shunt. Augmentation of flow is obtained by manual compression of the forearm, or upper arm; alternatively, asking the patient to clench their fist will increase venous flow. If there is a suspicion of a possible venous compression syndrome, the arm veins can be examined with the limb in different positions of abduction; comparison of flow on the two sides can be of value.

DIAGNOSIS OF DEEP VEIN THROMBOSIS

The diagnosis of normal or thrombosed veins is based on the compressibility of the veins, the appearance of the veins and the changes which occur to the spectral and colour Doppler findings. The main changes associated with deep vein thrombosis are shown in Table 5.3. The lower limb is examined for possible thrombosis much more frequently than the upper limb, although the features described are also applicable to the arm veins.

Compressibility

As noted above, a normal vein is easily compressible with only mild to moderate pressure from the transducer, so that the lumen is completely obliterated. A vein filled with thrombus will be held open, although it must be remembered that fresh thrombus has the consistency of jelly, so that it can be compressed to some extent by strong pressure.

Table 5.3 Signs of deep vein thrombosis.
- Absent or reduced compressibility
- Thrombus in the vein: static echoes, incomplete colour fill-in, expansion of the vein
- Static valve leaflets
- Absent flow on spectral or colour Doppler
- Impaired or absent augmentation of flow
- Loss of spontaneous flow and respiratory variation
- Increased flow in collateral channels

Appearances of the vein and the vein lumen

The lumen of a normal vein is usually anechoic and, on colour Doppler, the whole lumen of the vein should be filled with colour, particularly on augmentation of flow. Although fresh thrombus is anechoic, or hypoechoic, it becomes increasingly echogenic as it matures. In addition fresh thrombus has a tendency to expand the vein and make it look rounder and fuller than a normal vessel. This is accentuated at the upper end of the thrombus where the patent lumen above the clot may be relatively poorly filled with blood due to the distal obstruction by the thrombus (Fig. 5.9).

Fresh thrombus is not particularly adherent to the vein wall, so that some blood may be seen around the periphery of the clot in the vein. Another appearance which may be seen in early thrombosis is that of a thin tail of thrombus extending up the vein from its origin and lying free in the lumen of the vein (Fig. 5.10). Older thrombus becomes increasingly echogenic, adherent to the vein wall and contracts as it becomes more organized and fibrotic. This may result in the vein being reduced to a relatively small echoic structure that may be difficult to locate. Alternatively, the thrombus may retract to one side of the vein, resulting in an asymmetric lumen.

An exception to the rule that flowing blood is not echogenic is seen in pregnancy, or any other situation where there is slow venous flow and a tendency to hyperviscosity. In these individuals faint, mobile echoes are seen moving up the vein on real-time imaging; these accelerate on augmentation of flow. These echoes are produced by clumps, or aggregates of red cells, and do not usually cause any significant difficulties in diagnosis with modern, real-time, colour Doppler equipment.

Normal valves may be seen moving gently in the currents from blood passing them, particularly in the larger thigh veins (Fig 5.11). One of the earliest sites of deep vein

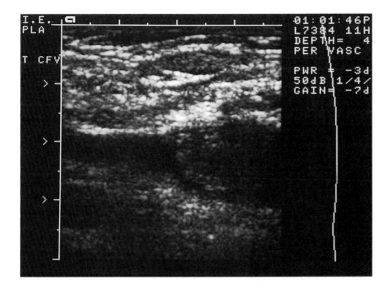

Fig. 5.9 A vein containing thrombus: low-level echoes are seen in the clot and there is a degree of collapse of the underfilled patent lumen above the thrombus.

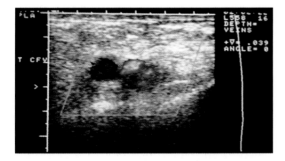

Fig. 5.10 A small tail of thrombus extending up the vein which is not sufficiently large to produce any obstruction to flow and could be overlooked if visualization of this area was poor.

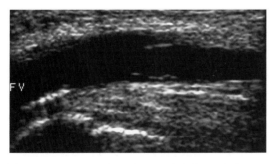

Fig. 5.11 A normal valve in the superficial femoral vein.

thrombus formation is in the sinus above a valve cusp, so that apparent rigidity or fixation of a cusp should raise the suspicion of possible early deep vein thrombosis and a careful examination of the area should be undertaken.

The walls of a normal vein are smooth and unobtrusive. Following recanalization after a deep vein thrombosis, they become irregular, thickened and echogenic; calcification may also occur in a small number of cases.

Doppler findings

Spontaneous flow and respiratory variation

Even at rest and with some head-up tilt there should still be spontaneous flow along the vein which shows some respiratory variation or phasicity. This variation is produced by the intra-abdominal pressure changes on respiration. On inspiration the diaphragm descends and the intra-abdominal pressure rises; this results in decreased flow from the leg veins into the abdomen. On expiration the intra-abdominal pressure decreases and flow from the legs increases. Similarly, if the patient holds their breath, flow in the leg veins slows and may cease until the patient relaxes, when there is relatively high flow from the legs.

If there is thrombus occluding the vein there will not be any flow detected in the vein lumen at the level of the thrombus. Sometimes thrombosis is segmental, with a segment of iliac vein or superficial femoral vein occluded but with patent veins below this level; there is a higher incidence of this in pregnant patients and patients with pelvic tumours. Patent segments below the thrombus may show some slow antegrade flow, particularly if collateral channels are adequate, but this does not show any respiratory variation and the augmentation response is damped.

Augmentation

Normal venous flow is slow and can be improved by compression distal to the point of assessment. There are various techniques for achieving this which are discussed further in the section on chronic venous insufficiency, but for the assessment of possible deep venous thrombosis manual compression of the calf is usually sufficient. The muscles of the calf are squeezed rapidly and firmly in order to propel blood up the veins. In a normal venous system there will be a rapid rise and fall in the frequency shift; whereas if there is a thrombosed segment in the veins, this will increase resistance to flow with damping, or absence, of the augmentation response (Fig. 5.12). It should be remembered that increased resistance to flow anywhere in the vein above the point of compression will result in impaired augmentation the thrombus may be above or below the point of examination. Therefore, the demonstration of impaired augmentation should lead to a careful search for thrombus in that limb; particularly in the calf or iliac segments. The squeeze of the calf muscles should not be violent, or excessive, as patients will often have tender or painful calves; in addition there is a small potential risk of

dislodging a fresh friable thrombus, producing a pulmonary embolus. The risk of this is small and reports of this type of event are few[10].

Flow in collateral channels

When the normal venous channels are occluded, blood may be seen in collateral veins. In the acute stage, intramuscular channels will not have developed significantly but increased velocity and flow may be seen in the two saphenous veins, or the profunda femoris vein, which provide ready-made collateral pathways. Over a period of several weeks the intramuscular venous channels will develop and these may be apparent on colour Doppler; therefore their presence indicates a thrombus of some age, rather than fresh thrombus, unless there has been rethrombosis in a segment of clearing clot.

Distinction of acute from chronic thrombus

The features which suggest older, rather than fresh, thrombus are given in Table 5.4. However, it is not always possible to define the age of a thrombus and, in these cases the management of the patient must be based on the clinical picture.

Fresh thrombus is hypoechoic or anechoic. It is not attached to the wall around the whole circumference of the vein but if it fills the vein, the vein is a little expanded[11]. Increased flow may be detected in the profunda femoris vein, or saphenous veins. As thrombus matures it becomes increasingly echogenic and starts to contract as it becomes organized. Longitudinal studies of thrombosed veins show that some 64% of veins will recanalize completely, or in part, by one year after thrombosis, although valvular incompetence will be found at some level in the majority of these[12]. The remaining veins will show varying degrees of recanalization, with a

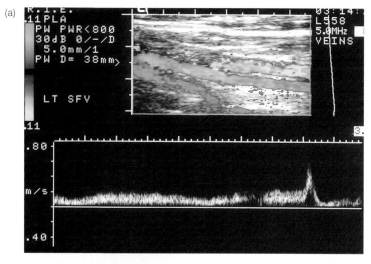

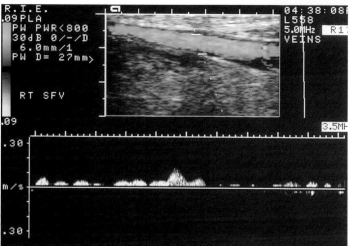

Fig. 5.12 (a) A normal augmentation response to squeezing the calf; there is a rapid rise and fall in the velocity of blood past the transducer. (b) Abnormal augmentation, with damping of the response as a result of thrombus impeding the flow of blood up the vein.

Table 5.4 Distinction between acute and chronic thrombus.

Acute	Chronic
Anechoic or hypoechoic	Increasingly echogenic
Expansion of the vein	Contraction of the vein
Some compression possible	Incompressible
Thrombus 'tail' in lumen	Clot adherent around the wall of the vein
Absent or minimal collaterals	Collateral channels in the tissues

thickened irregular wall around an uneven lumen; or remain as fibrotic, permanently occluded structures. Abnormal collateral venous channels will develop in the soft tissues around any segments which are significantly obstructed for any length of time.

PROBLEMS AND PITFALLS IN THE DIAGNOSIS OF DEEP VEIN THROMBOSIS

Some of these have been discussed already; however, the value of ultrasound as a technique for the diagnosis of deep vein thrombosis

101

depends on the operator performing a careful, complete examination, being aware of potential pitfalls and recognizing when a less than adequate examination has been performed. The main problem areas which should be remembered are shown in Table 5.5.

The essential requirement for a satisfactory examination is good ultrasound access to the veins of the limb. Many patients with a possible diagnosis of deep vein thrombosis have swollen or oedematous legs; this situation is aggravated if the patients are also obese. If visualization is poor then it is possible to miss significant thrombus unless the situation is recognized and appropriate care is taken with the examination and machine settings, as well as with the selection of an appropriate transducer.

Dual superficial femoral veins may be overlooked unless they are actively sought with transverse scanning. If they are not recognized, then one component may be patent and seen on colour Doppler, whereas the other component may contain thrombus and be overlooked (Fig. 5.13).

Similarly, non-occlusive thrombus may be missed if the vein is not seen adequately. If there is only a small amount of thrombus in

Table 5.5 Problems and pitfalls in the diagnosis of deep vein thrombosis.

- Swollen/oedematous/fat legs
- Dual thigh and popliteal veins
- Non-occlusive thrombus
- Segmental calf vein thrombus
- Segmental iliac vein thrombus
- Pregnant patients

the vein then good flow signals will be obtained on spectral and colour Doppler and the presence of the thrombus may not be recognized (Fig 5.10). This is particularly important in obese or oedematous legs.

The calf veins are multitudinous in number and variable in their anatomy. Even with a careful, patient, time-consuming examination it is difficult to exclude completely the presence of a small segmental thrombus in a calf vein or muscular sinus. In a mobile patient with a little calf tenderness or swelling this is not a problem, as the body's normal thrombolytic mechanisms will probably clear this. However, in a patient who is immobile following surgery or a stroke, a small segmental calf thrombus indicates that the clotting cascade has been

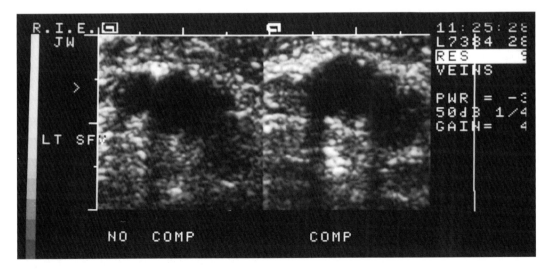

Fig. 5.13 Transverse scan of the superficial femoral vessels showing a dual segment of superficial femoral vein. One of the components is occluded by thrombus and the other is patent. Compression fails to obliterate the venous component on the right of the image which contains thrombus.

activated and there is a possibility that this small thrombus may increase in size, resulting in a significant, occlusive thrombus. Therefore a follow-up scan should be considered in these patients in order to identify any progression of thrombus from the calf.

The accuracy of Doppler in the detection of asymptomatic thrombus is less impressive than that for symptomatic thrombus[4, 13], and the technique is therefore inadequate as a screening tool for the detection of asymptomatic thrombus. This is probably because asymptomatic thrombi are more likely to be small and non-occlusive; in addition, there is a higher incidence of distal thrombi in the calf veins, which may be more difficult to demonstrate with ultrasound[3].

The external and common iliac veins may not be demonstrated in their entirety due to obesity or overlying bowel gas. Care must be taken to exclude segmental iliac vein thrombosis, especially if this is a possibility following pelvic surgery; however, it is very rare for iliac thrombosis not to include the common femoral vein[14]. The internal iliac veins are difficult to assess but any thrombus arising in these, which extends into the common iliac vein and significantly impedes blood flow, may be suggested by an impaired augmentation response in the femoral veins, or loss of respiratory variation on deep breathing or panting. However, non-occlusive thrombus which is insufficient to produce this effect may be overlooked; transvaginal scanning may be of value in difficult cases. It is important that the proximal extent of any thrombus is defined so that any subsequent extension can be appreciated. In addition, insertion of a caval filter might be considered and it is important to know if access is possible from the groin through the iliac veins. Once a filter has been inserted, the subsequent patency of the cava and iliac veins can be assessed using ultrasound (Fig. 5.14)[15].

Some of the features of thrombosis associated with pregnancy have already been

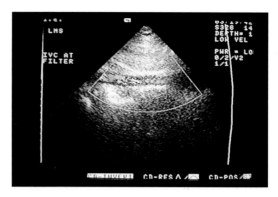

Fig. 5.14 A caval filter in place. Note the change in colour due to the alteration in direction of flow in relation to the transducer.

discussed. In addition to problems in diagnosis related to the uterus compressing the pelvic veins, there is an increased tendency to develop segmental proximal thromboses in the iliac and upper femoral veins. This is more common on the left side[16], perhaps reflecting the additional potential compression from the right common iliac artery, which crosses the left common iliac vein just beyond the aortic bifurcation. In addition, pregnancy produces changes in blood viscosity and coagulation which result in an increased tendency to develop blood clots. Patients who have undergone caesarean section have a higher risk of developing a deep vein thrombosis.

Other causes of leg swelling, pain or tenderness

Unlike venography, ultrasound allows examination of other structures in the pelvis and leg. Other pathologies may be seen which account for the patient's symptoms of a swollen, or painful, tender leg; these are given in Table 5.6. It is important to remember that, even if a ruptured popliteal cyst is seen, or a superficial thrombophlebitis is demonstrated (Fig. 5.15), the deep veins must still be examined carefully, as a coexistent deep vein thrombosis may otherwise be overlooked.

Table 5.6 Other causes of leg swelling, pain or tenderness.

- Popliteal cysts
- Haematoma
- Superficial thrombophlebitis
- Iliac nodes/pelvic masses
- Arteriovenous fistula
- Lymphoedema

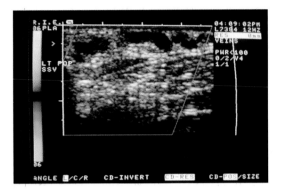

Fig. 5.15 Thrombosis of the superficial veins is easily recognized but the deep veins should still be examined.

ACCURACY IN RELATION TO OTHER TECHNIQUES

Despite these potential problems, ultrasound is a good non-invasive method for the diagnosis of symptomatic deep vein thrombosis, especially between the lower popliteal region and the groin[3]. The key to its value in any given department is that the sonographers must not only be well trained in the technique, but must also be able to recognize an inadequate examination so that appropriate further measures, such as venography or a repeat scan, can be arranged. Should venography be required to clarify areas of doubt, this can be focused on the area of concern identified at the ultrasound examination and only a limited examination may be required.

Many studies have shown that, in comparison to venography, ultrasound is an accurate technique for the diagnosis of symptomatic deep vein thrombosis in the femoropopliteal segments, even in the absence of colour Doppler[3]. Used alone, compression is an accurate method for detecting deep vein thrombosis, with sensitivities of 89% and specificity of 100% being reported for proximal thrombosis[17], and sensitivities of 86–92% and specificities of 96–100% for careful examination of the calf veins[18]. The additional use of colour Doppler allows very accurate diagnosis of deep vein thrombosis, particularly in the femoropopliteal segments. With the development of colour Doppler techniques, further studies have shown the value of ultrasound and that the calf veins can be examined satisfactorily in most cases (Table 5.7)[19]. The need for an adequate examination must be emphasized. In one study, the initial results in the calf were significantly less accurate than the results for the femoropopliteal segment, but when the examinations were reviewed and only those which were technically adequate were considerd, the overall accuracy improved markedly and reached a similar level to that obtained in the upper part of the limb[20] (Table 5.7).

It is important to draw a distinction between the accuracy of ultrasound for the diagnosis of

Table 5.7 Results of Doppler ultrasound in the diagnosis of symptomatic deep vein thrombosis.

Author	No. of patients	Sensitivity (%)	Specificity (%)	Regions studied
Rose *et al* (20)	75	96	100	Iliac and femoropopliteal
	75	92	100	Femoropopliteal only
	75	73	86	Calf only (all studies)
	45	95	100	Adequate calf vein studies
Baxter *et al* (19)	40	100	100	Femoropopliteal
	40	95	100	Calf only

symptomatic thrombus and asymptomatic thrombus. The results for the latter are less good as, almost by definition, asymptomatic thrombus will be non-occlusive in many cases and therefore easier to miss. Weinmann *et al* noted an overall sensitivity in six reported series of only 59% for proximal thrombus, although the specificity was 98%[3]. In addition, asymptomatic thrombus may be small, or involve one or only a few calf vein segments. A further review by Wells of 17 screening studies in orthopaedic patients showed a sensitivity of 62%, specificity of 97% and a positive predictive value of 66% in those studies which had been carried out with an adequate scientific method[21].

RECURRENT VARICOSE VEINS AND CHRONIC VENOUS INSUFFICIENCY

The venous system of the lower limb is relatively fragile and easily damaged by a variety of insults including thrombosis, trauma and inflammation. Previous thrombosis may not clear completely, resulting in chronic obstruction and damage to the valves. In limbs affected by deep vein thrombosis, 69% had at least one segment of incompetent vein which was more likely to occur in the previously thrombosed segment[22]. This damage results in loss of the protective action of the valves so that a continuous column of blood is present between the heart and the tissues of the calf, ankle and foot. In the erect position this may extend over 1.25 m and the hydrostatic pressure exerted on the tissues interferes with the circulation of blood in the capillaries, the transfer of nutrients and waste matter between blood and the tissues and may also promote local inflammatory responses in the tissues. These changes result in the development of varicose veins, varicose eczema and, ultimately, varicose ulceration. Treatment options include standard varicose vein surgical techniques, pressure stockings, dressings and, more recently, venous reconstruction tech-

niques. The pattern of damaged and incompetent veins can be defined using Doppler ultrasound to examine the deep and superficial veins in order to identify thrombosed or partially recanalized veins. Incompetent venous segments, together with incompetent perforating veins, can be mapped out and appropriate surgical or medical techniques applied. Approximately 1% of the population will have venous leg ulceration at some point in their lives[2], and up to 22% will have evidence of chronic venous insufficiency[5].

Recurrence of varicose veins after surgery or sclerotherapy may occur. Three main patterns of recurrence have been described[23]. A patent long saphenous vein may be present, suggesting that it has been missed at the time of the operation. Small collateral veins along the line of the long saphenous vein may enlarge to reconstitute the path of the vein. Finally, drainage can occur through venous collaterals which pass along a variety of courses remote from the normal line of the vein.

Technique of examination

The patient is best examined standing, or with a large degree of head-up tilt if the couch can be elevated, otherwise inadequate pressure will be exerted on the valves to test their competence. As the examination may be time-consuming – particularly if both legs are being examined – it is useful if the patients have some means of supporting themselves, such as a handle or rail on the wall; this enables them to stand in reasonable comfort with their weight on the leg that is not being examined and with slight flexion of the leg under examination. Alternatively, they may support themselves by holding the side of the ultrasound machine. It is useful if they are asked to stand on a low plinth, as this makes examination of the popliteal and calf regions less uncomfortable for the examiner.

Various techniques can be used to assess competence or incompetence of a venous

5

segment. The most convenient method for general assessment is to squeeze firmly the patient's calf, or lower thigh, to promote forward flow. Incompetent valves will allow reverse flow back through them after forward flow has ceased (Fig. 5.16), whereas competent valves will stop any reverse flow. Pressure cuffs that can be inflated and deflated rapidly can be used to produce a similar effect and produce a more standardized stimulus than manual compression[24]. They can also be used to compress a segment of leg in order to squeeze out the venous blood and then released suddenly so that any incompetent segments will show up by reversed filling from above. Alternatively, proximal compression may be applied to induce reverse flow. Getting the patient to perform a Valsalva manoeuvre will also show incompetent segments but there are two disadvantages to this technique. First, the

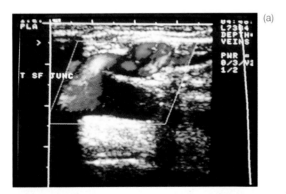

(a)

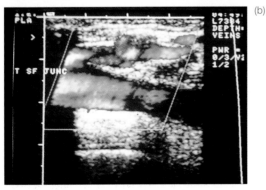

(b)

Fig. 5.16 Reflux occurring at the saphenofemoral junction on colour Doppler: (a) forward flow; (b) reverse flow.

effect will only demonstrate reverse flow as far as the first competent valve, so that any incompetent segments below this will not be demonstrated. Second, it is quite difficult to explain to many patients the exact nature and method for performing a Valsalva. Asking the patient to blow into a high-resistance spirometer circuit can produce the desired sudden increase in intra-abdominal pressure and is easier for many patients to understand. In some patients reflux will be seen simply with inspiration.

Reflux can be defined as reverse flow occurring after the cessation of forward flow. It is generally held to be significant if it lasts for more than 0.5 s [25], although the time taken for reflux to cease does not correlate particularly well with the severity of reflux as measured by air plethysmography[26]. Shorter periods of reversed flow may be seen in normal veins and represent the short period as the valve cusps come together and blood in the venous segment settles under the influence of gravity. Reflux should not be confused with the reversed flow which occurs with turbulence, particularly in the common femoral vein and popliteal veins. The difference is usually apparent on colour Doppler, and turbulence is seen on spectral Doppler as reverse flow occurring at the same time as forward flow.

The examination begins in the groin, where the common femoral vein, profunda femoris vein and saphenofemoral junction are identified and assessed. If there is a history of previous venous surgery the details are sometimes uncertain, or even wrong, and the region of the saphenofemoral junction should be examined carefully to assess the type of surgery, whether it was successful and whether there are any significant collaterals, or recanalized segments which are incompetent. The loss of the normal smooth curve of the long saphenous vein as it passes laterally and deeply towards the common femoral vein is suggestive of previous surgery with subsequent recanalization or collateral formation.

The patency and competence of the deep and superficial veins of the thigh are then assessed down to the level of the knee. Whilst examining the long saphenous vein the presence of incompetent perforators should be sought, especially if the vein becomes incompetent at a level below the saphenofemoral junction. These can be identified most easily by scanning down the vein transversely whilst applying recurrent compression to the calf or lower thigh. The commonest of these perforating veins is in the lower thigh at the level of the junction of the middle and lower thirds and is called the mid-thigh perforator vein (Figs 5.2 and 5.17). The use of tourniquets may help clarify difficult cases but this is not usually required with colour Doppler.

The patient is then turned so that the popliteal region can be examined. The veins in the popliteal fossa are assessed and the saphenopopliteal junction is examined. The level of the saphenopopliteal junction should also be noted, especially if this is not in the expected location. As with the saphenofemoral junction, recurrence after surgery can alter the anatomy and pattern of flow so that care is needed in defining the situation.

Examination of the calf veins may also be performed, although the findings tend to be more variable and their significance more diffi-cult to interpret. Incompetence may be seen in a similar fashion to that demonstrated more proximally. Sometimes the veins appear dilated and it is felt that they should be incompetent, but it is very difficult, or impossible, to induce significant forward flow in the vessels, or any subsequent reflux. The anatomy and function of the calf veins and the calf perforator veins may have important implications for the development of varicose changes, and this area is the subject of continuing research.

If necessary, varices can be traced proximally in order to identify the point of communication with the deep or superficial segments. This is usually best done with the transducer at right angles to the line of the vein being followed, judicious compression of lower varices will show the course of the veins on colour Doppler and confirm the presence of reflux, where appropriate. Care must be taken not to compress superficial veins with excessive transducer pressure when following the veins.

SAPHENOUS VEIN MAPPING

The long saphenous vein is the preferred conduit for arterial bypass grafting in the coronary arteries and lower limb. If there is any doubt concerning the suitability of the vein for the procedure, ultrasound can be used to assess

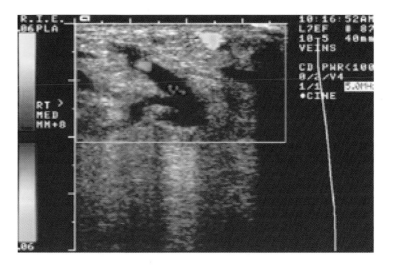

Fig. 5.17 An incompetent calf perforating vein.

the calibre and available length of the vein. Ideally the vein should be more than 3–4 mm wide for much of its length and more than 2 mm at the ankle if a long, femorodistal graft is being considered[27]. The aim of the examination depends on the surgical procedure being contemplated. If the vein is to be removed for a coronary artery or reversed lower limb arterial graft, then the examination can be limited to confirming the presence of the vein and assessing its calibre over the required length. If an *in situ* lower limb arterial graft is to be performed then a much more detailed examination is required in order to identify perforating veins and superficial branches communicating with the main vein, as these must be ligated during the operation to stop arteriovenous fistulae developing.

Technique

The examination is performed with the patient standing, if possible, as this produces distension of the vein, allowing easier location due to dilatation and a better estimation of the calibre of the vessel. If the patient is unable to stand they can be examined sitting with their legs over the side of the couch; if this is not possible then they can be assessed lying supine with a low-pressure tourniquet applied in order to produce distension of the superficial veins.

One of the problems associated with this examination is that ultrasound gel gums up fibre-tipped markers, making it impossible to mark the course of the vein on the skin, or the location of perforators. In order to avoid this problem the skin should not be covered with gel in the normal manner but the gel should be applied to the transducer and this then placed in the region of the saphenofemoral junction. Once the vein has been located the transducer is aligned along its course, the skin is marked over the vein at the lower end of the transducer. The transducer is then moved so that its upper end is on the skin mark, aligned along

the vein, and a further mark put at the location of the vein at the new position of the lower end of the transducer. The course of the vein is followed down the limb, with skin markings being made at each transducer length. Care must be taken in the calf, where the long saphenous vein has two main components: the anterior branch usually passes down to the front of the lateral malleolus and is the larger component, with the posterior branch running posteriorly to the posteromedial aspect of the calf.

Once the main marks have been applied, the location of the saphenofemoral junction, together with any other perforator veins, dual segments and tributaries, can be identified and marked. This is usually more easy to achieve by scanning transversely along the line of the long saphenous vein with regular augmentation of flow from squeezing the calf. The calibre of the vein is measured in the transverse plane, taking care not to compress the vessel with pressure from the transducer.

CONCLUSIONS

Providing care and attention are paid to examination technique then colour Doppler ultrasound is a reliable method for the diagnosis of deep vein thrombosis in symptomatic patients. The technique has become the first-line investigation for deep vein thrombosis in many centres, allowing any subsequent venography to be restricted to the area of doubt or concern on the ultrasound examination. It is important to recognize that the technique has some limitations and that several pitfalls exist.

Ultrasound also provides a non-invasive technique for the investigation of patients with chronic venous disease, or recurrence of varicose veins following surgery, enabling an accurate assessment of the pattern of incompetence or recurrence to be established and allow an appropriate surgical approach to be developed.

The long saphenous vein can be assessed for

its suitability as a bypass conduit for arterial or coronary artery bypass procedures. In addition, ultrasound provides a method for examining the central veins prior to central venous line insertion if problems are anticipated in locating a suitable channel for line insertion.

REFERENCES

1. Anderson FA Jr, Wheeler HB, Goldberg RJ *et al* (1991) A population-based perspective of the hospital incidence and case-fatality rates of deep vein thrombosis and pulmonary embolism: the Worcester DVT study. *Archives of Internal Medicine* **151**: 933–938
2. Callam MJ, Ruckley CV (1996) The epidemiology of chronic venous disease. *A Textbook of Vascular Medicine*, pp 562–579. London: Arnold
3. Baxter GM (1997) The role of ultrasound in deep vein thrombosis. Editorial. *Clinical Radiology* **52**: 1–3
4. Weinmann EE, Salzman EW (1994) Deep vein thrombosis: a review. *New England Journal of Medicine* **331**: 1630–1641
5. Phillips GWL, Paige J, Molan MP (1995) A comparison of colour duplex ultrasound with venography and varicography in the assessment of varicose veins. *Clinical Radiology* **50**: 20–25
6. Da Silva A, Widmer LK, Martin H, Mall Th, Glaus L, Schneider M (1974) Varicose veins and chronic insufficiency: prevalence and risk factors in 4376 subjects of the Basle Study II. *VASA* **3**(2): 118–125
7. Gordon AC, Wright I, Pugh ND (1996) Duplication of the superficial femoral vein: recognition with duplex ultrasonography. *Clinical Radiology* **51**: 622–624
8. Basmajian JV (1952) Distribution of valves in femoral, external iliac and common iliac veins and their relationship to varicose veins. *Surgery in Gynaecology and Obstetrics* **85**: 537–542
9. Linton RR (1938) The communicating veins of the lower leg and the operative technique for their ligation. *Annals of Surgery* **107**: 582–593
10. Perlin SJ (1992) Pulmonary embolism during compression US of the lower extremity. *Radiology* **184**: 165–166
11. Zwiebel WJ, Priest DL (1990) Colour duplex sonography of extremity veins. *Seminars in Ultrasonography, Computed Tomography and Magnetic Resonance* **11**: 136–137
12. Franzeck UK, Schalch I, Jager KA, Schneider E, Grimm J, Bollinger A (1996) Prospective 12-year follow-up study of clinical and haemodynamic sequelae after deep vein thrombosis in low-risk patients (Zurich study). *Circulation* **93**: 74–79
13. Davidson BL, Elliot CG, Lensing AWA (1992) Low accuracy of colour Doppler ultrasound in the detection of proximal leg vein thrombosis in asymptomatic high-risk patients. *Annals of Internal Medicine* **117**: 735–738
14. Rose SC, Zwiebel WJ, Miller FJ (1994) Distribution of acute lower extremity deep venous thrombosis in symptomatic and asymptomatic patients. *Journal of Ultrasound in Medicine* **13**: 243–250
15. Smart LM, Redhead DN, Allan PL, Ruckley CV (1992) Follow-up study of Gunther and LGM inferior vena cava filters. *Journal of International Radiology* **7**: 115–118
16. Polak JF, Wilkinson DL (1991) Ultrasonographic diagnosis of symptomatic deep venous thrombosis in pregnancy. *American Journal of Obstetrics and Gynecology* **165**: 625–629
17. Cronan JJ, Dorfman GS, Scola FH, Schepps B, Alexander J (1987) Deep venous thrombosis: US assessment using vein compression. *Radiology* **162**: 191–194
18. Atri M, Herba MJ, Reinhold C *et al* (1996) Accuracy of sonography in the evaluation of calf deep vein thrombosis in both postoperative surveillance and symptomatic patients. *American Journal of Radiology* **166**: 1361–1367
19. Baxter GM, Duffy P, Partridge E (1992) Colour flow imaging of calf vein thrombosis. *Clinical Radiology* **46**: 198–201
20. Rose SC, Zwiebel WJ, Nelson BD *et al* (1990) Symptomatic lower extremity deep venous thrombosis: accuracy, limitations and role of colour duplex flow imaging in diagnosis. *Radiology* **175**: 639–644
21. Wells PS, Lensing AW, Davidson BL, Prins MH, Hirsh J (1995) Accuracy of ultrasound for the diagnosis of deep vein thrombosis in asymptomatic patients after orthopaedic surgery. A meta-analysis. *Annals of Internal Medicine* **122**: 47–53
22. Markel A, Manzo RA, Bergelin RO, Strandness DE Jr (1992) Valvular reflux after deep vein thrombosis: incidence and time of occurrence. *Journal of Vascular Surgery* **15**: 377–384
23. Stonebridge PA, Chalmers N, Beggs I, Bradbury AW, Ruckley CV (1995) Recurrent varicose veins: a varicographic analysis leading to a new, practical classification. *British Journal of Surgery* **82**: 60–62
24. van Bemmelen PS, Bedford G, Beach K, Strandness DE (1989) Quantitative segmental evaluation of venous valvular reflux with duplex ultrasound scanning. *Journal of Vascular Surgery* **10**: 425–431
25. Iafrati MD, Welch H, O'Donnell TF, Belkin M, Umphrey S, McLaughlin R (1994) Correlation of venous non-invasive tests with the Society for Vascular Surgery/International Society for Cardiovascular Surgery clinical classification of

5

chronic venous insufficiency. Journal of Vascular Surgery **19**: 1001–1007

26. Rodriguez AA, Whitehead CM, McLaughlin RL, Umphrey SE, Welch HJ, O'Donnell TF (1996) Duplex-derived valve closure times fail to correlate with reflux flow volumes in patients with chronic

venous insufficiency. *Journal of Vascular Surgery* **23**: 606–610

27. Leopold PW, Shandall A, Kupinski AM *et al* (1989) Role of B-mode venous mapping in infrainguinal *in situ* vein arterial bypasses. British Journal of Surgery **76**: 305–307

The aorta and inferior vena cava

6

PAUL L. ALLAN

Doppler examination in the abdomen is associated with specific problems which are not encountered in peripheral vascular examinations, and these are particularly relevant to examinations of the aorta, inferior vena cava and their associated vessels.

Respiratory motion and cardiac pulsation impair the examination, but getting the patient to suspend respiration for any length of time results in relative hypoxia and subsequently increased respiratory movement. It is therefore better to scan as much as possible during quiet respiration, asking the patient to hold their breath only for short periods in order to obtain a spectral trace. In most cases only two or three cardiac cycles are needed for assessment.

Many vessels will always seem to be orientated at right angles to the scan plane, especially with sector or curved linear transducers. Different angles of approach and repositioning of both transducer and patient may be required in an attempt to improve the Doppler angle.

Bowel gas is also a problem as it can obscure a vessel, or produce distracting motion artefacts as it bubbles past; scanning after an overnight fast may improve the situation, as may an injection of hyoscine. It has been suggested that patients should receive bowel preparation as for an enema, but this author feels that this is not usually justified for the small advantage it may occasionally confer.

Abdominal Doppler examinations are performed on vessels which lie more deeply than the peripheral vessels and this has several consequences. First, lower-frequency transducers are used and this limits the size of Doppler shift which will be obtained for a given velocity. Second, longer-pulse repetition intervals are required to allow the sound to travel the greater distances; this also limits the size of Doppler shift which can be measured as a result of the Nyquist limit (see Chapter 1). Operators should therefore seek to minimize the scan depth and use the highest-frequency transducer compatible with adequate visualization.

THE AORTA

Anatomy

The aorta enters the abdomen at the level of T12 and runs down the posterior abdominal wall to the left of the midline, with the inferior vena cava to its right side (Fig. 6.1). It divides into the common iliac arteries at the level of L4, which is about the level of the iliac crests. Para-aortic nodes are distributed anteriorly and on both sides of the vessel.

The abdominal aorta gives branches to the abdominal organs and to the abdominal wall. The parietal branches to the wall are not usually large enough to be seen regularly using

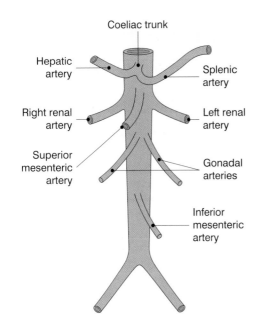

Fig. 6.1 The abdominal aorta and its major branches.

colour Doppler and will not be considered further. The visceral branches supply the liver, kidneys, adrenal glands, gonads, spleen, bowel and pancreas. The vessels to the adrenals and gonads are also usually too small to be seen reliably on ultrasound; the renal and hepatic arteries have been covered elsewhere.

The splanchnic arteries supply the bowel and associated organs. The *coeliac trunk* arises from the anterior aspect of the aorta just after it has entered the abdomen. The trunk is only about 1 cm long and divides into three branches: the common hepatic artery, the splenic artery and the left gastric artery. The *common hepatic artery* passes to the right over the head of the pancreas, where it gives of the gastroduodenal artery which can be seen passing inferiorly between the head of the pancreas and the margin of the duodenum; the other branches from this segment of the hepatic artery are not usually apparent on ultrasound. The artery ascends in the lesser omentum as the proper hepatic artery, in company with the portal vein and common bile duct, to the porta of the liver, where it divides into right and left hepatic arteries. The *splenic artery* passes to the left and runs along the superior margin of the body of the pancreas to the hilum of the spleen. It has a tortuous course and an arterial loop may be mistaken for a small cyst in the pancreas if the situation is not recognized; colour Doppler allows quick identification of the true nature of the 'cyst'. The right gastric artery arises from the splenic artery but is not usually seen on ultrasound.

The *superior mesenteric artery* arises 1–2 cm below the coeliac trunk and supplies the small bowel and colon to the distal transverse colon. The superior mesenteric vein is seen on the right side of the upper portion of the artery and can be followed to its confluence with the splenic vein, forming the portal vein. The individual branches of the artery are not usually seen clearly on ultrasound. The *inferior mesenteric artery* arises from the anterior aorta about 3–4 cm above the bifurcation. The inferior mesenteric vein may be seen on the left of the artery but diverges as it passes up to join the splenic vein.

Several variations in the anatomy of the splanchnic arteries are well recognized. The most important one in relation to ultrasound is the origin of the right hepatic artery from the superior mesenteric artery. Occasionally the coeliac trunk is absent with its branches arising separately from the aorta; the left hepatic artery may arise from the left gastric artery and accessory hepatic arteries may arise from the superior mesenteric artery or other arteries in the region.

Scanning technique

Aorta

The upper abdominal aorta can nearly always be examined through the left lobe of the liver; the coeliac trunk and superior mesenteric arteries are also visible from this approach. A 3 or 5 MHz transducer is used depending on the build of the patient. The patient should fast for 8 hours prior to the examination, for two reasons: first, fasting will improve visualization of the aorta and its branches; second, splanchnic blood flow will be in the basal fasting state, rather than the dynamic postprandial state.

If the aorta is the main object of the investigation it is followed distally to its bifurcation. The vessel should be scanned both longitudinally and transversely, taking note of the overall diameter, the presence of any aneurysmal dilatation and any para-aortic masses or pathology. If visualization from an anterior approach is impaired, then scanning in a coronal plane through the right lobe of the liver will allow the upper aorta to be visualized; scanning in a coronal oblique plane from a left posterolateral approach can provide a view of the mid- and lower aorta, together with the bifurcation. The calibre of the vessel is measured from the outer aspect of the vessel wall, ideally during systolic expansion. The systolic anteroposterior diameter is the easiest and most repeatable measurement to make and this is therefore used for follow-up of aneurysm patients. It is important to ensure that the true anteroposterior diameter is measured, particularly in ectatic, tortuous arteries, as oblique measurements will result in falsely high measurements. Colour Doppler and spectral Doppler are used to assess any potential disturbances of flow which may result from atheroma or dissection.

Splanchnic arteries

The coeliac trunk and its main branches are examined using colour and spectral Doppler. The main trunk is short but it is directed towards the transducer so that an excellent Doppler angle is achieved. The proximal hepatic and splenic arteries, together with the superior mesenteric artery, are often orientated almost at right angles to the scan plane with an anterior approach (Fig. 6.2), so that some

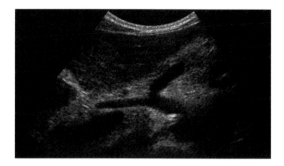

Fig. 6.2 Transverse view of the coeliac axis showing the splenic artery on the right and the hepatic artery on the left.

experimentation with points of access is required to get acceptable Doppler angles. The hepatic artery is followed to the right and the gastroduodenal artery can be identified beside the head of the pancreas. The proper hepatic artery is traced towards the porta where it divides into the right and left hepatic arteries. The origin of the superior mesenteric artery is examined (Fig. 6.3) and the vessel traced as far distally as it remains visible. Firm pressure with the transducer may help in displacing bowel gas from in front of the vessel, but care must be

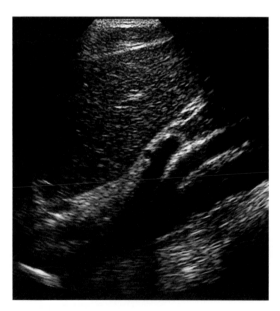

Fig. 6.3 Longitudinal scan showing the origin of the coeliac axis superiorly and the superior mesenteric artery just below this.

taken not to compress the artery and produce a spuriously high Doppler shift. Colour Doppler is used to identify any abnormal areas of flow, including 'visible bruits', or tissue vibrations, which may be seen in cases of severe stenosis. Power Doppler is of less value in the abdomen than in peripheral vessels as arterial pulsation, respiratory movement and bowel gas motion can all cause marked motion artefacts which obscure the signal from the vessel.

The inferior mesenteric artery is sometimes difficult to locate. It can be found by scanning transversely up from the bifurcation and it may be identified just to the left of the aorta, 2–4 cm above the bifurcation (Fig. 6.4).

Normal and abnormal findings

Aorta

The calibre of the normal aorta varies with the age, sex and build of the patient, being larger in men, older patients and tall patients. The calibre also varies with the level in the abdomen. Goldberg *et al* found an average diameter of 22 mm above the renal arteries, 18 mm just below the renal arteries and 15 mm above the bifurcation[1]. The normal Doppler waveform in the aorta also varies with location. In the upper aorta there is a narrow, well-

defined systolic complex with forward flow during diastole; below the renal arteries the diastolic flow is much reduced and above the bifurcation it is absent, or reversed diastolic flow may occur, with a waveform similar to that seen in the lower limb arteries (Fig. 6.5)[2].

The main abnormalities affecting the aorta are atheroma, aneurysm, dissection and para-aortic masses. *Atheroma* can affect the aorta and produce stenosis or occlusion; aortic disease, unless severe is usually overshadowed clinically by symptoms arising from the peripheral or the coronary arteries. Sometimes there is uncertainty as to whether aortic disease seen on arteriography is clinically significant. In these cases velocity ratios taken from above and at the stenosis can be used to assess the degree of haemodynamic compromise. However, accurate criteria have not been

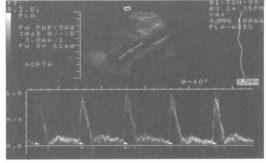

(a)

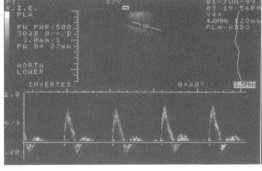

(b)

Fig. 6.5 (a) The aortic waveform in the upper abdomen showing diastolic flow. (b) The aortic waveform above the bifurcation with absent diastolic flow and a waveform similar to that seen in the lower limb arteries.

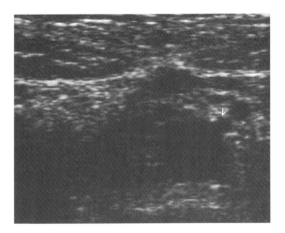

Fig. 6.4 Transverse scan showing the inferior mesenteric artery and vein lying adjacent to the aorta.

developed for aortic stenosis, as is the case for carotid and peripheral Doppler examinations, but a significant increase in the velocity and the velocity ratio by a factor of two or more would indicate a severe stenosis[3]. If the stenotic area is clearly seen, a direct measurement of diameter or area stenosis can be obtained; colour or power Doppler is of value in defining the margins of the residual lumen.

An *aneurysm* of the abdominal aorta can be defined as an increase of the anteroposterior diameter over 3 cm, or a localized increase of 1.5 times the diameter of the adjacent normal aorta. Aneurysms may extend into the abdomen from the thoracic aorta, or may arise within the abdominal aorta, usually affecting the infrarenal segment. Aneurysms are nearly always true aneurysms secondary to degeneration of the connective tissue in the vessel wall. Occasionally mycotic aneurysms secondary to infection, or pseudo-aneurysms secondary to trauma, may be seen. Ultrasound diagnosis is normally straightforward, the cardinal measurement is the anteroposterior diameter, which is best obtained by scanning transversely with the ultrasound beam at right angles to the long axis of the vessel, in order to ensure a true anteroposterior measurement. It is also important to locate the upper and lower margins of the aneurysmal segment, particularly in relation to the renal arteries. If these cannot be identified with certainty it should be remembered that the main renal arteries usually arise from the aorta 1–2 cm below the superior mesenteric artery, and this vessel can therefore be used as an approximate marker for the renal vessels.

Colour and spectral Doppler may show turbulent flow within the aneurysm, or indeed very slow flow with very little forward movement of the blood. However, examination of normal-calibre vessels below the aneurysm will show rapid reconstitution of the waveform as the pressure wave is constrained by the narrower calibre. Doppler can also be used to confirm renal blood flow, particularly after surgery, if there is any question that this has been cut off.

Ultrasound is used to monitor the rate of increase in size of the aneurysm over time. However, it should be remembered that the calibre of the aorta increases slowly with age and this should be borne in mind when assessing the significance of any alteration in the size of smaller aneurysms. Measuring any change in the calibre of the adjacent normal aorta may be helpful in assessing the significance of any change in the diameter of an aneurysm. The main complication arising from an aneurysm is leakage or rupture. Ultrasound can be used to identify any retroperitoneal haematoma which would indicate a leak but computed tomography (CT), if available, provides a more accurate overall assessment of the situation, providing the patient's condition is sufficiently stable to allow investigation. Rarely, an aortocaval or aortoduodenal fistula may develop; high-volume pulsatile flow in the inferior vena cava is seen on Doppler in cases of caval fistula (Fig. 6.6).

Dissection of the abdominal aorta nearly always results from the extension of a dissection of the thoracic aorta extending into the abdomen. Rarely, it may originate in the abdominal aorta, or result from trauma. The aorta is usually dilated to some extent but dissection can occur in the presence of a normal-calibre aorta. The flap may be visible depending on its orientation in relation to the ultrasound beam, and if a dissection is suspected the aorta should be examined from several different approaches in an effort to show the flap (Fig. 6.7). Spectral and colour Doppler will show the presence and character of any flow in the true and false lumens and, even if a flap is not visible, the different flows in the two channels may be apparent on Doppler; reversed flow may be seen in the non-dominant channel due to compression in systole. Doppler can also be used to assess

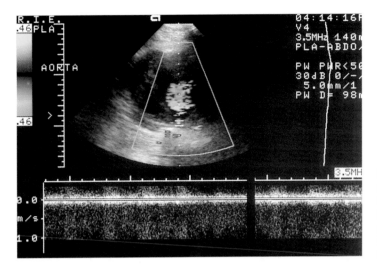

Fig. 6.6 Colour Doppler image of an aortocaval fistula in a patient with an aortic aneurysm. The spectral Doppler gate is on the fistula and the spectral display shows a turbulent signal which is largely off the spectral range at these settings.

blood flow in the major branches supplying the bowel, liver, kidneys and lower limbs[4].

Splanchnic arteries

Blood flow in the superior and inferior mesenteric arteries varies depending on whether the patient is fasting, or has recently eaten. In the fasting state the flow is typical of a relatively high-resistance vascular bed with low diastolic flow. Following the ingestion of food there is a reduction in the peripheral resistance of the mesenteric vessels, resulting in increased diastolic flow, together with an increase in peak systolic velocity (Fig. 6.8).

The main indication for examination of blood flow in the splanchnic arteries is the investigation of possible *intestinal ischaemia*. This is usually subacute or chronic ischaemia, as significant acute ischaemia presents as an acute abdomen and is managed accordingly. The splanchnic circulation is capable of developing multiple collateral channels and this makes the assessment of possible gut ischaemia difficult. The demonstration of stenosis of two of the three splanchnic arteries is strongly suggestive of the diagnosis and, in the appropriate clinical situation, the demonstration of severe stenosis in one vessel with occlusion of another is also

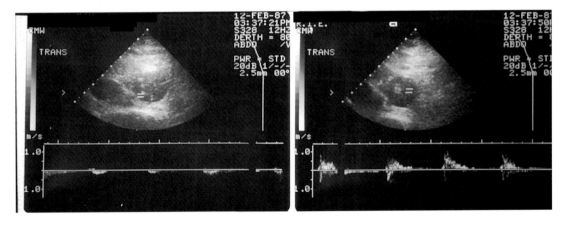

Fig. 6.7 Transverse views of abdominal aorta showing a dissection flap and spectral displays of the flow in the two channels.

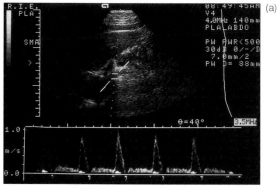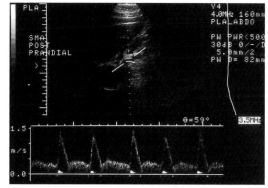

Fig. 6.8 Flow in the superior mesenteric artery (a) before and (b) after food.

supportive of the diagnosis. Colour Doppler is of value in identifying the abnormal segment (Fig. 6.9), although care must be taken not to mistake a high shift resulting from disease with the high shift from normal velocity flow, which is seen due to the low Doppler angle resulting from the orientation of the coeliac trunk and proximal superior mesenteric artery to the ultrasound beam. In addition, colour Doppler may show a visible tissue bruit. The proximal 2–3 cm of the vessels is the most common site for disease and a peak velocity of more than 2.8 m s^{-1} in the coeliac trunk or proximal superior mesenteric artery correlates well with a stenosis of more than 75% diameter reduction[5].

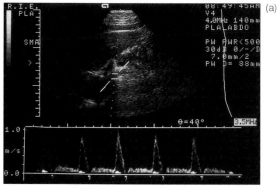

Fig. 6.9 Colour Doppler image of the coeliac axis and superior mesenteric artery in a patient with a stenosis of the coeliac axis.

Indirect signs of intestinal ischaemia include oedema of the mucosa and bowel wall and also reduced peristalsis. In severe cases gas bubbles may be seen in the portal vein flow; these produce a characteristic popping sound on spectral Doppler (Fig. 6.10).

The problems associated with the diagnosis of mesenteric ischaemia are illustrated by the fact that 18% of patients over 60 years without symptoms of mesenteric ischaemia have been shown to have significant disease on Doppler[6]. This emphasizes the need to assess the findings in the light of the clinical situation.

Other applications

The nature of para-aortic masses can be clarified using colour Doppler and masses can be distinguished from aneurysms.

An aorta which is prominent but of normal calibre in a thin patient, or the aorta in a patient with a marked lumbar lordosis, may be mistaken clinically for a mass or aneurysm. Ultrasound can confirm the normal calibre of the vessel and the lack of pathology in these patients.

Blood flow in the coeliac and mesenteric arteries is also responsive to a variety of pharmacological agents such as glucagon and somatostatin, or pathological states such as cirrhosis and Crohn's disease. Doppler

117

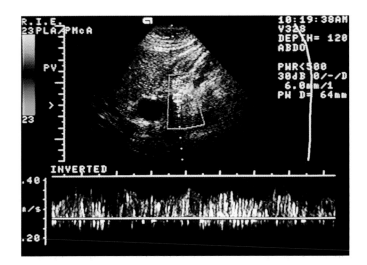

Fig. 6.10 The spectral display from the portal vein of a patient with severe ischaemia showing the characteristic echoes from bubbles of gas in the blood.

ultrasound can show flow changes associated with these situations and may hold some promise for the future in the assessment of disease activity, or response to treatment.

THE INFERIOR VENA CAVA

Anatomy

The inferior vena cava is formed by the confluence of the common iliac veins at the level of the 5th lumbar vertebra and runs cranially to the right of the midline. It passes through the diaphragm at the level of the 8th thoracic vertebra and enters the right atrium. In the embryo there is a complex arrangement of venous sinuses which form during embryogenesis, and several of these contribute to the inferior vena cava; this means that there are many variations of anatomy which may be seen. The most common variation is that the common iliac veins continue cranially as paired 'venae cavae', with the left component crossing to join the right side at the level of the left renal vein. Many other variations have been recorded; these are more easily assessed using contrast-enhanced CT than ultrasound, but may cause some confusion if they are seen during an ultrasound examination and not recognized.

Technique

The inferior vena cava can be examined using the techniques described for the abdominal aorta. However, in the supine position the vessel may be narrow in the anteroposterior plane and difficult to define. Scanning transversely with colour Doppler and using the aorta as a guide may allow localization of the vein in these circumstances; or elevation of the leg(s) by an assistant will increase flow and the calibre of the vein, thus making it more visible. The calibre of the cava will vary with the state of hydration of the patient. In a well-hydrated patient it will be distended, whereas in a dehydrated patient it will be collapsed, narrow and more difficult to visualize. Excessive transducer pressure applied in an effort to disperse bowel gas will also compress the cava, therefore a balance must be sought in order to visualize segments of the vessel in some patients.

Normal and abnormal findings

Flow in the inferior vena cava is slow and varies with both respiration and cardiac pulsation (Fig. 6.11). On inspiration the diaphragm descends. This results in negative pressure in the chest and increased pressure in the

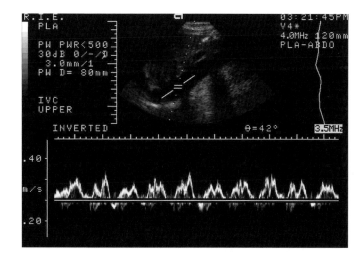

Fig. 6.11 The inferior vena cava in the upper abdomen showing the variations in flow which occur with respiration and cardiac activity.

abdomen, and blood therefore flows from the abdomen to the chest; the reverse occurs on expiration. Superimposed on this is the more rapid periodicity resulting from cardiac activity; this is seen particularly in the upper abdomen. The prominence of the caval waveform also depends on the degree of hydration of the patient. A dehydrated patient's cava will be narrow and difficult to see below the renal veins, whereas in fluid overload the cava is dilated and there is cardiac periodicity detectable down into the iliac veins.

One of the most common indications for specific examination of the inferior vena cava is to assess whether *thrombus* from a pelvic or lower limb deep vein thrombosis has extended up into the cava. Thrombus may fill the lumen of the cava and even produce some expansion of the vessel; alternatively, a tongue of thrombus may be seen lying free in the lumen, extending up towards the right atrium (Fig. 6.12).

Caval filters are inserted in some patients who are at risk of pulmonary embolus from more distal thrombus. There are several types but all are inserted in the mid- or lower cava,

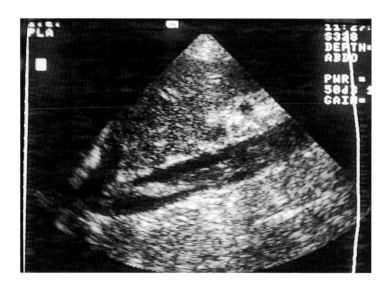

Fig. 6.12 A tongue of thrombus extending up into the upper inferior vena cava in a patient with deep vein thrombosis behind the left lobe of the liver.

below the renal veins. Identifying a metallic, echogenic structure within the inferior vena cava above the level of the renal veins may indicate migration of the filter. There is a small risk that thrombus may extend past the filter, or develop at the site of the filter. Colour Doppler is a quick and easy method for confirming patency of the cava around and above the filter[7]. The metal struts of the filter can be recognized within the lumen of the cava and colour Doppler, or power Doppler, will show blood flow past the level of the filter (Fig. 6.13).

Renal tumours and hepatocellular carcinoma are two tumours which have a tendency to invade venous channels and, as a result, *tumour thrombus* may extend into the cava from the renal or hepatic veins. Compromise of the venous drainage of the liver or kidneys is shown by loss of the normal cardiac and respiratory periodicity of the waveform. Some tumours in the retroperitoneum may compress or directly invade the inferior vena cava causing obstruction to the venous return from the lower abdomen and legs. Although the caudal segments of the inferior vena cava and the iliac veins usually remain patent, they will often be dilated, flow will be sluggish or reversed, the flow profile will be flat, and there will be an absence of the normal Valsalva response.

Following *liver transplantation* the cava should be assessed to ensure satisfactory flow. The appearances will depend on the type of anastomosis performed. In the past, the segment of donor cava attached to the new liver replaced the equivalent segment of native cava, which had been removed with the diseased liver. Many surgeons now perform a 'piggyback' technique, where the native cava is left in place, the inferior end of the donor caval segment is oversewn and the upper end anastomosed to the native cava. This results in a postoperative appearance which can be confusing if it is not recognized, as there will appear to be two cavae associated with the transplanted liver (Fig. 6.14).

Other postoperative problems which may occur in relation to the cava following transplantation include compression, if the new liver is relatively large; distortion of the cava may also occur if there is relative twisting of the caval channel as a result of fitting the donor liver into the native abdomen. In the longer term stenosis may develop at the sites of anastomosis.

Retroperitoneal and other abdominal *masses* may compress or occlude the inferior vena cava. The situation is usually apparent, especially with colour Doppler, which shows the cava entering the mass and becoming narrowed or occluded with absent flow. Congenital *webs* can occur, particularly at the upper end of the cava. These

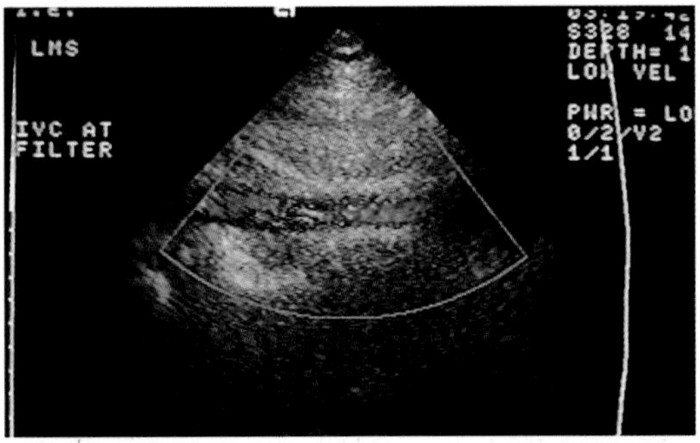

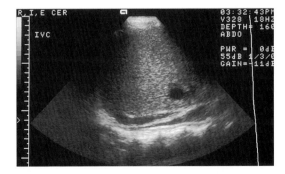

Fig. 6.13 Colour Doppler image of the inferior vena cava in a patient with a caval filter in place. The change in colour reflects the changing Doppler angle as the blood flows through the sector scan.

Fig. 6.14 An image of the upper caval region in a liver transplant patient with a 'piggyback' caval anastomosis, showing the donor and the native vessels.

may produce a variable degree of caval narrowing and in some cases may predispose to hepatic vein thrombosis.

Fistulae involving the cava may rarely occur spontaneously, often secondary to an aortic aneurysm (Fig. 6.6), or they may be surgically created as is the case with portocaval shunts. In the case of aortocaval fistulae, colour Doppler may show a visible tissue bruit with pulsatile flow in the cava above the level of the fistula; sometimes the fistula itself is difficult to identify. Surgical portocaval shunts are usually side-to-side shunts in the upper abdomen at the level where the proximal main portal vein passes close in front of the cava (Fig. 6.15). A tissue bruit may be apparent and the shunt is more easily identified if the liver can be used as a window through to the point of anastomosis;

turning the patient up onto the left side may facilitate visualization.

CONCLUSION

The aorta and inferior vena cava, together with their major branches and tributaries, can be examined in most patients, provided that care and attention is spent in finding the best scan plane and ensuring that the system is set appropriately for the specific examination concerned, both in terms of imaging and Doppler settings. Helical CT and 3-D reconstruction is rapidly becoming the technique of choice for imaging the aorta, particularly if percutaneous stent/grafts are contemplated. However, ultrasound continues to have a significant role in relation to both initial diagnosis and follow-up of patients with aortic or caval disease.

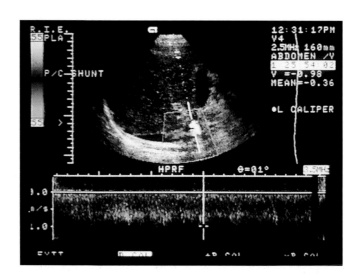

Fig. 6.15 Colour Doppler image of a portocaval shunt.

REFERENCES

1. Goldberg BB, Ostrum BJ, Isard HJ (1966) Ultrasonographic aortography. *Journal of the American Medical Association* **198**: 353–358
2. Taylor KJW, Burns PN, Woodcock JP, Wells PNT (1985) Blood flow in deep abdominal and pelvic vessels: ultrasonic pulsed Doppler analysis. *Radiology* **154**: 487–493
3. De Smet AA, Kitslaar PJ (1990) A duplex criterion for aortoiliac stenosis. *European Journal of Vascular Surgery* **4**: 275–278
4. Thomas EA, Dubbins PA (1990) Duplex ultrasound of the abdominal aorta – a neglected tool in aortic dissection. *Clinical Radiology* **42**: 330–334

5. Moneta GL, Yeager RA, Dawan R, Antonovic R, Hall LD, Porter JH (1991) Duplex ultrasound criteria for diagnosis of splanchnic artery stenosis or occlusion. *Journal of Vascular Surgery* **14**: 511–518

6. Roobottom CA, Dubbins PA (1993) Significant disease of the coeliac and superior mesenteric arteries in asymptomatic patients: predictive value of Doppler sonography. *American Journal of Radiology* **161**: 985–988

7. Smart LM, Redhead DN, Allan PL, Ruckley CV (1992) Follow-up study of Gunther and LGM inferior vena caval filters. *Journal of Interventional Radiology* **7**: 115–118

Doppler ultrasound of the liver

MYRON A. POZNIAK

The standard abdominal ultrasound examination should include a brief, but precise survey with spectral and colour Doppler[1-4]. This serves a twofold purpose. First, it adds valuable haemodynamic information to the evaluation of the abdominal organs, in most cases reinforcing normality, but occasionally revealing an unexpected finding. Second, by consistently integrating Doppler into the routine abdominal examination, sonologists will continually refine their Doppler skills so that significant haemodynamic abnormalities can be identified quickly and evaluated accurately. Although a cursory Doppler survey of the major vessels may add 2–3 min to an abdominal examination, regular practice enables the examiner to become more familiar with the equipment, more adept at perceiving abnormalities and more expert in analysing the results.

Sometimes altered blood flow may be the only abnormal finding to suggest the presence of pathology. The Doppler survey may reveal a subtle hypervascular lesion of which the examiner was otherwise unaware, or it may display hypervascularity of an observed lesion and awareness of a lesion's vascularity often increases diagnostic certainty. The use of colour Doppler in abdominal examinations also helps to differentiate vascular from non-vascular structures. Care must be taken, however, to ensure that equipment settings are appropriate: if gain, pulse repetition frequency and filtration are not optimized, slow flow can be missed in vascular structures or artifactual colour can be painted into non-vascular structures.

GENERAL ASPECTS

Some sonologists place considerable emphasis on the measurement of flow velocity but too great a dependence on this parameter may generate a false sense of security, or lead to diagnostic errors. Numerous systemic factors affect blood flow in abdominal vessels. These include the patient's state of hydration, cardiac output, blood pressure, vascular compliance, the interval since previous food and the haemodynamic effects of medications. These factors affect measured velocities in a variety of ways and to varying degrees, so that although the velocity may be above or below the normal levels expected in any individual vessel, it may not necessarily reflect focal disordered haemodynamics. Furthermore, defining flow within a vessel as normal or abnormal by simply comparing the measured velocity to a predetermined normal range is a poor method of establishing a diagnosis, as a few degrees difference in the angle of insonation, or improper angle correction, can significantly change the measured velocity. Assigning the proper degree of angle correction may be difficult if the vessel is poorly visualized, curved, or visualized only over a short segment.

Varying the width of the sample volume can be advantageous when examining the abdomen. If the examiner is screening for vascular patency, or trying to locate a specific vessel, a large sample volume is appropriate for rapid interrogation of a broad area; for example, when ruling out hepatic artery thrombosis in a liver transplant recipient. If, however, the examiner wants

to precisely characterize flow within a vessel and evaluate waveform detail, then the sample volume must be small and placed near the centre of the vessel, thereby interrogating the highest-velocity lamina (Fig. 7.1). A wide sample volume, by incorporating the slower lamina along the wall together with the faster central lamina, will broaden the spectral Doppler tracing and mimic turbulence (Fig. 7.2).

There is no specific acoustic window that is ideal for all patients and the operator must

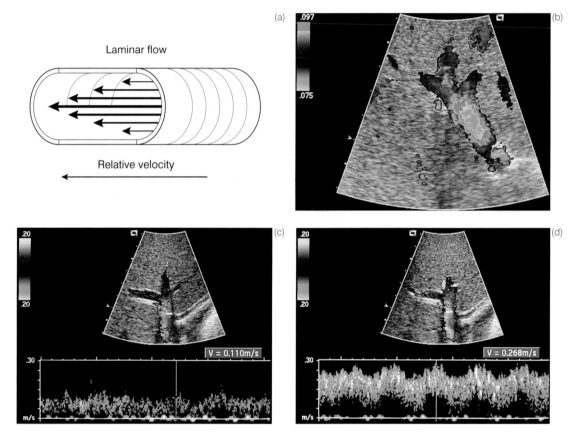

Fig. 7.1 (a) Schematic representation of normal laminar flow. The velocity along the wall of a vessel is slowed because of drag, therefore the relative velocity is less than that measured at the centre of the vessel. (b) Colour Doppler image of portal vein flow. A green tag was assigned to high-level velocities towards the transducer and the scale was set low to allow aliasing. Colour-encoding thus permits an accurate display of numerous lamina. Note the transition from the slowest velocities, red through orange, green and blue from the periphery to the centre of the vessel. The actual velocity displayed on a spectral tracing will be critically dependent on sample volume placement relative to these various velocity lamina. (c) Normal spectral Doppler tracing of portal vein flow. A small sample volume is placed near the vessel wall. The velocity as interrogated near the wall only measures approximately 0.11 m s^{-1}. (d) Spectral Doppler tracing of the same portal vein with the sample volume now placed more centrally interrogating the higher-velocity lamina. The measured velocity is now 0.27 m s^{-1}. Simply changing location of the sample volume is sufficient to cause a twofold change in measured velocity.

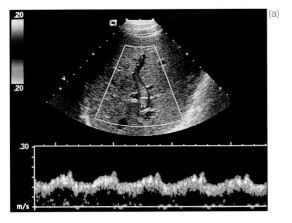
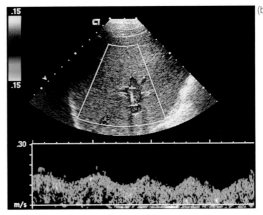

Fig. 7.2 (a) Spectral Doppler tracing of a portal vein with small, centrally placed sample volume. A thin lamina of flow is interrogated and, therefore, the displayed tracing shows a narrow range of velocities with a 'window' below the tracing. (b) The sample volume has been opened wide to incorporate all velocity lamina across this portal vein. Note the 'filling in' of the spectral tracing resulting in a perception of spectral broadening.

determine the best approach on an individual basis. This usually requires trying multiple windows at varying degrees of inspiration. During respiration, the upper abdominal organs move back and forth under the ultrasound transducer. When patients are able to cooperate, the operator should ask them to intermittently hold their breath during the Doppler examination and to breathe gently at other times. This improves the colour Doppler image and allows acquisition of longer spectral Doppler tracings. Patients who are unable to hold their breath can pose a significant problem and the operator may have to carefully 'ride' the vessel in real-time as it moves with respiration. An experienced sonologist may be able to 'rock' the transducer back and forth in synchrony with the patient's respiration, thus maintaining the sample volume over the area of interest and obtaining a longer tracing. If the patient is short of breath or unable to cooperate, short segments of spectral tracings are all that may be possible.

The presence of bowel gas is also an obvious impediment to a successful examination. Making the patient fast for 6–8 hours prior to an abdominal examination helps minimize the amount of abdominal gas, thereby increasing the likelihood that an appropriate sonographic window will be available for any particular vessel of interest. In addition, consistently scanning fasting patients decreases the risk of misinterpreting flow dynamics altered by a nutrient load.

Patient obesity is a severe limiting factor for an adequate Doppler examination. Delineation of anatomic detail is impaired when the examination is conducted at lower frequencies. During ultrasound imaging the operator may need to press firmly to displace some of the adipose tissue and position the transducer closer to the area of interest. Such a manoeuvre, however, is not appropriate during a Doppler examination, as pressure from the transducer compresses the underlying organ and its vasculature, thereby altering flow profiles and velocities. Compression of an organ or vessel with the transducer causes increased resistance to blood flow (especially diastolic), thereby elevating the perceived resistance to inflow (Fig. 7.3).

Terminology

In relation to Doppler ultrasound of the liver, it is important to be consistent in the use of terms

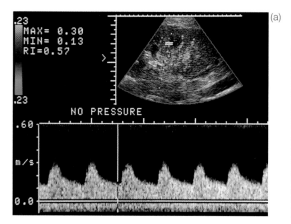
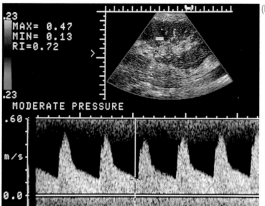

Fig. 7.3 (a) Spectral Doppler tracing of an interlobar renal artery. This tracing was obtained with gentle contact against the anterior abdominal wall. The resistive index measures approximately 57%. (b) The same vessel in (a) is now interrogated with moderate pressure applied with the transducer. Note the increased systolic velocity resulting in an elevation of resistive index to 72%. Pressure applied by the sonologist via the transducer can increase the resistance to arterial flow in any organ or vessel.

relating to blood flow. The term *pulsatility* refers to arterial flow; *phasicity* refers to changes in flow secondary to respiration; and the term *periodicity* is recommended when referring to velocity variation in the hepatic and portal veins secondary to cardiac activity.

Normal flow in the portal vein towards the liver is properly termed *hepatopetal* (as in centripetal force – not hepatopedal). Reversed portal vein flow is referred to as *hepatofugal* (as in centrifugal force).

INDICATIONS

A significant percentage of patients referred for right upper quadrant (RUQ) ultrasonography typically have elevated liver enzymes of unknown aetiology, incidentally detected on screening blood tests. Although sonographic imaging of the liver may reveal diffuse abnormality or focal disease, the majority of studies on these patients are often normal (Table 7.1). Doppler ultrasound should be applied to the portal vein, hepatic artery and the hepatic veins of these patients, and indeed in all RUQ examinations[5]; this may reveal flow alterations caused by inflammatory disease, neoplasm, or other disorders which are too subtle or too small to

cause imaging irregularities. Alterations in flow profiles and velocities in the hepatic vessels may be the result of either hepatic or cardiac disease, thereby helping to differentiate patients needing cardiac evaluation from those with liver disease who may benefit from liver biopsy, or require further hepatic imaging using computed tomography (CT), magnetic resonance imaging (MRI), or angiography.

When portal hypertension is suspected, Doppler ultrasound characterizes changes in portal haemodynamics and identifies pathways of portosystemic collateralization[6–7]. Doppler can confirm the patency of surgical or percutaneous shunts which have been performed in patients with bleeding oesophageal varices[8].

Identification and differentiation of bland thrombus from tumour thrombus within the

Table 7.1 Indications for Doppler ultrasound of the liver.

- Part of the routine examination of the liver and right upper quadrant
- Assessment of portal hypertension
- Pre- and postprocedural assessment of transjugular portosystemic shunt (TIPS) procedures
- Postoperative follow-up of liver transplants
- Assessment of focal liver disease

hepatic or portal veins by Doppler has significant implications for medical or surgical treatment planning.

Doppler ultrasound plays a key role in the postoperative monitoring of liver transplant recipients, confirming patency of the portal vein, hepatic artery and hepatic veins.

The role of Doppler in the characterization of parenchymal liver disease and screening for hepatocellular carcinoma is controversial. Marked alterations in flow profiles and velocities can be seen and have been described in the literature[9–18]. It is rare, though, to be able to precisely pinpoint a specific diagnosis based on Doppler findings, since there is considerable overlap in velocity and waveform alterations among various disease states[19].

SCAN TECHNIQUE

The patient is usually scanned while in a supine or left lateral decubitus position (Table 7.2). Depending on vessel orientation and patient body habitus, the portal vein and hepatic artery are best interrogated by either a subcostal approach pointing posterocephalad, or a right intercostal approach pointing medially. Since the portal vein and hepatic artery travel together in the portal triad, along with the common duct, these approaches should satisfactorily interrogate both vessels.

Scanning the left hepatic vein (and occasionally the middle hepatic vein) is best accomplished from a substernal approach. The transducer should be oriented transversely, pointing posterocephalad, and swept up and down across the liver. For the right hepatic

vein, a right lateral intercostal approach, with the transducer pointed cephalad is used. If the patient's liver extends below the costal margin during inspiration, a subcostal transverse view, angled cephalad, is useful (Fig. 7.4).

Some patients when asked to hold their breath perform a vigorous Valsalva manoeuvre. This results in increased intrathoracic pressure which may impede venous return, affecting flow profiles and velocities, particularly in the hepatic veins and inferior vena cava (IVC). This effect may alter the hepatic vein profile, creating the perception of hepatic venous outflow obstruction (HVOO). An attempt should be made to scan these patients in neutral breath-hold to avoid producing a misleading Doppler tracing.

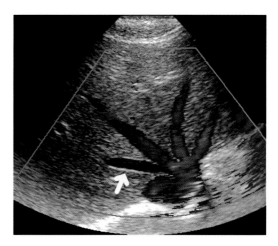

Fig. 7.4 Colour Doppler transverse view of the liver with a subcostal approach. This image was obtained during the brief burst of retrograde flow (the A wave). This colour crow's foot appearance of the three hepatic veins clearly confirms patency. Note the accessory right hepatic vein (arrow). Its orientation perpendicular to the interrogating beam prevents an accurate display of colour.

Table 7.2 Principles of the examination.

- General examination of liver parenchyma and abdomen
- Colour and spectral Doppler assessment of the portal vein, superior mesenteric and splenic veins, together with main intrahepatic portal branches
- Colour and spectral Doppler assessment of the hepatic artery from the coeliac axis to the porta, together with main intrahepatic branches
- Colour and spectral Doppler assessment of the main hepatic veins and the upper inferior vena cava

7

VASCULAR ANATOMY AND NORMAL FLOW PROFILES (Table 7.3)

Portal vein

The *portal vein* normally supplies approximately 70% of incoming blood volume to the liver. This relatively deoxygenated blood comes to the liver after perfusing the intestine and spleen. It is rich in nutrients after a meal, and arrives at the liver to be processed in the cells of the hepatic sinusoids. The portal vein is formed by the confluence of the splenic and superior mesenteric veins. It is accompanied by the hepatic artery and common bile duct to form the portal triad (Fig. 7.5); this has echogenic margins as it courses into the liver, due to the paraportal extension of Glisson's capsule and the presence of some perivascular fat. In the liver, these vessels progressively branch to supply the liver segments; anatomic variations of the portal vein are rare. The Couinaud system of segmental liver anatomy divides the liver vertically along the planes of the hepatic veins, and horizontally along the planes of the left and right portal veins. The

segmental branches of the portal vein enter the centre of the Couinaud segments, the ultrasound appearance of which has been described by LaFortune *et al*[20].

The typical portal vein flow profile has a relatively consistent velocity of approximately 18 cm s^{-1} ($\pm$5 cm s^{-1}) towards the liver (Fig. 7.6a)[21]. The flow velocity is uniform because cardiac pulsation is dampened by the capillaries of the intestine at one end of the portal system and by the liver sinusoids at the other end. Slight phasicity may be seen on the portal vein spectral tracing secondary to patient respiration, and a mild degree of periodicity may be present, due either to retrograde pulsation transmitted from the right heart via the hepatic vein (A wave), or to the inflow of blood during hepatic arterial systole[22]. Because these brief pressure surges into the liver transiently increase resistance to portal venous inflow, they effect a momentary slowing of antegrade flow in the normal portal vein (Fig. 7.6b)[23]. In studies of portal vein flow, Hosoki *et al*[24] and Wachsberg *et al*[25] reported the presence of some degree of periodicity in 7% and 64% of their respective normal study populations. Although some periodicity may be expected in portal vein flow, reversal of flow, even brief, should be considered an abnormal finding.

Table 7.3 Normal hepatic vessel velocities (fasting).

Hepatic artery	30–40 cm s^{-1} systolic, 10–15 cm s^{-1} diastolic
Portal vein	13–23 cm s^{-1}

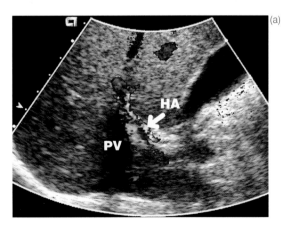 (a)

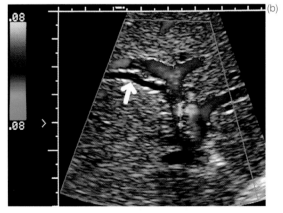 (b)

Fig. 7.5 (a) Oblique colour Doppler image of the portahepatis. The hepatic artery (HA) accompanies the portal vein (PV) and bile ducts. (b) Colour Doppler can easily differentiate the hepatic vasculature from a dilated biliary system (arrow).

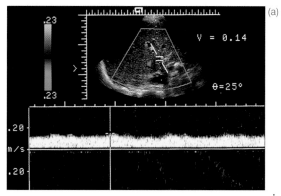

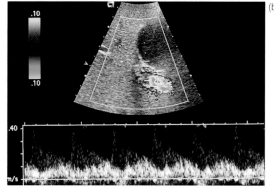

Fig. 7.6 (a) Spectral Doppler tracing of normal portal vein flow. Flow velocity of 0.14 m s^{-1} is relatively uniform and in a hepatopetal direction. (b) Spectral Doppler tracing of normal portal vein flow. Slight periodicity is present in this patient's portal vein tracing. The slight dip in antegrade velocity may coincide with the hepatic vein A wave or, as in this case, with hepatic arterial systole.

Hepatic artery

The arterial blood supply of the liver arises solely from the coeliac axis in approximately 76% of individuals. The *common hepatic artery* originates from the coeliac artery; after the origin of the gastroduodenal artery, it is called the *proper hepatic artery*. This then enters the liver alongside the portal vein where it divides into left and right hepatic arteries. There are numerous variants of hepatic artery anatomy. These include accessory vessels which exist in conjunction with normal branches of the hepatic artery, and replaced arteries, which make up the sole supply of a segment or lobe. For example, a replaced right hepatic artery arising from the superior mesenteric artery may be the sole blood supply to the entire right lobe of the liver; this situation occurs in approximately 11–25% of the population[26]. In a slender patient, colour Doppler ultrasound may be able to identify the replaced right hepatic artery behind the main portal vein as it courses towards the right lobe from the superior mesenteric artery (Fig. 7.7). The other variants occur

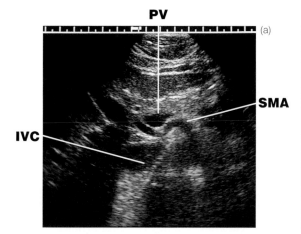

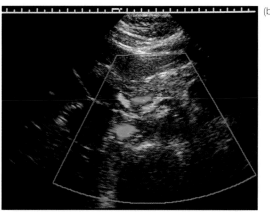

Fig. 7.7 (a) Transverse image of the mid-abdomen at the level of the superior mesenteric artery origin. A tubular structure is seen coursing from the superior mesenteric artery (SMA) to the right lobe of the liver, between portal vein (PV) and the inferior vena cava (IVC). (b) Colour Doppler identifies this tubular structure as a vessel. An arterial signal on spectral Doppler, identification of its SMA origin and a course towards the right lobe of the liver confirm this to be a replaced right hepatic artery.

less frequently and are more difficult to identify by Doppler ultrasound.

The normal hepatic artery in a fasting patient has a low-resistance Doppler flow profile (about 60–70% resistance index (RI)) (Fig. 7.8). During systole, the velocity is approximately 30–40 cm s^{-1}; while during diastole it normally slows to 10–15 cm s^{-1} which is usually less than the velocity of the portal vein flow. Technically, the best way to evaluate relative flow velocities in the hepatic artery and the portal vein is to increase the sample volume size so that both vessels are incorporated into the same tracing (Fig. 7.9).

Hepatic veins

The hepatic veins are relatively straight, anechoic, tubular structures that converge on the IVC approximately 1 cm below its confluence with the right atrium. The walls of the hepatic veins are relatively hypoechoic which helps to differentiate them from the portal veins in the more echogenic portal triads. There are no valves in the hepatic veins.

In most people the *right*, *middle*, and *left hepatic veins* enter the IVC in a 'crow's foot' configuration when viewed in the transverse plane (Fig. 7.4). The left and middle hepatic veins may enter as a common trunk along the

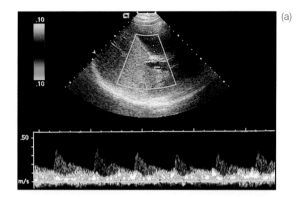

(a)

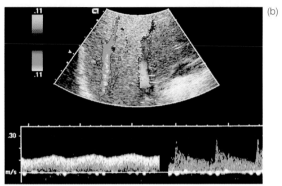

(b)

Fig. 7.9 Combined spectral Doppler tracing of the hepatic artery and portal vein. By opening the sample volume wide (a), or rocking the transducer between the hepatic artery and portal vein in the same tracing (b), the relative velocities between hepatic artery and portal vein can be directly compared. A normal velocity ratio between hepatic artery and portal vein is present in these patients. The hepatic artery diastolic velocity in a fasting patient is normally equal to or slightly less than portal vein velocity.

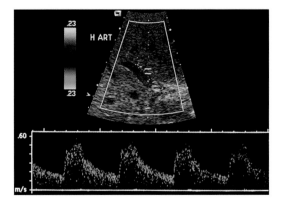

Fig. 7.8 Spectral Doppler tracing of a normal hepatic artery. Systolic upstroke is brisk, measuring less than 0.07 s. Resistive index measures approximately 70%. Velocity at end-diastole approximates 0.10 m s^{-1}.

left anterolateral aspect of the IVC. Approximately 30% of individuals have additional hepatic veins that may be identified by colour Doppler: a right superior anterior segmental vein may be seen draining into the middle hepatic vein; marginal hepatic veins may drain into the right and left hepatic veins; and a large accessory right hepatic vein may be seen entering the IVC several centimetres inferior to the junction of the three main hepatic veins in approximately 6–10% of people (Fig. 7.10). The venous drainage from the central portion of the liver parenchyma, including the caudate lobe, empties directly into the IVC and cannot

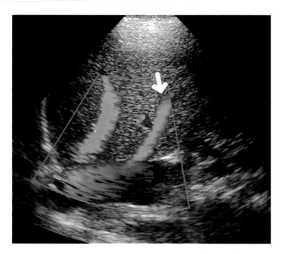

Fig. 7.10 Longitudinal colour Doppler image of the liver and inferior vena cava through the right flank. Note the prominent accessory hepatic vein (arrow) draining directly into the inferior vena cava from the posterior segment of the right lobe of the liver (Couinaud segment 6). This vein joins the inferior vena cava approximately 4 cm inferior to the junction of the right, middle and left hepatic veins.

be perceived by colour Doppler in the normal patient (Fig. 7.11). This separate drainage pathway is responsible for the unique behaviour of the caudate lobe in liver disease, and the distinctive enhancement pattern seen on

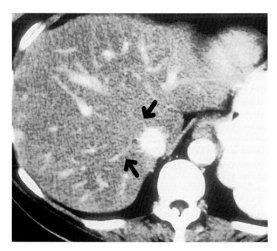

Fig. 7.11 CT scan through the mid-liver of a patient with severe fatty infiltration. Note several small hepatic veins (arrows) draining directly into the inferior vena cava. These veins are responsible for the altered appearance of the caudate lobe in patients with main hepatic vein thrombosis or cirrhosis.

contrast-enhanced CT scans of patients with hepatic vein thrombosis.

The hepatic vein waveform

The normal hepatic vein waveform is triphasic as a result of transmitted cardiac activity (Fig. 7.12) and is similar to the jugular vein waveform; indeed, the labels on the hepatic vein components have been transposed from the jugular vein pressure tracing. Most sonographic windows to the liver demonstrate the hepatic veins so that flow towards the heart is away from the transducer, which registers as flow below the baseline, but during right atrial systole blood is forced back into the liver and is therefore displayed above the baseline. These directions are best described as being *antegrade* (towards the heart) and *retrograde* (away from the heart).

This complicated tracing has been described and normal velocity measurements determined by Abu-Yousef[22]. Fig. 7.12b shows the hepatic venous waveform in conjunction with the ECG, tricuspid M-mode scan and atrioventricular status. The following stages can be identified:

1. The most distinctive feature is the retrograde A wave, which is the result of right atrial contraction and coincides with the P wave on the ECG. Since there is no valve between the right atrium and the IVC, a burst of reversed flow travels down the IVC and into the hepatic veins. This has a mean velocity of approximately 18 cm s^{-1}.

2. At the end of right atrial contraction, flow returns to the antegrade direction as the atrium relaxes. However, on right ventricular systole the tricuspid valve is slammed shut and actually bulges back into the right atrium. This creates its own pressure wave, the C wave, which may be perceived as a brief pause in the steadily increasing antegrade flow. This C wave coincides with the beginning of ventricular systole and occurs immediately after the QRS complex on the ECG.

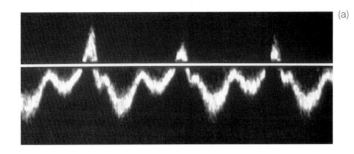

(a)

Fig. 7.12 (a) Normal hepatic vein spectral Doppler tracing. (b) Simultaneous tracings of an ECG, hepatic vein spectral Doppler tracing, and mitral valve M-mode tracing with correlation to atrial and ventricular systole and diastole. The divisions at the top of these tracings (1–5) correspond to the discussion in the text.

(b)

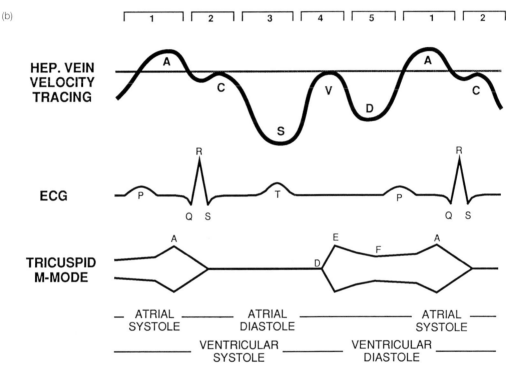

3. The right atrium continues to dilate and antegrade flow builds to a relatively high velocity of approximately 30 cm s^{-1}. Eventually, atrial filling approaches completion and antegrade flow starts to slow. This transition, known as the S wave, occurs during ventricular systole within 0.15 s of the QRS complex.

4. At the end of atrial filling, antegrade velocity decreases, or may even briefly reverse; this is known as the V wave and has a mean velocity of approximately −1.1 cm s^{-1}. In relation to the ECG, this occurs immediately following the T wave.

5. As the right ventricle enters diastole, the tricuspid valve opens and flow in the hepatic veins increases in the antegrade direction, as both the right atrium and right ventricle fill. Velocity builds to a mean of approximately 22 cm s^{-1} and this phase is referred to as the D wave. Eventually, the right heart chambers become filled passively and antegrade flow begins to slow. We then return to the A wave as the atrium again contracts to begin another cardiac cycle.

This waveform is seen in the hepatic veins and upper IVC in the vast majority of patients. Not all individuals, however, have a similar degree of periodicity within the hepatic veins. The percentage of patients that manifest a definite C wave is relatively small. The degree of flow reversal of the A wave and V wave may vary depending on the patient's cardiac status, state of hydration, heart rate, and the distance of Doppler interrogation from the heart. In a survey of a population of normal volunteers, a 9% incidence of a flattened hepatic vein flow profile has been reported[27].

Because the heart is located within the thorax, pressure changes caused by respiration affect the hepatic vein flow profile. When the patient forcefully exhales or bears down against a closed glottis, the elevated intrathoracic pressure resists antegrade flow, causing the S wave and D waves to be less prominent. The reversed component of flow increases so the A and V waves become more pronounced. Conversely, during forced inspiration and increasing negative intrathoracic pressure, the S wave and D wave become more prominent, while the A wave and V wave are less pronounced and may actually not manifest as reversed flow (Fig. 7.13).

ASSESSMENT OF DISEASE

Portal vein

Portal hypertension

In hepatocellular disease, the sinusoids are damaged, destroyed or replaced. As the volume of normally functioning liver parenchyma decreases, the resistance to portal venous flow increases, the portal vein dilates, and portal flow decreases and eventually reverses[6, 28–31]. There is an elevation in portal vein pressure, in excess of normal, by 5–10 mmHg, resulting in portal hypertension[32]. Use of the 'congestive index' has been recommended in helping to diagnose portal hypertension. This index is the ratio of the portal vein cross-sectional area (cm²) divided by the mean portal flow velocity (cm s⁻¹), thereby taking into account portal vein dilata-

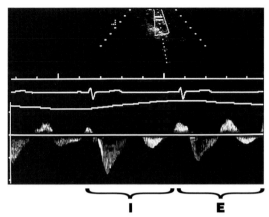

Fig. 7.13 Simultaneous hepatic vein spectral Doppler and respirometer tracings. Variations in the hepatic vein tracing can be perceived between inspiration and expiration. During inspiration (I) as the respirometer tracing is seen to rise, increased negative intrathoracic pressure causes air to be drawn into the lungs. This negative pressure is, however, also applied to the right atrium which draws blood from the inferior vena cava and hepatic vein with greater force. This is manifest in the hepatic vein tracing by a smaller, if not absent, regurgitant component of flow during the A wave and greater forward flow during the S and D waves. The converse is true during expiration (E), when intrathoracic pressure rises. This increased pressure results in a more prominent A wave. Forward flow towards the heart encounters the greater resistance as manifested by smaller S and D waves.

tion and decreased flow velocity, the two physiological changes associated with portal hypertension[33]. In normal subjects this ratio is less than 0.7.

As liver disease worsens, the periodicity in the portal vein may become more pronounced, with progressively increasing components of reversed flow, usually coinciding with hepatic arterial systole (Fig. 7.14)[28]. Finally, with end-stage liver disease, continuous hepatofugal flow is observed, usually with marked periodicity. Blood entering the liver in the hepatic artery normally passes through the hepatic sinusoids to the hepatic veins, but with increasing hepatocellular disease, scarring and fibrosis, the pathway of least resistance for the arterial inflow becomes the portal vein, with arterial blood being shunted to the portal vein via vasa vasorum, or via direct arteriovenous

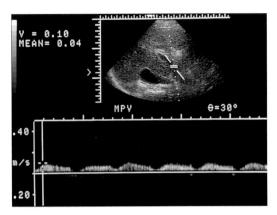

Fig. 7.14 Spectral Doppler tracing in a patient with severe alcohol-induced cirrhosis. Portal vein velocity has decreased although flow does remain hepatopetal through most of the cardiac cycle. Note the marked periodicity, however, which coincided with hepatic arterial systole.

shunting at the level of the sinusoids. Thus, the hepatofugal flow leaving the liver in the portal vein is arterial blood shunted from the hepatic artery (Fig. 7.15)[34].

Pronounced periodicity may be seen in the portal vein which does not coincide with hepatic arterial systole. This is usually due to cardiac disease, such as right ventricular dysfunction or tricuspid regurgitation, and is caused by a prominent reversed component of flow in the hepatic veins, either a 'cannon' A wave or a reversed S wave (Fig. 7.16)[35,36].

Varices

As portal hypertension progresses and pressure rises to 15 or 20 mmHg, sufficient pressure exists to cause the development of varices. These collateral pathways shunt blood from the portal to the systemic circulation. The more common channels are the short gastric, left gastric and coronary veins; recanalized paraumbilical veins and splenorenal-mesenteric anastomoses (Fig. 7.17). Other, less typical, pathways include pericholecystic, iliolumbar, gonadal, haemorrhoidal, and ascending retrosternal veins. Indeed, almost any vein in the abdomen may serve as a potential collateral to the systemic circulation and may be incorporated in a very convoluted shunt.

Short gastric varices coursing between the spleen and the greater curvature of the stomach are best imaged via the left flank, using the enlarged spleen as a window (Fig. 7.18). *Left*

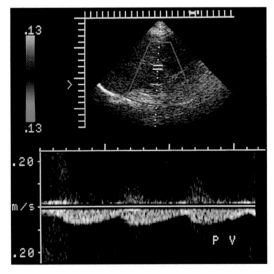

Fig. 7.15 Portal vein spectral Doppler tracing in a patient with severe hepatocellular damage secondary to paracetamol (acetaminophen) overdose. Portal vein flow is hepatofugal throughout the cardiac cycle.

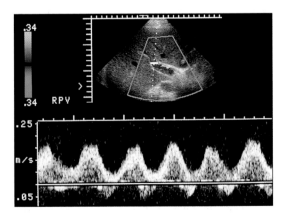

Fig. 7.16 Spectral Doppler tracing of portal vein flow in a patient with severe right ventricular dysfunction and tricuspid regurgitation. There is marked periodicity in the portal vein waveform. Hepatopetal flow decreases, and briefly reverses, coinciding with the large regurgitant component of hepatic vein flow during tricuspid regurgitation.

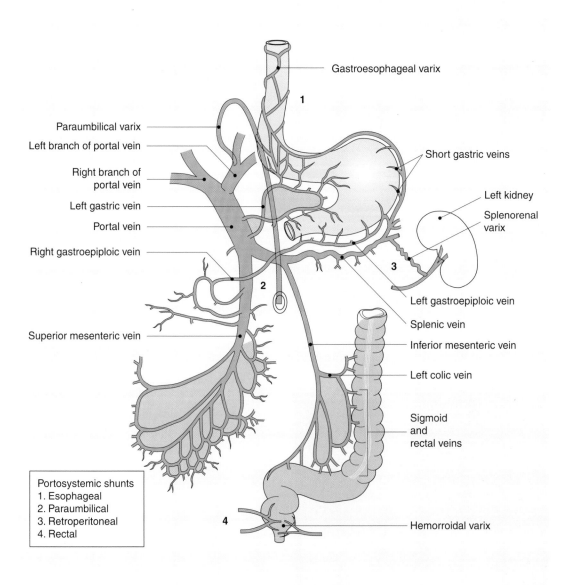

Fig. 7.17 Major portosystemic varices encountered in portal hypertension.

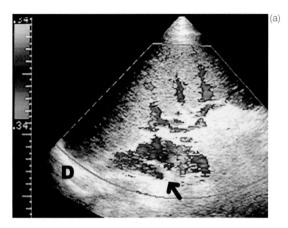 (a)

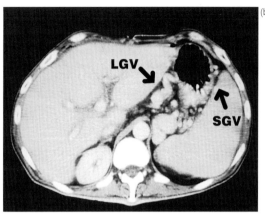 (b)

Fig. 7.18 (a) Longitudinal colour Doppler view of the left flank in a patient with portal hypertension. A tangled web of vessels (arrow) is seen at the splenic hilum and extends cephalad towards the diaphragm (D). These are short gastric varices coursing from splenic veins to the stomach and from there to the systemic circulation via esophageal varices. (b) Contrast-enhanced CT of a patient with portal hypertension. Short gastric varices (SGV) are best imaged from the left flank using the spleen as a sonographic window. The left gastric varix (LGV) is best imaged through the left lobe of the liver.

gastric, or *coronary vein varices* running from the splenic or portal vein to the lesser curvature of the stomach are best imaged through the left lobe of the liver (Figs. 7.18b and 7.19). Both sets of varices then converge on the gastro-oesophageal junction. From there, blood flow proceeds upwards through oesophageal varices

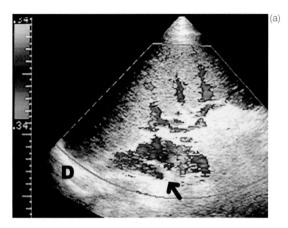

Fig. 7.19 Longitudinal colour Doppler image in the midline of a patient with portal hypertension. A large tortuous left gastric varix is seen coursing from the region of the coeliac axis towards the gastro-oesophageal junction. Whereas short gastric varices tend to be a plexus of small vessels, the left gastric varix is typically a single large tortuous vessel.

to eventually communicate with the azygous vein and the systemic circulation. Because of the potential lethal risk from spontaneous, brisk haemorrhage from these varices, a variety of endoscopic, surgical or percutaneous procedures may be employed to divert blood away from them[37].

In utero, oxygenated blood flows from the placenta up the umbilical vein to the left portal vein and through the ductus venosus into the IVC and right atrium. After birth, this pathway involutes and the umbilical vein is represented by the ligamentum teres in the falciform ligament. In portal hypertension, *paraumbilical veins* in this ligament can dilate and carry blood from the left portal vein along the anterior abdominal wall to the umbilical region (Fig. 7.20)[38]. From the umbilicus, the blood may pass to the superior or inferior epigastric veins, or through subcutaneous veins in the anterior abdominal wall – a 'caput medusae' – to reach the systemic venous system. Because inferior epigastric varices run just deep to the rectus muscles, they are not apparent on clinical examination but easily identified by colour Doppler (Fig. 7.21). Patients with known portal hypertension who present with an umbilical hernia

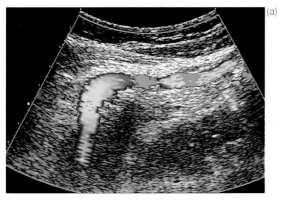
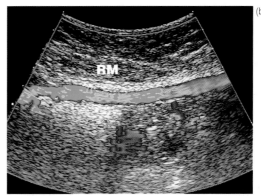

Fig. 7.20 (a) Longitudinal colour Doppler image of a patient with portal hypertension. A large vein carries flow from the left portal vein towards the transducer. It courses along the falciform ligament and then turns caudad along the anterior abdominal wall. (b) Midline longitudinal colour Doppler image. Flow in this recanalized paraumbilical vein courses towards the umbilicus, deep to the rectus muscles (RM).

should undergo imaging evaluation prior to surgery, as the hernia may contain a dilated varix, rather than bowel (Fig. 7.22).

Splenorenal-mesenteric collaterals are typically quite large and very tortuous. They are seen in the left flank coursing between the splenic hilum and the left renal vein (Fig. 7.23).

Occasionally, this pathway can communicate via mesenteric veins in the pelvis to a gonadal vein and then back to the renal vein and the systemic circulation.

Pericholecystic varices can occur in the gall bladder wall and are associated with portal vein thrombosis. Ultrasound imaging may reveal

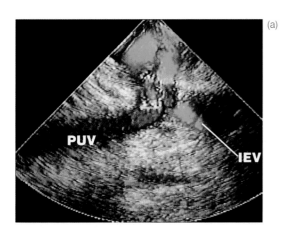
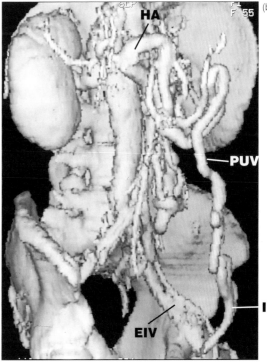

Fig. 7.21 (a) Longitudinal colour Doppler image directly over the umbilicus. A recanalized paraumbilical vein (PUV) carries blood towards the umbilicus. No caput medussa was present in this patient since flow continues from the umbilical region via the inferior epigastric vein (IEV). (b) 3-D CT angiogram in a patient with portal hypertension. Note the large recanalized paraumbilical vein (PV) coursing towards the umbilicus. From there flow continues back to the systemic circulation via the left inferior epigastric vein (IEGV) to the left external iliac vein (EIV).

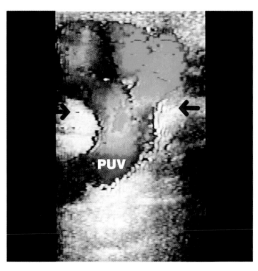

Fig. 7.22 Longitudinal linear colour Doppler image directly over the umbilicus. A recanalized paraumbilical vein (PUV) courses deep to the rectus sheath (arrows). At the umbilicus, however, the vessel passes through the sheath and herniates into the subcutaneous tissues.

cystic or tubular structures in the gall bladder wall. These should not be confused with the Rokitansky–Aschoff sinuses of hyperplastic cholecystosis and colour Doppler is useful to show flow within these vessels; the spectral tracing is that of portal venous flow (Fig. 7.24). From the gall bladder, subhepatic collaterals communicate to the abdominal wall and

subcostal veins. Haemorrhoidal collaterals are not routinely studied by Doppler.

Portal vein thrombosis

This must be considered when no Doppler signal is detected within the portal vein and may be due to blood clot, or to tumour invasion. However, the examiner should first review the system set-up and re-evaluate scale, gain and filtration settings. If these are found to be set appropriately and there is still no perceptible flow, the patient should be asked to perform a Valsalva manoeuvre. This elevates intrathoracic and right atrial pressure, transmitting higher pressure to the IVC, hepatic veins, and subsequently into the liver parenchyma. This increased pressure causes even greater resistance to portal venous inflow and may convert stagnant portal flow to hepatofugal flow (Fig. 7.25). One may also consider the use of an intravenous ultrasonographic contrast agent to enhance perception of very slow flow.

Early *thrombosis* of the portal vein may be difficult to visualize with ultrasound since fresh clot can be markedly hypoechoic[39]. As clot matures, it becomes more echogenic and retracts, allowing partial recanalization of the

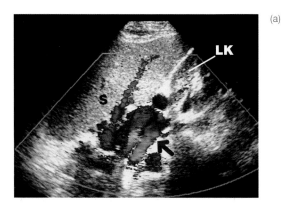

(a)

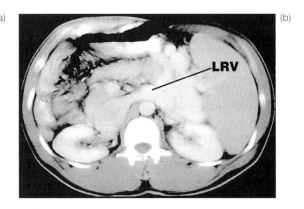

(b)

Fig. 7.23 (a) Longitudinal colour Doppler image of the left flank in a patient with portal hypertension. A large complex varix is seen extending from the splenic hilum (S) and left kidney (LK). Note the increase in left renal vein calibre (arrow) where it is joined by the varix. (b) Axial contrast-enhanced CT image at the level of the left renal vein. The large complex varix is medial to the enlarged spleen and flows into the left renal vein (LRV).

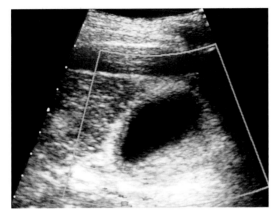

Fig. 7.24 Colour Doppler image of the gall bladder in a patient with portal hypertension and portal vein thrombosis. Numerous vessels are identified in the gall bladder wall. Spectral Doppler revealed a portal vein waveform as would be expected in varices and not an arterial waveform as would be seen in the cystic artery.

portal vein (Fig. 7.26). Patients with long-standing portal vein thrombosis may develop collateral flow into the liver via a lace-like network of veins. This is known as cavernous transformation of the portal vein or a cavernoma[40–41]. Grey-scale imaging alone can seldom visualize these vessels because of their small size, but colour Doppler reveals a web of numerous serpiginous small veins which typically involve a fairly wide area of the liver hilum (Fig. 7.27). Spectral Doppler shows portal flow in the branches of the cavernoma.

Neoplastic invasion

Hepatocellular carcinoma has the propensity to invade the portal and hepatic veins. Intravascular tumour is classified as stage IV disease and is considered unresectable. Involvement of the portal vein by tumour may cause an increase in its cross-sectional area and a decrease in portal vein flow. Tumour in the portal vein will receive its blood supply from the hepatic artery and spectral Doppler of the 'thrombus' will show an arterial waveform, which usually projects in a hepatofugal direction, supplying the tumour as it grows out of the liver. A bland thrombus will not manifest such a tracing on Doppler, so that invasive tumour can be differentiated from bland thrombus and the diagnosis of stage IV

(a)

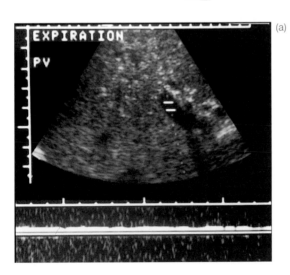

(b)

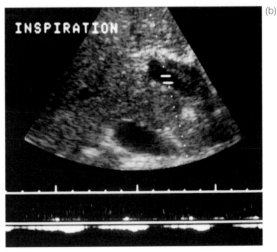

Fig. 7.25 Spectral Doppler tracings of a patient with end-stage liver disease being considered for liver transplantation. (a) In expiration, with lower intrathoracic pressure, flow in the portal vein is seen to be thready, but nevertheless hepatopetal. (b) This tracing was obtained after the patient was instructed to take a deep breath in and bear down. The elevated intrathoracic pressure transmitted via the IVC to the hepatic veins and liver parenchyma causes increased resistance to portal inflow. This results in a change in portal vein direction from hepatopetal to hepatofugal.

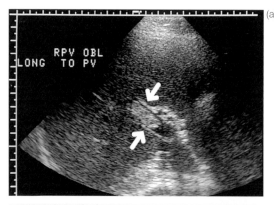

(a)

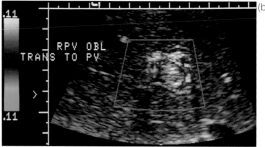

(b)

Fig. 7.26 (a) Oblique image of the portal vein in a patient with hypercoagulability. Echogenic thrombus is seen adherent to the portal vein wall (arrows).(b) Colour Doppler image transverse to the portahepatis. Flow is seen coursing past the partially occluding thrombus in a hepatopetal direction.

hepatocellular carcinoma with vascular invasion confirmed (Fig. 7.28)[42].

Portal vein aneurysm

Aneurysm of the portal vein has been reported but it is extremely rare. The vein may enlarge to a diameter of 3 cm or larger. Spectral Doppler should be applied to confirm a portal vein waveform and rule out hepatic artery aneurysm, since the latter carries a much higher incidence of complications and rupture[43].

Portal vein gas

Gas may be seen in the portal vein and its branches in a variety of gastrointestinal disorders such as sepsis, obstruction with distension, necrotizing enterocolitis, infarction or ulceration. Numerous tiny hyperechoic foci can be seen in the portal vein, flowing into the liver. Since these bubbles are moving fairly rapidly, their perception is improved by increasing scanner temporal resolution by limiting the

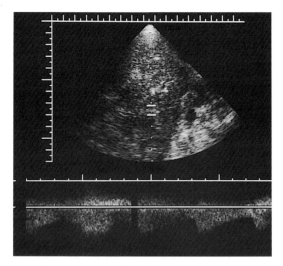

Fig. 7.27 Oblique colour Doppler image of the portohepatis. A normal portal vein could not be visualized. Instead there is a plexus of small vessels with hepatopetal flow. After portal vein thrombosis this web of small vessels reconstitutes portal flow to the liver and is known as cavernous transformation of the portal vein.

Fig. 7.28 Spectral Doppler tracing over the portal vein in a patient with hepatocellular carcinoma. An arterial waveform is present in the plug of tissue identified in the portal vein. This represents hepatocellular carcinoma extending into the portal vein. Reproduced with permission from Pozniak and Baus[42].

field of view to the area of the portal vein and minimizing, or turning off, frame averaging. The spectral Doppler tracing reveals sharp bidirectional spikes superimposed on the Doppler tracing of the portal vein[44]. These spikes do not reflect a higher velocity of the air bubble but represent an artefact resulting from the system being set to display the Doppler shift of red blood cells, so that the much more intense echoes from the air bubbles register as spikes of noise on the tracing (Fig. 7.29).

Hepatic artery

A comparison of hepatic arterial velocities with those of the portal vein may be used as an indicator of liver disease. The normal portal vein velocity in a fasting patient is about 18 cm s^{-1}, the normal systolic velocity in the hepatic artery is 30–40 cm s^{-1}, and 10–15 cm s^{-1} in diastole. If the waveforms of the hepatic artery and portal vein can be captured simultaneously on a Doppler tracing, the normal hepatic arterial diastolic velocity will therefore be seen to dip just below that of the portal vein (Fig. 7.9).

Almost all liver disease processes receive their blood supply primarily from the hepatic artery. As the process becomes more severe, or involves

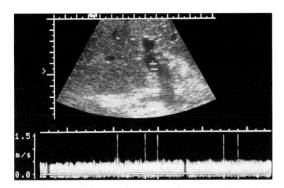

Fig. 7.29 Spectral Doppler tracing of the portal vein in a patient with pneumatosis intestinalis. The spikes present in this spectral Doppler tracing are caused by air bubbles in the portal vein. These bubbles are travelling at the same velocity as the rest of the blood in the portal vein. With the spectral gain set for blood, the intense sound reflection caused by the passing air bubbles creates spikes of noise.

a larger area of liver, hepatic artery flow increases. As liver disease worsens, the portal venous inflow encounters progressively increasing resistance, resulting in decreased hepatopetal portal velocity. Therefore, if the Doppler examination shows hepatic arterial diastolic velocities greater than that of the portal vein, the liver parenchyma should be carefully evaluated to rule out focal or diffuse liver disease[6]. This finding, however, is non-specific and can be seen with neoplasm (both primary and metastatic) and infection (viral, bacterial, parasitic or fungal) (Fig. 7.30). Benign conditions (e.g. haemangioma, fatty infiltration), however, do not perceptibly affect main hepatic artery or portal vein flow (Fig. 7.31).

Hepatic artery resistance has been studied in several disease states. Alterations in resistance may be observed but, to date, have not been shown to be sufficiently specific or sensitive in the diagnosis of any one particular condition[45]. Rapid onset of oedema or inflammation of the liver may produce a substantial amount of congestion, leading to higher resistance to hepatic arterial inflow and elevation of the resistance index. Hypervascular disorders, especially those with arterial venous shunting, such as neoplasm, can lower the arterial resistance. A tardus parvus waveform and low resistance flow may also be perceived downstream from significant hepatic artery stenosis, or a diaphragmatic crus defect of the coeliac axis (Fig. 7.32).

Hepatic artery aneurysm

Aneurysm of the hepatic artery is usually extrahepatic and may be congenital or acquired. Pancreatitis, trauma or liver biopsy are the most common aetiologies. Mycotic aneurysms can be seen in immune-compromised patients, those with bacterial endocarditis, or those abusing intravenous drugs. Sonography demonstrates a rounded area with swirling flow on colour. An arterial spectral tracing may be perceived but is usually quite distorted due to turbulence.

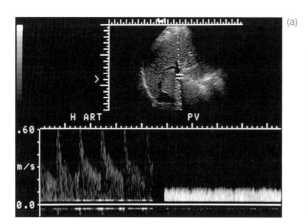
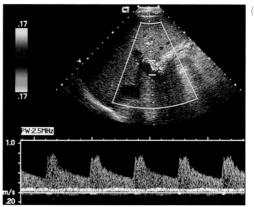

Fig. 7.30 (a) Spectral Doppler tracing at the portahepatis of a patient with hepatitis B-induced cirrhosis. Hepatic arterial velocities are markedly increased with a relative decrease in the portal vein velocity. (b) Combined Doppler tracing of the hepatic artery and portal vein in this HIV patient with acute fulminant hepatitis. A marked increase in hepatic arterial velocities with combined decrease in portal vein velocity is demonstrated. The large sample volume over the portahepatis allows superimposition of the tracings.

Clot may eventually develop within the aneurysm or pseudoaneurysm (Fig. 7.33). Communication may develop from the aneurysm to the portal vein or hepatic vein converting the aneurysm to an arteriovenous fistula. Spectral Doppler flow profiles show bounding arterial inflow velocities, swirling turbulent flow within the aneurysm and arterialization of the venous outflow[46,47].

Hereditary haemorrhagic telangiectasia (Osler–Rendu–Weber disease)

This disease is characterized by multiple small aneurysmal telangiectases distributed over the skin, mucous membranes, alimentary tract, liver, brain and spleen. These patients have a tendency for frequent haemorrhages requiring transfusion. Vascular lesions in the liver can evolve into arterial venous fistulas and aneurysms[48,49]. Ultrasound may reveal large

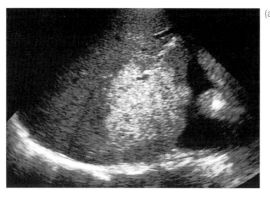
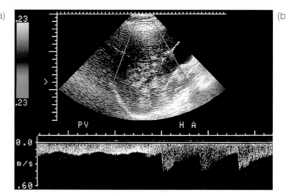

Fig. 7.31 (a) Transverse ultrasound image of the right lobe of the liver. There is a bright, somewhat rounded, echogenic mass in the inferior aspect of the right lobe. (b) Spectral Doppler of the right hepatic artery and portal vein supplying the mass. Portal vein and hepatic artery velocities are relatively normal. The ratio of flow is not altered. Biopsy proved the mass to be focal fatty infiltration.

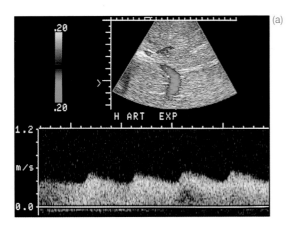 (a)

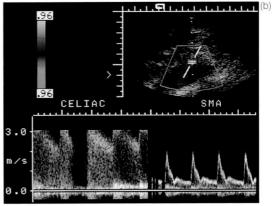 (b)

Fig. 7.32 (a) Spectral Doppler tracing of the hepatic artery in a young patient with upper abdominal pain. A markedly tardus parvus waveform is seen with slow upstroke in systole and very low resistance. (b) Combined spectral Doppler tracing of the coeliac artery and superior mesenteric artery (SMA) shows normal flow velocity in the SMA. The coeliac artery shows a turbulent waveform with high velocity greater than 3 m s^{-1}. MR angiography confirmed coeliac artery compression by the arcuate ligament of the diaphragm.

hepatic arteries feeding large, ectatic, serpiginous arteriovenous malformations, which in turn feed large draining veins[49].

Hepatic veins

Hepatic venous outflow obstruction (HVOO)

The term Budd–Chiari syndrome is usually

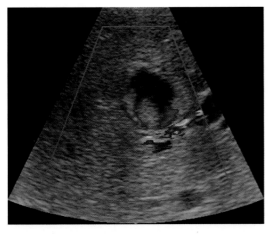

Fig. 7.33 Transverse colour Doppler image of the mid-liver. A rounded lesion is present with some internal debris. Flow is seen around this debris. An arterial spectral Doppler waveform was present in the feeding vessel. Angiography confirmed a partially thrombosed intrahepatic hepatic artery aneurysm.

taken to refer to hepatic vein thrombosis. Budd–Chiari, however, refers to liver dysfunction due to any cause of compromised hepatic vein outflow, both thrombotic and non-thrombotic. Ludwig *et al* have recommended that the term hepatic venous outflow obstruction (HVOO) should be used instead of Budd–Chiari syndrome[50]. This is appropriate since spectral and colour Doppler are capable of identifying numerous non-thrombotic causes of HVOO and differentiating them from hepatic vein thrombosis[51]. The clinical presentation of HVOO will vary, depending upon how rapidly it develops and the degree of obstruction. Approximately 50% of patients first present with RUQ pain and hepatomegaly. Almost all develop ascites, while a few may develop mild jaundice. Patients with chronic, partial obstruction may develop cirrhosis and portal hypertension. If the obstruction progresses to complete occlusion, then shock, hepatic coma and death may ensue.

Sonographic imaging features of HVOO may include echogenic intraluminal material (either thrombus or tumour), diffuse narrowing and compression of the veins from generalized liver swelling, or focal vascular compromise by a mass. Doppler findings include complete absence of hepatic vein flow (Fig. 7.34) or localized flow disturbances due to focal partial obstruction. In addition, the central portions of the hepatic veins (distant from the IVC) that remain patent will display low-velocity continuous flow, rather than the normal flow pattern with periodicity. Finally, liver congestion due to HVOO will also cause flow abnormalities in portal vein flow, such as diminished hepatopetal, bidirectional or hepatofugal (reversed) flow. The diagnosis of complete thrombosis by ultrasound imaging is difficult since the echogenicity of the clot is often similar to that of the adjacent liver parenchyma. Because the identification of absent blood flow by Doppler is an exclusionary diagnosis, it is difficult to determine with absolute certainty that the cause is thrombosis. Occasionally thrombosis may be limited to one or two hepatic veins. This results in a unique shunt of blood from the affected lobe of the liver to another via hepatic vein collaterals.

HVOO may be seen in three disease categories: hepatic vein thrombosis; non-thrombotic focal compromise of hepatic vein drainage (e.g. stricture, web or neoplasm); or reduced compliance of liver parenchyma (e.g. hepatitis, cirrhosis or transplant rejection).

Hepatic vein thrombosis most commonly occurs in patients with a hypercoagulation disorder and the use of oral contraceptives increases the risk of hepatic vein thrombosis two and a half times. Hepatic vein injury and phlebitis may also be associated with thrombosis but in approximately two thirds of cases, the cause is idiopathic. The caudate lobe has a separate venous drainage to the IVC, which is usually spared from thrombosis, resulting in caudate enlargement and normal enhancement on contrast-enhanced CT (Fig. 7.35). Occasionally, thrombosis may be limited to one or two of the hepatic veins, resulting in shunting of blood from the affected lobe to the unaffected side through hepatic venous collaterals (Fig. 7.36). A strategically located mass (either benign or malignant) may expand and press upon the ostia of the hepatic veins, resulting in impaired venous drainage. Renal cell carcinoma can extend from the renal vein into the IVC in 5% of cases; rarely this may extend up to the right atrium and compromise the hepatic vein ostia, and this may result in elevation of the liver enzymes (Fig. 7.37). Renal carcinoma

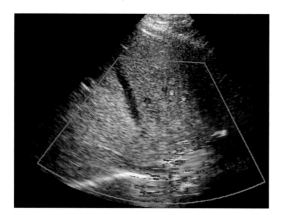

Fig. 7.34 Colour Doppler transverse image of the upper liver. Even with maximized Doppler sensitivity, no flow was perceived in the middle hepatic vein of this patient. The hepatic vein had become thrombosed when a central line was inadvertently advanced through the heart into the inferior vena cava and up into the middle hepatic vein.

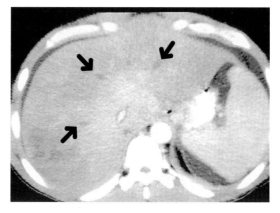

Fig. 7.35 Contrast-enhanced axial CT scan of the mid-liver. Note the uniform enhancement centrally in the caudate lobe but peripherally the enhancement is decreased and irregular. The three hepatic veins (arrows) are seen as low-attenuation structures consistent with thrombosis.

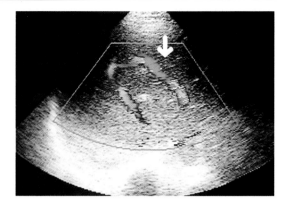

Fig. 7.36 Transverse colour Doppler view of the mid-liver in a patient with catheter-related inferior vena cava thrombus. The flow in the right hepatic vein is reversed and coursing towards the transducer. A prominent collateral vein then carries flow to the middle hepatic vein (arrow) and back towards the heart. Note the aliasing in the more distal hepatic vein due to the higher velocity caused by the increased volume of flow.

liver metastases maintain this propensity for vascular invasion (Fig. 7.38).

Membranous obstruction (fibrous web) of the IVC has been reported as one of the major causes of HVOO in South Africa and Asia[52, 53]. The aetiology of these is probably acquired since chronic hepatitis B infection is common in these patients, and up to 50% may develop hepatocellular carcinoma. There is some support, however, for a congenital hypothesis. The obstruction is usually at, or just above, the level of the hepatic vein ostia; this results in damping of cardiac pressure changes into the IVC and the hepatic veins, and flattening of the Doppler waveform. The obstruction may eventually lead to hepatic vein thrombosis.

Diffuse hepatic parenchymal disease resulting in a reduction of liver compliance can easily compromise hepatic venous drainage as these are a low-pressure system (basically the same as the right atrium, i.e. −2 to +7 mmHg). Both oedema from acute inflammation and fibrosis from chronic parenchymal disease (Fig. 7.39a) can compromise the hepatic veins, producing a relative HVOO. Some periodicity may be perceived in close proximity to the

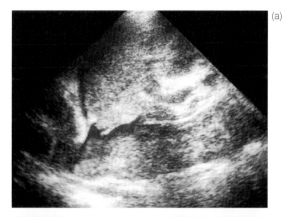

(a)

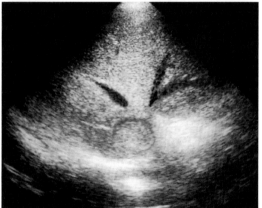

(b)

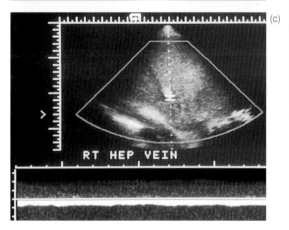

(c)

Fig. 7.37 (a) Longitudinal view of the inferior vena cava in a patient with renal cell carcinoma. A large plug of tumour thrombus is seen extending in the inferior vena cava up to the level of the heart. (b) Transverse view of the liver. The inferior vena cava tumour thrombus obstructs the hepatic vein ostia. Note the distention of the hepatic veins. (c) Spectral Doppler tracing shows flattening of the hepatic vein profile and complete absence of periodicity. A triphasic waveform is not seen, since cardiac retropulsation cannot get beyond the tumour thrombus.

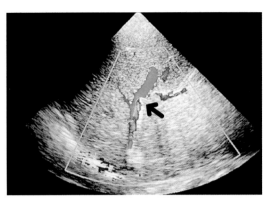

Fig. 7.38 Oblique view of the right hepatic vein in a patient with renal cell carcinoma metastatic to the liver. A small knuckle of tumour is extending from the large echogenic mass in the right lobe (arrow) into the right hepatic vein. Note distention of the hepatic vein above the tumour thrombus and the disordered flow with aliasing below that level.

junction of the hepatic veins with the IVC, but it quickly dampens as the sample volume is moved further away from the heart (Fig. 7.39b).

Hepatic veno-occlusive disease

Non-thrombotic occlusion of small hepatic veins can occur in bone marrow transplant recipients with alkaloid toxicity or secondary to chemotherapy or radiation therapy. The obstruction of terminal hepatic venules by connective tissue and collagen presents as jaundice, hepatomegaly, pain, ascites and altered liver functions. The associated coagulopathy usually precludes biopsy for diagnosis[54]. Spectral Doppler of the hepatic veins typically shows a normal flow profile. Portal vein flow, however, is typically decreased and may actually reverse[55]. Hepatic artery flow typically shows increased resistance[56].

Altered or increased hepatic vein periodicity

Near the heart, the normal spectral Doppler tracing of the hepatic vein has a small retrograde component of flow above the baseline, the A wave. It is relatively small when compared to the antegrade components below the baseline, the S and D waves. The ratio of retrograde to antegrade flow decreases during inspiration (which lowers intrathoracic pressure) or when the Doppler sample volume is moved further from the heart (Fig. 7.13). A consistently large component of retrograde flow is an abnormal finding, and if identified, the examiner should consider the presence of cardiac or pulmonary disease. Distortion of the triphasic hepatic vein waveform can occur with many different

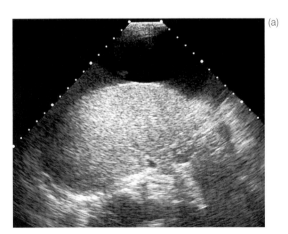

(a)

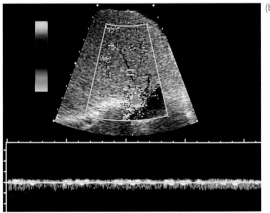

(b)

Fig. 7.39 (a) Transverse image of the liver in a patient with severe cirrhosis. The liver is small, nodular and very echogenic. (b) Spectral Doppler tracing of the hepatic vein within the liver. Patency of the vessel is confirmed by colour Doppler but flow is markedly compromised by compression of this vessel. There is complete absence of periodicity and a relatively slow velocity.

cardiac disorders, including cardiomyopathy, constrictive pericarditis, tamponade, tricuspid or pulmonary valve disease, atrioventricular dissociation, atrial fibrillation and right ventricular dysfunction. Pulmonary hypertension and massive pulmonary embolism may also distort the hepatic vein waveform.

Specific patterns of hepatic vein velocity profiles have been described in *restrictive cardiomyopathy*, *pericardial constriction*, and *tamponade*. A dramatic increase in D wave amplitude in patients with restrictive cardiomyopathy reflects increased right atrial pressure and rapid early diastolic filling, characteristic of restriction. Reversal of the A wave is seen in pericardial constriction and tamponade, and represents impaired late diastolic filling of the right ventricle. It is greatest during forced expiration due to the increased intrathoracic pressure transmitted to the pericardium.

Tricuspid regurgitation results in large volumes of blood leaking back through an incompetent or diseased tricuspid valve. In mild tricuspid regurgitation, the hepatic vein flow profile is characterized by attenuation of the S wave and a relative increase in V wave amplitude. In severe tricuspid regurgitation, systolic reversal of the S wave and fusion of the S and V waves is seen. Instead of forward flow filling the atrium during atrial diastole, the relatively high ventricular systolic pressure forces blood back through the tricuspid valve into the IVC and the hepatic veins (Fig. 7.40)[57].

In *atrioventricular dissociation*, the atrial and ventricular electromechanical events occur independently of each other. With complete heart block, atrial contraction against the closed tricuspid valve can result in a markedly accentuated A wave. Clinically, the increased jugular vein pulsations are described as 'cannon' A waves. The same phenomenon can occur in patients with premature ventricular ectopic beats which follow atrial contraction.

With *atrial arrhythmias*, the A wave may have a varying relationship to the S wave due

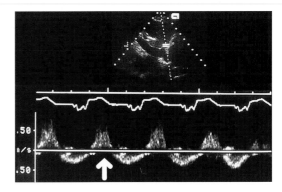

Fig. 7.40 Spectral Doppler hepatic vein tracing in a patient with severe tricuspid regurgitation. Note the striking S wave reversal (arrow) and fusion with the V wave. Particularly note the high ratio of retrograde flow (above the baseline) as compared to antegrade (below the baseline) flow.

to premature atrial contraction or a variable PR interval as seen in Mobitz I heart block. In atrial flutter, multiple small amplitude A waves may be present. The lack of organized atrial activity in atrial fibrillation leads to the loss of distinct A waves in the hepatic vein tracing.

In patients with moderate to severe *right ventricular dysfunction*, hepatic vein Doppler flow profiles fall into three basic patterns. The first Doppler indication of right ventricular dysfunction is accentuation of the atrial A wave, due to reduced right ventricular compliance which cannot accommodate all of the right atrial output. Further deterioration of right ventricular function results in attenuated systolic forward flow (S wave) due to a decrease in the descent of the base of the right ventricle. There is increased early diastolic forward flow (D wave), because of increased early diastolic filling of the right ventricle and increased A wave amplitude. Patients with severe right ventricular dysfunction usually have associated tricuspid insufficiency. This results in S wave reversal. S wave amplitude changes may also reflect reduced right atrial compliance, reduced right ventricular systolic function, or tricuspid insufficiency. A wave amplitude changes indicate reduced right ventricular compliance or increased right atrial inotropy (Fig. 7.41).

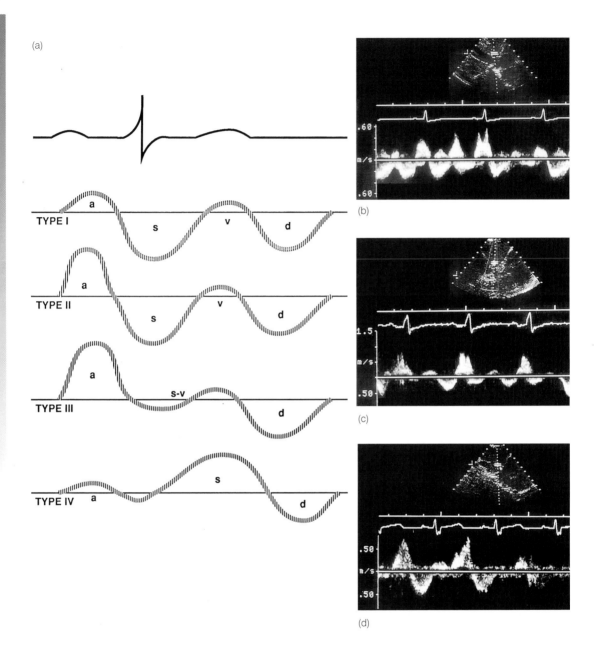

Fig. 7.41 (a) With progressively worsening right ventricular dysfunction the hepatic vein spectral Doppler tracings become more distorted. Hepatic vein flow profiles have been characterized into four different types:

Type 1 normal pattern (see Fig. 7.12a). The retrograde component of flow (A wave) follows soon after the P wave on the ECG tracing. (b) *Type 2* pattern has an accentuated A wave. Greater reversal of flow is likely secondary to reduced right ventricular compliance and/or increased atrial systolic force. (c) *Type 3* pattern shows an attenuated systolic forward flow (S wave). This is due to a decrease in the descent of the base of the right ventricle. Also, increased early diastolic forward flow is seen in the D wave due to increased early diastolic filling of the right ventricle. Again, note the increased A wave amplitude. (d) *Type 4* pattern is seen with severe right ventricular dysfunction, which is usually accompanied with severe tricuspid insufficiency. Note that the dominant reversed component of flow now occurs well after the QRS. It is not related to the P wave.

Arterialized hepatic vein flow

An arterial waveform within the hepatic veins is an extremely rare finding. It may be seen with a fistula from the hepatic artery to the hepatic vein following biopsy or surgery. Rarely, erosion of a hepatic artery aneurysm into the hepatic vein will produce arterial pulsations in the veins.

Focal liver lesions – malignant

Hepatocellular carcinoma

Hepatocellular carcinoma is the most common primary malignant neoplasm of the liver. It most frequently occurs in patients with underlying chronic liver disease such as hepatitis B infection, less commonly with alcoholic cirrhosis. Ultrasound imaging is relatively poor for the detection of hepatocellular carcinoma, with a sensitivity of only 50% for the sonographic identification of malignancy in cirrhotic livers[58]. The distorted echo-texture of the liver parenchyma, together with the tumour's variable sonographic appearance, make it difficult to distinguish the neoplasm.

Hepatocellular carcinoma is typically a hypervascular neoplasm and several authors have promoted the use of spectral and colour Doppler in helping to diagnose it[59, 60]. The tumour typically shows abundant neovascularity, resulting in decreased vascular impedence and resistance. Arterioportal venous shunting also occurs through the tumour[61]. The Doppler waveform in these tumours therefore typically manifests increased diastolic flow with a low resistance flow profile (Fig. 7.42). A basket pattern of flow within the lesion on colour Doppler has been described as characteristic for hepatocellular carcinoma[60]; the internal branching vessels within the tumour, combined with the network of surrounding vessels, being responsible for this appearance. However, similar findings occur in other conditions (Fig. 7.43). A low-RI, high-velocity flow with systolic frequency shifts approximating 3 m s[-1] may be seen in the main hepatic artery, but metastases to the liver, especially from hypervascular primaries, can manifest similar changes in the hepatic artery flow profile.

Peripheral portal vein flow alteration has been suggested by some investigators to be valuable in differentiating benign from malignant lesions. Hepatofugal flow can be perceived on spectral and colour Doppler in proximity to hepatocellular carcinoma or metastatic disease. Miller *et al*[62], however,

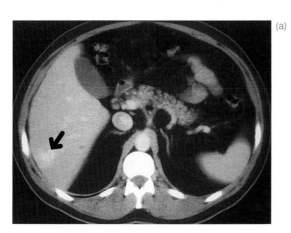

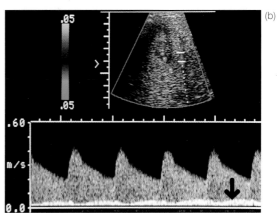

Fig. 7.42 (a) Contrast-enhanced axial CT scan in a patient with biopsy-proven hepatocellular carcinoma. A brightly enhancing lesion is identified in the periphery of the right lobe (arrow). (b) Spectral Doppler tracing of the right hepatic artery and right portal vein shows changes characteristic of liver disease and neoplasm. Note the relative high diastolic flow with low resistance. Note the attenuated portal vein flow (arrow).

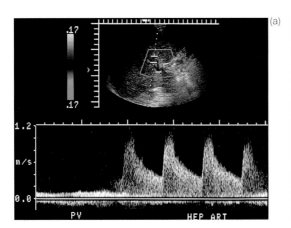
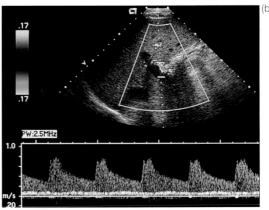

Fig. 7.43 (a) Spectral Doppler tracing at the porta hepatis in a patient with biopsy-proven chemical hepatitis. This tracing was obtained by a slight change in orientation of the transducer during the scan traversing from portal vein to the hepatic artery. Hepatic arterial velocities are markedly increased with low resistive index and high diastolic flow. Portal velocity is decreased. (b) Combined hepatic artery and portal vein tracing at the portahepatis in a patient with HIV. In contrast to (a) this tracing was obtained with the sample volume open wide and included both flow profiles simultaneously. Similar alteration in velocities is perceived with bounding arterial flow and diminished portal vein inflow.

showed that this kind of flow profile can also be identified in proximity to large haemangiomas, subcapsular haematomas and other benign conditions[62]. Therefore, this finding cannot alter the standard differential diagnosis based on grey-scale findings.

Low sensitivity and specificity unfortunately limits the value of ultrasound imaging and Doppler in diagnosing hepatocellular carcinoma. Biphasic CT is now considered the most accurate tool for the early detection of the tumour, where a brightly enhancing hepatic lesion during the arterial phase of contrast injection is considered to be hepatocellular carcinoma until proven otherwise.

Metastases

Metastatic liver lesions occur with a frequency approximately 20 times greater than primary hepatic neoplasms. Their sonographic appearances are markedly variable but these do not correlate with cell type. One of the more frequently occurring appearances is that of the target pattern, or halo sign. The hypoechoic rim surrounding the lesion is caused by

compressed liver parenchyma, or by proliferating tumour at the edge of the lesion.

Colour Doppler may reveal displacement of normal liver vasculature by the expanding metastatic lesion. Little if any flow is usually seen in the metastasis itself. Spectral Doppler can reveal low-resistance, high-velocity flow in the hepatic artery. However, this is not consistent enough to be of value in characterizing an unknown lesion. If metastasis is suspected, this change in the hepatic artery spectral Doppler waveform can be considered strongly suggestive, but it does not obviate the need for biopsy.

Focal liver lesions – benign

Hepatic steatosis (fatty liver)

In response to hepatocellular disease, the liver can accumulate triglycerides within the hepatocytes. This reversible cellular response may be seen with obesity, alcoholic liver disease, diabetes, parenteral nutrition and numerous other disorders[63]. Ultrasound commonly reveals a bright echogenic liver with poor through transmission. The central vasculature is often poorly visualized due to compression of these vessels by surrounding fat-laden parenchyma. It is well known that fatty infiltration can be patchy and irregular. Occasionally the appearance can be nodular but most often it is non-spherical in shape, with geometric margins or wedge-shaped segmental distribution. Doppler ultrasound typically shows no change in the hepatic haemodynamics, or distribution of vessels. Hepatic artery and portal vein velocities maintain a normal ratio. This is in contrast to malignancy which usually shows an increased hepatic arterial velocity. Absence of this velocity alteration may be helpful in further reinforcing the impression of benign fatty infiltration in cases where the imaging appearance is confusing (Fig. 7.44). If significant doubt exists CT, magnetic resonance (MR) scintigraphy or biopsy may be necessary to clinch the diagnosis[64, 65].

Haemangiomas

These are the most common solid benign neoplasms of the liver. They are hyperechoic when small (<3 cm) but the echogenicity of larger haemangiomas can be variable. Colour Doppler adds little to the diagnosis of haemangioma as the flow is typically too slow to register, even at the most sensitive settings. Flow may be demonstrated occasionally with power Doppler (Fig. 7.45). Unfortunately, this may only serve to confuse the diagnosis, as the classic teaching is that flow in haemangiomas is imperceptible. In common with other benign masses there is rarely any alteration to the hepatic arterial inflow on spectral Doppler. Further evaluation with scintigraphy, or MR, may be necessary to clinch the diagnosis.

Focal nodular hyperplasia

Focal nodular hyperplasia is a relatively rare hepatic lesion seen in young to middle-aged women. It is believed to be hormone dependent and not premalignant. Ultrasound often reveals a solitary, small lesion (<3 cm), often at the periphery of the liver. The echogenicity is varied with hypo-, hyper-, and isoechoic focal nodular hyperplasia reported with equal frequency. A central scar has been reported as a dominant feature of the lesion; however, it is seldom seen sonographically, but even if seen, it does not help clinch a benign diagnosis. Focal nodular hyperplasia is typically hypervascular with a prominent central artery and radiating branches in a stellate or spokewheel configuration with centrifugal flow; this is a unique characteristic of this lesion (Fig. 7.46). If doubt still exists in the diagnosis, then a technecium-99 sulphur

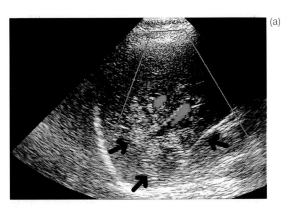 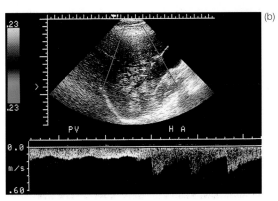

Fig. 7.44 (a) Transverse colour Doppler image of the right lobe of the liver. A geographic area of increased echogenicity is seen in the mid-right lobe (arrows). This was an unsuspected finding in a patient with normal liver function tests. (b) Spectral Doppler tracing of the right hepatic artery and right portal vein shows a normal flow velocity ratio. Biopsy revealed the echogenic lesions to be focal fatty infiltration.

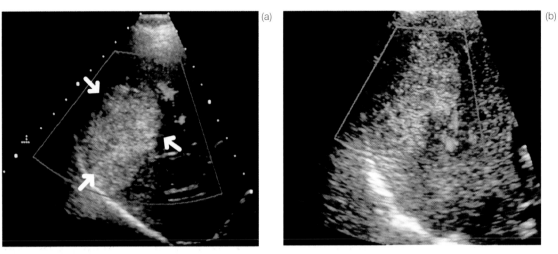

Fig. 7.45 (a) Transverse colour Doppler image of the right lobe of the liver. A large echogenic mass is seen occupying the majority of the right lobe (arrow). No flow is perceived within the mass by colour Doppler despite settings at the most sensitive level. (b) Power Doppler image of the lesion shows a lace-like pattern of subtle flow within the mass. Biopsy confirmed the lesion to be a haemangioma.

colloid study should be performed as the presence of Kupffer cells within the lesion can successfully differentiate focal nodular hyperplasia from other pathology[66–68].

Adenoma

Hepatic adenoma, a rare benign liver tumour, is being seen with increasing frequency. In females it is related to oral contraceptive use, in males to anabolic steroids[69]. Adenomas appear as solid masses with variable echogenicity due to differences in fat content or haemorrhage. Doppler has not shown utility in their differentiation from other liver masses.

Infantile haemangioendothelioma

Infantile haemangioendothelioma is a rare liver tumour of infancy. It commonly presents as

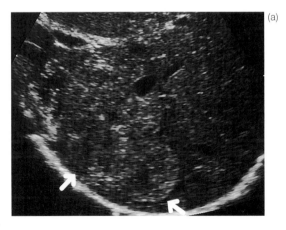
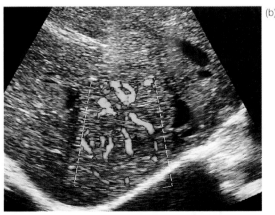

Fig. 7.46 (a) Transverse grey-scale image of the right lobe of the liver. A rounded lesion of slightly increased echogenicity is identified (arrows). (b) Power Doppler image through the lesion shows a stellate configuration of radiating branch vessels. Biopsy revealed focal nodular hyperplasia. Images courtesy of Dr William Middleton.

multiple lesions scattered throughout the liver with areas of infarction, haemorrhage and occasionally calcification. The tumour is composed of anastomosing vascular channels lined by one or more layers of endothelial cells. The incidence of congestive heart failure is high because of arterial venous shunting within the masses. It is considered a benign tumour and most gradually regress after presentation. Some children, however, succumb to the congestive heart failure associated with the high degree of arterial venous shunting. The ultrasound appearance of these lesions usually shows mixed or variable echogenicity. Large feeding arteries and draining veins (Fig. 7.47) can be perceived by colour Doppler with turbulent flow noted on spectral Doppler[70–72].

MONITORING TREATMENT OF LIVER DISEASE

Surgical portosystemic shunts

Numerous variants of surgical shunting have been devised over the years, including mesocaval, distal splenorenal (Warren shunt), proximal splenorenal, portocaval and mesoatrial shunts[73]. As with any surgical anastomosis,

stenosis and eventual thrombosis may develop. Imaging of shunt integrity by Doppler ultrasound is sensitive but because the shunt is usually retroperitoneal in location it can be extremely difficult to visualize. It is mandatory that the sonographer knows the exact type and location of the shunt in order to focus the examination in the correct region. Brisk hepatofugal flow in the main portal vein is a secondary finding that indicates shunt patency but the definitive diagnosis is made by direct visualization of the shunt with colour Doppler[74] (Fig. 7.48).

Transjugular intrahepatic portosystemic shunts

Interventional diversion of portal flow, as an alternative to surgery or sclerotherapy, was first proposed in 1969[75]. Transjugular intrahepatic portosystemic shunt (TIPS) placement involves the percutaneous creation of a link between the high-pressure portal system of a cirrhotic patient and the low-pressure hepatic veins. A transparenchymal track is created between the hepatic vein and the portal vein. This is dilated and a stent is then inserted to maintain patency. Although the TIPS is most

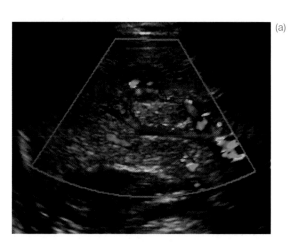
(a)

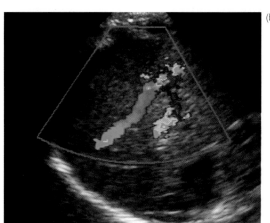
(b)

Fig. 7.47 (a) Oblique colour Doppler views of the right lobe of the liver. The large feeding vessels are identified with flow going into a large tangled vascular malformation. (b) From there flow is seen draining into a large hepatic vein. Infantile haemangioendothelioma was confirmed at autopsy.

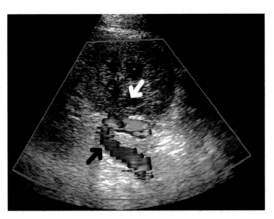

Fig. 7.48 Oblique longitudinal view of the left flank focused at the upper pole of the left kidney. The large venous structure with flow coursing towards the transducer is the splenic vein (black arrow). The patient is status post-splenectomy and anastomosis of the distal splenic vein to the renal vein. The anastomosis is widely patent with turbulent flow and aliasing noted at the point of anastomosis (white arrow).

often placed between the right hepatic vein and the right branch of the portal vein, a left hepatic vein to left portal vein route may be selected for technical or anatomic reasons.

Preprocedural assessment

Ultrasound and Doppler evaluation should be performed before TIPS placement to confirm patency of the portal vein and hepatic veins, rule out thrombosis, measure vessel size and search for the presence of portosystemic varices. Preprocedural assessment also allows a better appreciation of the results of the procedure in relation to the haemodynamic effects, changes in spleen size and the amount of ascites. The presence of varices (especially paraumbilical veins) should be identified prior to the procedure so that these vessels may be occluded by coil placement.

Postprocedural assessment

Unfortunately, TIPS complications are very common, the most significant being stenosis with eventual thrombosis and occlusion.

Clinical monitoring of TIPS function is insensitive. Doppler sonography is performed to monitor the TIPS, the adjacent hepatic veins, as well as the main, right and left portal veins, in order to ensure early detection of shunt compromise and allow timely revision. Prompt identification of a stenosis with timely intervention may prevent progression to thrombosis. A recently thrombosed TIPS may be recanalized successfully, but if it is mature thrombus then treatment usually requires the placement of a second TIPS.

Routine Doppler monitoring after shunt placement should be considered mandatory as it is an excellent non-invasive modality for sequential monitoring of TIPS patency. An evaluation of the TIPS should be performed within 24 hours after its creation to confirm patency and establish baseline flow directions and velocities. Subsequent evaluation is conducted just prior to discharge of the patient and then periodically thereafter; the frequency varies among centres but most re-examine the shunt at approximately 3-month intervals.

Optimum scanning parameters and normal ultrasound findings following TIPS have been described by a number of investigators[76–80]. Transducers of 2.25–3.5 MHz are usually necessary because of the frequently increased echogenicity and sound-attenuating features of the cirrhotic liver, along with the fact that the shunt is usually fairly deep within the body. The Doppler gain should be set as high as possible, without encountering noise. The transducer is focused at the level of the shunt or vessel of interest, the sample volume is placed in the centre with an angle of insonation less than 60° when feasible. This may be difficult to accomplish, especially in the middle segment of the shunt, where the direction of flow frequently runs perpendicular to the insonating beam. The pulse-repetition frequency is set as low as possible, but avoiding aliasing. Optimizing the scanning parameters will help minimize the chances of making a false-positive diagnosis of shunt thrombosis[76, 80].

Normal findings

A complete TIPS evaluation includes a survey of the abdomen to quantify ascites. The radiologist should also look for intrahepatic, perihepatic or subcapsular haematomas; intraperitoneal bleeding (as indicated by increased volume or echogenicity of the ascites); biliary obstruction; and echogenic contents in the common bile duct or gall bladder that suggest haemobilia[78, 81]. The shunt is then located between the right portal vein and right hepatic vein. The stent is highly echogenic and appears as two parallel, curvilinear lines, usually uniform in diameter in the parenchyma but slightly flared at the portal and hepatic venous ends (Fig. 7.49). The shunt diameter is easily measured[79], but a curved TIPS that passes obliquely through the plane of insonation may appear artificially narrowed[78]. The stent should extend from within the portal vein, across the parenchyma

and into the hepatic vein. Imaging sometimes reveals malposition of the stent as a result of inappropriate deployment, or subsequent migration down into the portal vein, or up into the hepatic vein and right atrium (Fig. 7.50).

Flow within the stent is then evaluated by Doppler ultrasound. The presence of blood flow is easily confirmed, as the entire shunt lumen fills with colour due to the relatively fast, turbulent flow (Fig. 7.51). Assuming a right portal to

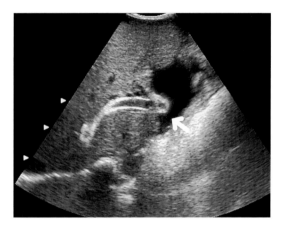

Fig. 7.50 A transverse view of the TIPS at its junction with the inferior vena cava shows the open end of the stent projecting into the right atrium (arrow).

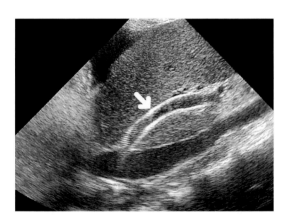

Fig. 7.49 Grey-scale longitudinal image of the right lobe of the liver. The TIPS catheter is seen coursing from the portahepatis region to the junction of the right hepatic vein with the inferior vena cava. This long shunt is composed of two stent elements. Note the subtle narrowing at the mid-shunt and the increased echogenicity of the shunt wall where the two stent elements overlap (arrow). A subtle serrated appearance to the shunt is seen near the IVC where the echo reflects off the individual wire elements of the stent.

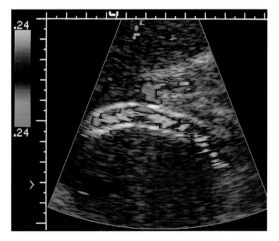

Fig. 7.51 Oblique colour Doppler image of the TIPS. The entire lumen saturates with colour indicating patency. Note the non-uniformity of the colour encoding – a function of the turbulence within this tract.

155

right hepatic vein TIPS, the velocity, flow direction and waveform are then checked at the portal vein end, mid-shunt and hepatic vein end. The main portal vein and the left portal vein are assessed and the right hepatic vein is checked both proximal to and just beyond its junction with the stent (Fig. 7.52). Spectral Doppler evaluation should verify that the direction of flow in the shunt is from the portal vein to the hepatic vein. Flow through the normal shunt is non-pulsatile, but flow in a widely patent shunt may show periodicity throughout the shunt due to right atrial pressure changes being transmitted back through the shunt, against the direction of flow (Fig. 7.53). Periodicity is most prominent near the hepatic venous end[80]. In one study, half of the patients with patent TIPS demonstrated some periodicity at the hepatic venous end of the shunt, while the other half had high-velocity turbulent flow[79]. Periodicity may be accentuated within the shunt in patients with tricuspid valve disease or congestive heart failure[76].

Flow velocities in the shunt vary widely, ranging from approximately 50 to 270 cm s^{-1} [77, 79, 80]. Velocities can also be quite variable through the shunt itself, usually increasing from the portal venous end to the hepatic venous end of the shunt. The mean velocity of patent shunts has been reported as 95 cm s^{-1} in the shunt near the portal venous end[76] and 120 cm s^{-1} in the middle segment of the shunt[77]. Flow across the shunt is usually quite turbulent, especially when multiple stent components are used, when overriding stents can cause a relative narrowing of the shunt lumen. Normal velocities in the main portal vein are variable. Following TIPS insertion, the mean portal vein velocity has been reported to increase from 7 to 24 cm s^{-1} in one study[79] and from 20 to 38.4 cm s^{-1} in another[80]. Hepatic arterial flow has also been shown to increase after TIPS, presumably because the shunt diverts the portal venous inflow away from the liver[78].

In a properly functioning TIPS, flow direction in the portal system is towards the portal vein end of the stent. Therefore, flow in the main portal vein is hepatopetal and its velocity is typically quite brisk (between 20 and 50 cm s^{-1}). It must be kept in mind that velocities measured in

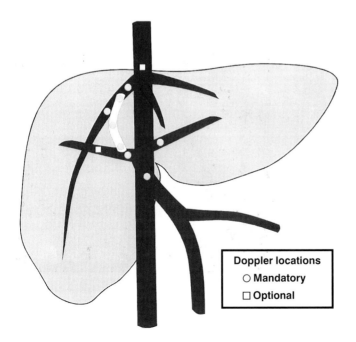

Doppler locations
○ **Mandatory**
□ **Optional**

Fig. 7.52 The TIPS and related vasculature in the standard right hepatic vein to right portal vein TIPS configuration. The blue circles indicate those points at which a Doppler tracing should be obtained in a complete TIPS evaluation. Figure courtesy of Gerald Mulligan, MD.

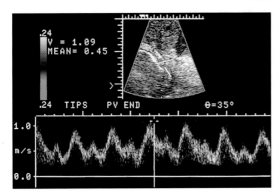

Fig. 7.53 Doppler tracing obtained at the portal vein end of a TIPS. Note the marked periodicity of the flow within the TIPS. The waveform is that commonly seen in the hepatic veins and inferior vena cava. Identification of this marked degree of periodicity at the portal vein end of the shunt is a confident indicator of a widely patent shunt.

the stent-bearing portion of the portal vein represent flow in the portal vein, not in the shunt[78]. Flow in the left and right portal veins usually becomes hepatofugal – flowing out of the diseased liver and towards the inflow of the shunt (Fig. 7.54)[76]. Depending on the diameter of the shunt and the severity of the liver disease,

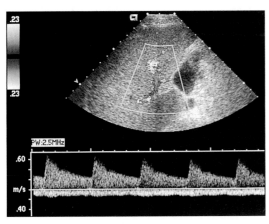

Fig. 7.54 Combined spectral Doppler tracing of the left portal vein and left hepatic artery in a patient with an appropriately functioning TIPS. The sample volume is opened wide and positioned so that both vessels can be interrogated in the same tracing. Note flow in the hepatic artery is towards the transducer, therefore into the left lobe of the liver. Left portal vein flow, however, is away from the transducer, therefore hepatofugal, towards the inflow of the shunt.

however, flow may continue to be hepatopetal into the parenchyma. If the patient has patent paraumbilical vein collaterals, these will continue to shunt blood away from the liver. Flow in the left portal vein, therefore, continues in a hepatopetal direction despite normal TIPS function. If portal branch flow changes direction over time from hepatofugal to hepatopetal, a significant flow-limiting lesion is assumed to be present in the TIPS.

The Doppler data are recorded and maintained in a table format for follow-up (Fig. 7.55). Serial documentation provides the best means of identifying any variations in velocity and/or flow direction over time and these changes are the best early indicator of shunt compromise.

Shunt stenosis

The two most common causes of TIPS compromise are *neointimal hyperplasia* throughout the shunt, or a focal stenosis at the hepatic vein end. Most TIPS will have some degree of neointimal hyperplasia but this may progress to the point where it limits flow through the TIPS. At the point of maximum stenosis within the TIPS the increased velocity may be perceived by Doppler (Fig. 7.56). Other components of the TIPS and the portal system, however, will show decreased velocities. With sufficient compromise, flow in the branch portal veins becomes hepatopetal and flow in the main portal vein may become hepatofugal.

Focal *hepatic vein stenosis* can occur where the end of the TIPS abuts the hepatic vein caused by focal irritation of the vein wall by the stent. This results in decreasing velocities throughout the shunt[78]. A key Doppler finding of this focal stenosis is the presence of post-stenotic flow disturbances with a high-velocity jet and turbulence in the hepatic vein or IVC[82]. The sonologist must therefore evaluate flow beyond the end of the stent, sometimes even as

Name: ID:

Date	VELOCITIES				DIRECTIONS		Comments
	PV End	Mid	HV End	Main PV	Lt PV	HV ↑ TIPS	

Fig. 7.55 TIPS data sheet. Each patient receiving a TIPS should have a data sheet maintained with velocities and flow directions documented at each visit. Progressive compromise of a TIPS can then be more easily diagnosed as progressive changes in velocities or a change in direction of flow become manifest. Velocity measurements in the mid-TIPS tend to be the most erratic. A persistent decrease in main portal vein velocity over a sequence of studies is the most definitive indicator of shunt compromise.

far as the right atrium. Flow in all three hepatic veins is normally towards the heart but a stenosis at the junction of the TIPS and the hepatic vein can cause flow compromise peripherally in the vein with damping of periodicity, or segmental flow reversal (Fig. 7.57).

Several investigators have attempted to determine flow velocities which define the presence of TIPS stenosis[76–78, 83] but reported findings have varied considerably. In one study, a velocity of <50 cm s⁻¹ at the portal venous end was 100% sensitive and 93% specific[76]. In another study, a velocity of <50 cm s⁻¹ in the middle segment of the TIPS was 78% sensitive and 99% specific, with a positive predictive value of 96%, negative predictive value of 91%, and accuracy of 92%[77]. When these investigators used a velocity of <60 cm s⁻¹ as the criterion, sensitivity increased to 84% but specificity dropped to 89% and accuracy to 87%. At <70 cm s⁻¹, sensitivity was 89% but specificity was 83% and accuracy was 85%. In another study, a velocity of 90 cm s⁻¹ was applied but the sensitivity was only 87.5% with specificity of 95%[84]. These varied findings underscore the fact that flow velocities vary widely from patient to patient, and that the best method for TIPS evaluation is to use individual patient baseline velocities obtained soon after TIPS placement[85]. A change in velocity of

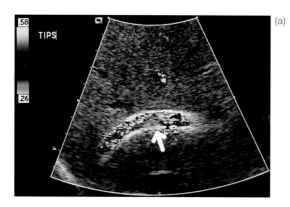 (a)

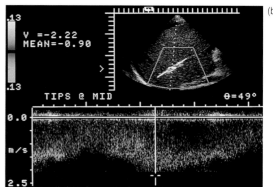 (b)

Fig. 7.56 (a) Oblique colour Doppler image along the length of the TIPS shunt. Turbulent flow is seen in the majority of the shunt; however, a focal area of thrombus and/or neo-intimal hyperplasia is perceived in the mid-TIPS (arrow). (b) Spectral Doppler tracing at the mid-TIPS shows turbulent flow and a high velocity of 2.2 m s⁻¹, well above the normal anticipated mean velocity of 1.2 m s⁻¹ in the mid-TIPS.

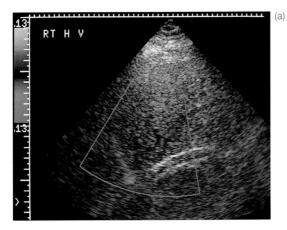 (a)

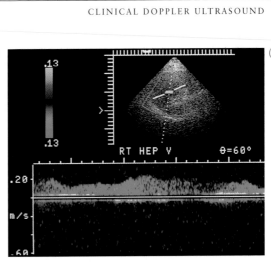 (b)

Fig. 7.57 (a) Longitudinal colour Doppler image including the right hepatic vein and TIPS shunt. Note that colour does not fill the entire lumen of the TIPS shunt. The colour signal from the right hepatic vein shows flow coursing towards the transducer, that is, away from the inferior vena cava. This indicates focal stenosis at the hepatic vein junction with the TIPS shunt, resulting in reversed right hepatic vein flow. (b) Spectral Doppler tracing of the right hepatic vein confirms flow away from the IVC and back into the liver. This reversed flow will continue via transparenchymal collateral pathways and shunt to the middle or left hepatic vein, thereby returning blood flow to the heart.

±50 cm s⁻¹ from baseline has been proposed as the threshold value for predicting haemo-dynamically significant shunt compromise[58].

If there is significant flow compromise through the TIPS, main portal vein velocity decreases. Flow in the left portal vein may change back to a hepatopetal direction (Fig. 7.58), representing a reversion to pre-TIPS haemodynamics[78, 80, 82] (Table 7.4).

Shunt occlusion

If no flow can be detected in the shunt and flow velocity and direction in the portal vein is the same as it was prior to TIPS placement, shunt occlusion must be considered. The absence of flow by colour Doppler within the TIPS is a highly specific indicator of shunt thrombosis[75, 76]. Before concluding that the stent is occluded, however, meticulous scanning for slow flow should be performed, since flow velocity may be extremely low in a shunt that is highly stenosed but still patent. Colour Doppler settings (including pulse repetition frequency, gain and filtration) need to be optimized to differentiate true occlusion from very slow flow. A properly

functioning TIPS, however, is not a low-flow system, so misinterpretation of thrombosis for technical reasons is rarely a problem. Identifying low flow, however, has the same implication as occlusion, and that is the need

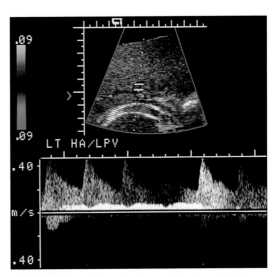

Fig. 7.58 Spectral Doppler tracing of the left hepatic artery and portal vein including a colour Doppler image of the TIPS. Absence of colour signal within the shunt indicates TIPS thrombosis. This is further confirmed by the presence of hepatopetal flow in the left portal vein. This is in contrast to the normal left portal vein and hepatic artery flow directions, as illustrated in Fig. 7.54.

Table 7.4 Criteria for compromised TIPS function.

- Shunt velocity of <50 cm s–1
- Increase or decrease in shunt velocity of >50 cm s–1 compared with initial postprocedure value
- Focal region of increased velocity in the shunt or hepatic vein
- Hepatopetal flow in right and left portal vein branches (in the absence of a recanalized paraumbilical vein)
- Hepatofugal flow in main portal vein

for TIPS revision. Indeed, repeat interventions are the key to long-term success of TIPS[86].

Liver transplantation

Over 20 000 liver transplants have been performed in the world since 1988. The current 1-year graft survival rate in the United States is approximately 79% with 1-year patient survival rate of approximately 87%[87]. Improved surgical techniques, development of effective immunosuppressive medications, human leukocyte antigen typing for recipient matching, and establishment of coordinated transplant sharing systems have greatly improved the success rate in liver transplantation. Graft survival statistics are further enhanced by prompt identification of liver transplant dysfunction and rapid intervention when appropriate.

Preoperative assessment

Preoperative assessment consists of confirmation of vascular patency, mapping native vascular anatomy, quantification of diseased liver volume, identification of vascular collaterals secondary to portal hypertension and a search for intra- or extrahepatic malignancy. There are many ways to accomplish this, including angiography and ultrasound, but currently CT with CT angiography in the arterial phase and portal phase is the favoured method.

Postoperative assessment

The major complications of liver transplantation are rejection, vascular stenosis or thrombosis, biliary leak or obstruction, and malignant disease. Acute rejection is best monitored by serum liver enzymes, bilirubin, and ammonia levels and diagnosis is established by biopsy. Ultrasound and Doppler have little to offer in the diagnosis of acute rejection. Doppler ultrasound, however, plays a key role in monitoring for potential vascular complications.

Evaluation of the newly transplanted liver requires a precise understanding of the surgical anatomy. Many variations are possible including segmental or reduced-size transplantation, especially in the paediatric population[88, 89]. Variations of the arterial anastomoses are necessary when the donor hepatic arterial anatomy is anomalous. Variations of venous anastomoses are necessary when the recipient portal vein is thrombosed. The sonologist must be aware of any variations so that a thrombosed accessory hepatic artery or a stenotic jump graft is not missed.

The liver transplant ultrasound examination should include a general survey of the abdomen and pelvis in order to identify and quantify any haematomas or fluid collections. The liver parenchyma is then examined to rule out any focal abnormality, specifically any fluid collection, area of infarction, or possible neoplasm. The biliary system should be evaluated to rule out obstruction or sludge accumulation, especially in a patient with hepatic artery thrombosis. The intra- and extrahepatic hepatic arteries are checked to confirm patency and the waveforms are analysed to rule out stenosis. Patency of the portal vein is confirmed and the Doppler waveform analysed, particularly across the anastomosis. Patency of the three hepatic veins is confirmed and their waveforms are evaluated. Finally, the IVC is checked with special attention to the upper anastomosis.

Abnormal findings

The *hepatic artery* anastomosis is technically the most difficult to create and problems such as stenosis, thrombosis and fistula formation have the most significant impact on liver transplant success, as they predispose to infarction, intrahepatic abscess, biliary stricture and biloma. Doppler findings indicating hepatic artery stenosis include an intrahepatic tardus parvus waveform with low-resistance flow and a high-velocity jet with turbulence at the point of stenosis. A focal high-velocity jet just beyond the hepatic artery anastomosis in excess of 200 cm s[-1] or greater than three times the velocity in the prestenotic hepatic artery is highly indicative of a clinically significant stenosis[90]. The identification of an intrahepatic tardus parvus waveform with low resistance (<50% RI) flow, and a prolonged upstroke in systole (>0.08 s)[90] with rounding of the systolic peak, should force a careful survey in the anticipated region of the anastomosis for the high-velocity jet (Fig. 7.59)[90, 91]. Although

an intrahepatic arterial tracing may be demonstrated, it should be remembered that a severe stenosis may still lead to biliary ischaemia, or may progress to complete thrombosis.

Absence of an arterial signal along the main portal vein and its branches on spectral and colour Doppler ultrasound indicates hepatic artery thrombosis. Since this is a diagnosis based on an absence of flow, great care must be taken to ensure proper Doppler settings. Scanning by a second experienced sonologist is encouraged, since this ultrasound diagnosis routinely leads to arteriography. Use of ultrasound echo-enhancing agents is recommended to improve perception of a weak arterial signal and decrease the rate of false-positive diagnosis of hepatic artery thrombosis.

In cases of hepatic artery thrombosis which are treated conservatively, collaterals will develop and an intrahepatic arterial signal can be detected by Doppler ultrasound as early as 2 weeks after the thrombosis. This typically manifests as a thready tracing with a tardus parvus appearance and can be seen in as many as 40% of patients with documented hepatic artery thrombosis, especially children[92].

In the early postoperative period, the hepatic artery tracing can be quite variable but often

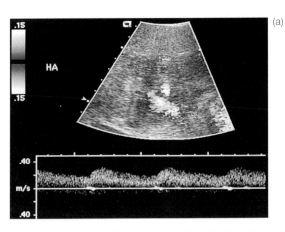
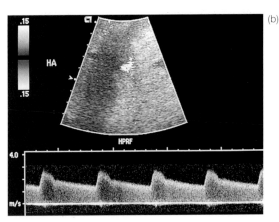

Fig. 7.59 (a) Spectral Doppler tracing of the intrahepatic hepatic artery. The tracing shows a slow upstroke in systole and very low resistance. After identifying a tardus parvus waveform, the examiner should evaluate along the course of the main hepatic artery, specifically the region of the anastomosis, for a high-velocity jet. (b) Spectral tracing of the main hepatic artery at the anastomosis reveals a high-velocity jet (>2.5 m s[-1]) with marked turbulence, indicating hepatic artery stenosis.

shows a relatively high-resistance flow. This is a relatively common manifestation of the anoxia and traumatic insult sustained by the liver during harvesting, handling, preservation and surgery. The high-resistance flow typically resolves within a few days of transplantation[93]. A delayed finding of high resistance is a poor prognostic indicator and some of these patients go on to develop thrombosis[94]. The exact cause of thrombosis is not always apparent and in numerous cases is presumed to be secondary to immunological causes and rejection.

Arteriovenous fistulae are a rare complication of transplantation and are most often the result of a biopsy. Imaging rarely reveals an abnormality but colour Doppler often shows a localized flash artefact. When Doppler settings are adjusted for high velocities, the feeding artery and draining vein are better visualized. Spectral Doppler reveals a low-resistance arterial waveform with high diastolic velocity (Fig. 7.60)[95, 96].

The donor *portal vein* is usually anastomosed end-to-end with the recipient portal vein. Variations may be required if the recipient portal vein is thrombosed, hypoplastic or of insufficient length. Because the vessel is relatively large, colour Doppler findings can be rather striking. Not all flow disturbances perceived by colour Doppler are haemo-

dynamically significant and compromise of portal vein flow is relatively rare. When it occurs, it may be due to a mismatch between the sizes of the recipient and donor portal veins, or to an excessive length of vessel causing a kink, or to a stenosis. If portal vein stenosis is suspected, the velocity gradient across the anastomosis should be measured by spectral Doppler; a velocity gradient of less than fourfold is unlikely to be significant (Fig. 7.61)[97]. Posttransplantation portal vein thrombosis is quite rare and most often attributable to technical factors. If slow velocity is identified in the portal vein (<1 m s^{-1}), it may be due to increased intrahepatic resistance from rejection, or to reduced inflow as can be seen with the collateral steal phenomenon, which can occur when large varices remain unligated, shunting blood from the portal system to the systemic circulation, bypassing the liver[98, 99].

The donor *inferior vena cava* has a long intrahepatic course and is therefore transplanted along with the liver. The IVC may be inserted in-line with both supra- and infrahepatic anastomoses; the native intrahepatic IVC is excised with the diseased liver. The surgical technique which is currently favoured retains the native IVC of the recipient in place and the upper end of the donor IVC is anastomosed

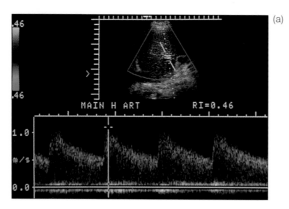 (a)

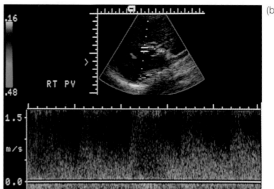 (b)

Fig. 7.60 (a) Spectral Doppler tracing of the main hepatic artery of a liver transplant recipient. A high-velocity and relatively low-resistance waveform is identified but flow is relatively non-turbulent. (b) Spectral Doppler tracing in an area of flash artefact within the right lobe of the liver. A very turbulent, high-velocity, arterial waveform is present as would be expected with an arterial venous fistula. This fistula was presumed the sequela of a prior biopsy.

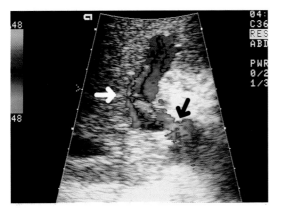 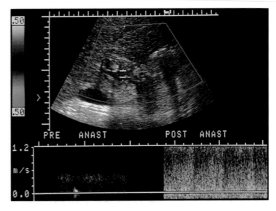

Fig. 7.61 (a) Colour Doppler image of the portal vein in the region of the anastomosis. Note the area of relative narrowing at the point of anastomosis (black arrow). A high-velocity jet is seen (white arrow). Further along the course of the portal vein, eddy currents are identified. These occur secondary to the disordered flow caused by the stenosis. (b) Spectral Doppler tracing obtained on either side of the portal vein anastomosis. The pulse repetition frequency was set low to be able to project the relatively slow preanastomotic portal vein flow. As a result, the postanastomotic (poststenotic) tracing shows a high degree of aliasing due to the high-grade stenosis. Moving the sample volume across the anastomosis in a single tracing allows a direct, accurate comparison of pre- and postanastomotic velocities.

end-to-side to the native IVC. The lower end of the donor IVC is oversewn, which functionally converts it into a hepatic vein. This type of anastomosis is commonly referred to as a 'piggyback'[100]. Any compromise of the upper caval anastomosis, from either stenosis or kinking, may cause hepatic venous outflow obstruction. Ultrasound findings include marked damping, or complete flattening of the hepatic vein velocity profile with complete loss of periodicity, distension of the hepatic veins and a high-velocity jet with turbulence just above the caval anastomosis (Fig. 7.62). Loss of periodicity may also be due to compression of the hepatic veins by the surrounding liver tissue by oedema in the early postoperative period, typically due to preservation injury, or by oedema in the later postoperative period related to rejection[92, 101]. Due to the relatively large size of the IVC and the potential for a size mismatch between the donor and recipient cavae, a greater than fourfold velocity gradient at the anastomosis is required to confidently diagnose a haemodynamically significant stenosis.

In those patients with an in-line IVC, compromise of the lower anastomosis may present as lower extremity oedema and renal failure. Ultrasound and colour Doppler imaging of the anastomosis may reveal a kink or focal stenosis with a relatively high-velocity jet. As with a piggyback procedure, a size mismatch between the donor and recipient vessels may produce a relatively high-velocity jet, and a less than threefold velocity increase at the anastomosis is seldom clinically significant. A three- to fourfold gradient is likely to be significant and should be correlated with the clinical findings. A greater than fourfold gradient must be considered haemodynamically significant.

Several authors have studied the possibility of predicting acute liver transplant rejection by identifying changes in the *hepatic vein* waveform. During rejection, hepatocellular oedema and inflammatory infiltration increase the pressure within the confining capsule of the liver. This reduces the compliance of the liver and results in a dampened hepatic vein waveform. The theory is appropriate but other causes of hepatocellular oedema, such as

163

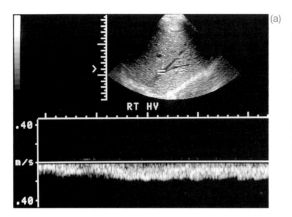

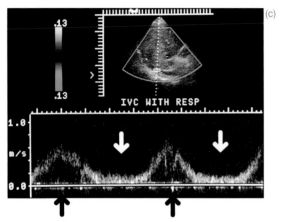

Fig. 7.62 (a) Spectral Doppler tracing of the right hepatic vein in a liver transplant recipient. There is no periodicity identified on this tracing despite easy visualization of the hepatic vein. (b) Combined colour and spectral Doppler tracing at the point of IVC anastomosis. A very high-velocity jet is perceived just above the anastomosis. Effects of cardiac pulsation cannot work past this relative narrowing. Therefore, this results in flattening of the hepatic vein tracing. (c) Spectral Doppler tracing obtained at the upper IVC anastomosis during active respiration. The transducer is positioned just below the costal margin and angled cephalad. During inspiration, downward movement of the diaphragm causes the sample volume to interrogate the high-velocity jet above the stenosis (black arrows). During expiration, upward movement of the diaphragm carries the sample volume into the substenotic IVC, therefore the relative velocity is considerably slower (white arrow).

cholangitis, hepatitis and upper IVC anastomotic stenosis, produce similar damping, thereby limiting the specificity of this finding. The diagnosis of rejection is best made by needle biopsy. Ultrasound and Doppler guidance can be used to guide the biopsy needle into the liver but away from the large central vessels[102].

REFERENCES

1. Rao BK (1991) Colour flow Doppler sonography of the abdomen. *Current Opinion in Radiology* 3: 225–229
2. Czembirek H (1987) Value of abdominal pulsed duplex sonography. *Radiologe* 27: 98–105
3. Mostbeck G, Mallek R, Gebauer A, Tscholakoff D (1992) Duplex ultrasound and colour-coded Doppler ultrasound of visceral blood vessels in abdominal diseases. *Wiener Klinische Wochenschrift* 104: 227–233
4. Grant EG, Schiller VL, Millener P *et al* (1992) Colour Doppler imaging of the hepatic vasculature. *American Journal of Radiology* 159: 943–950
5. Ralls PW (1990) Colour Doppler sonography of the hepatic artery and portal venous system. *American Journal of Radiology* 155: 517–525
6. Iwao T, Toyonaga A, Oho K *et al* (1997) Value of Doppler ultrasound parameters of portal vein and hepatic artery in the diagnosis of cirrhosis and portal hypertension. *American Journal of Gastroenterology* 92: 1012–1017
7. Harada A, Nonami T, Kasai Y, Nakao A, Takagi H (1988) Systemic haemodynamics in non-cirrhotic portal hypertension – a clinical study of 19 patients. *Japanese Journal of Surgery* 18: 620–625
8. Grant EG, Tessler FN, Gomes AS *et al* (1990) Colour Doppler imaging of portosystemic shunts. *American Journal of Radiology* 154: 393–397

9. Sacerdoti D, Merkel C, Bolognesi M, Amodio P, Angeli P, Gatta A (1995) Hepatic arterial resistance in cirrhosis with and without portal vein thrombosis: relationships with portal haemodynamics. *Gastroenterology* **108**: 1152–1158

10. Zironi G, Gaiani S, Fenyves D, Rigamonti A, Bolondi L, Barbara L (1992) Value of measurement of mean portal flow velocity by Doppler flowmetry in the diagnosis of portal hypertension. *Journal of Hepatology* **16**: 298–303

11. Ohta M, Hashizume M, Kawanaka H *et al* (1995) Prognostic significance of hepatic vein waveforms by Doppler ultrasonography in cirrhotic patients with portal hypertension. *American Journal of Gastroenterology* **90**: 1853–1857

12. Pierce ME, Sewell R (1990) Identification of hepatic cirrhosis by duplex Doppler ultrasound value of the hepatic artery resistive index. *Australasian Radiology* **34**: 331–333

13. Iwao T, Toyonaga A, Shigemori H *et al* (1996) Hepatic artery haemodynamics responsiveness to altered portal blood flow in normal and cirrhotic livers. *Radiology* **200**: 793–798

14. Vilgrain V, Lebrec D, Menu Y, Scherrer A, Nahum H (1990) Comparison between ultrasonographic signs and the degree of portal hypertension in patients with cirrhosis. *Gastrointestinal Radiology* **15**: 218–222

15. Shikare SV, Bashir K, Abraham P, Tilve GH (1996) Hepatic perfusion index in portal hypertension of cirrhotic and non-cirrhotic aetiologies. *Nuclear Medicine Communications* **17**: 520–522

16. Leen E, Goldberg JA, Anderson JR *et al* (1993) Hepatic perfusion changes in patients with liver metastases: comparison with those patients with cirrhosis. *Gut* **34**: 554–557

17. Moriyasu F (1993) Doppler ultrasound in diagnosis of liver tumour and portal hypertension. *Radiology Medicin* (Torino) **85**: 44–55

18. Yasuhara K, Kimura K, Nakamura H, Iwadare M, Ohto M, Matsuzaki O (1995) Doppler velocity histogram analysis of hepatocellular carcinoma. *Journal of Clinical Ultrasound* **23**: 225–231

19. Gorka W, Kagalwalla A, McParland BJ, Kagalwalla Y, al Zaben A (1996) Diagnostic value of Doppler ultrasound in the assessment of liver cirrhosis in children: histopathological correlation. *Journal of Clinical Ultrasound* **24**: 287–295

20. Lafortune M, Madore F, Patriquin H, Breton G (1991) Segmental anatomy of the liver: a sonographic approach to the Couinaud nomenclature. *Radiology* **181**: 443–448

21. Zwiebel WJ (1995) The liver: diffuse disease and vascular disorders. *Seminars in Ultrasound* **16**: 34

22. Abu-Yousef MM (1992) Normal and respiratory variations of the hepatic and portal venous duplex Doppler waveforms with simultaneous electrocardiographic correlation. *Journal of Ultrasound in Medicine* **11**: 263–268

23. Gallix BP, Taourel P, Dauzat M, Bruel JM, Lafortune M (1997) Flow pulsatility in the portal venous system: a study of Doppler sonography in healthy adults. *American Journal of Radiology* **169**: 141–144

24. Hosoki T, Arisawa J, Marikawa T *et al* (1990) Portal blood flow in congestive heart failure: pulsed duplex sonographic findings. *Radiology* **174**: 733–736

25. Wachsberg RH, Needleman L, Wilson DJ (1995) Portal vein pulsatility in normal and cirrhotic adults without cardiac disease. *Journal of Clinical Ultrasound* **23**: 3–15

26. Lippert H, Pabst R (1985) *Arterial variations in man*, pp 32–33. Munich: JF Bergmann

27. Shapiro RS, Winsberg F, Maldjian C, Stancato-Pasik A (1993) Variability of hepatic vein Doppler tracings in normal subjects. *Journal of Ultrasound in Medicine* **12**: 701–703

28. Westra SJ, Zaninovic AC, Vargas J, Hall TR, Boechat MI, Busuttil RW (1995) The value of portal vein pulsatility on duplex sonograms as a sign of portal hypertension in children with liver disease. *American Journal of Radiology* **165**: 167–172

29. Gibson PR, Gibson RN, Donlan JD, Ditchfield MR, Bhathal PS (1991) Duplex Doppler ultrasound of the ligamentum teres and portal vein: a clinically useful adjunct in the evaluation of patients with known or suspected chronic liver disease or portal hypertension. *Journal of Gastroenterology and Hepatology* **6**: 61–65

30. Kuo CH, Changchien CS, Tai DI, Chen JJ (1995) Portal vein velocity by duplex Doppler ultrasound as an indication of the clinical severity of portal hypertension. *Chan Keng I Hsueh* **18**: 217–223

31. Kozaiwa K, Tajiri H, Yoshimura N *et al* (1995) Utility of duplex Doppler ultrasound in evaluating portal hypertension in children. *Journal of Paediatric Gastroenterology and Nutrition* **21**: 215–219

32. Gorg C, Schwerk WB, Gorg K *et al* (1991) Focal involvement of malignant lymphoma in the liver. *Bildegebung* **58**: 67

33. Moriyasu F, Nishida O, Ban N *et al* (1986) Congestion index of the portal vein. *American Journal of Radiology* **146**: 735–739

34. Rector WG, Hoefs JC, Hossack KF, Everson GT. (1988) Hepatofugal portal flow in cirrhosis: observations on hepatic haemodynamics and the nature of the arterioportal communications. *Hepatology* **8**: 16–20

35. Abu-Yousef MM, Milam SG, Farner RM (1990) Pulsatile portal vein flow: a sign of tricuspid regurgitation on duplex Doppler sonography. *American Journal of Radiology* **155**: 785–788

36. Loperfido F, Lombardo A, Amico CM *et al* (1993) Doppler analysis of portal vein flow in tricuspid regurgitation. *Journal of Heart Valve Disease* **2**: 174–182

37. Wachsberg RH, Simmons MZ (1994) Coronary vein diameter and flow direction in patients with portal

hypertension: evaluation with duplex sonography and correlation with variceal bleeding. *American Journal of Radiology* **162**: 637

38. Saddekni S, Hutchinson DE, Cooperberg PL (1982) The sonographically patent umbilical vein in portal hypertension. *Radiology* **145**: 441

39. Parvey HR, Raval B, Sandler CM (1994) Portal vein thrombosis; imaging findings. *American Journal of Radiology* **162**: 77

40. Raby N, Meire HB (1988) Duplex Doppler ultrasound in the diagnosis of cavernous transformation of the portal vein. *British Journal of Radiology* **61**: 586–588

41. Weltin G, Taylor KJ, Carter AR, Taylor CR (1985) Duplex Doppler: identification of cavernous transformation of the portal vein. *American Journal of Radiology* **144**: 999–1001

42. Pozniak MA, Baus K (1991) Hepatofugal arterial signal in the main portal vein – an indicator of intravascular tumour spread. *Radiology* **180**: 663–666

43. Vine HS, Sequira JC, Widrich WC *et al* (1979) Portal vein aneurysm. *American Journal of Radiology* **132**: 557

44. Merritt CRB, Goldsmith JP, Sharp MJ (1984) Sonographic detection of portal venous gas in infants with necrotizing enterocolitis. *American Journal of Radiology* **143**: 1059

45. Joynt LK, Platt JF, Rubin JM, Ellis JH, Bude RO (1995) Hepatic artery resistance before and after standard meal in subjects with diseased and healthy livers. *Radiology* **196**: 489–492

46. Ramchandani P, Goldenberg NJ, Soulen RL *et al* (1983) Isobutyl 2-cyanoacrylate embolization of a hepatoportal fistula. *American Journal of Radiology* **140**: 137

47. Falkoff GE, Taylor KJW, Morse S (1986) Hepatic artery pseudoaneurysm: diagnosis with real-time and pulsed Doppler ultrasound. *Radiology* **158**: 55

48. Cloogman HM, DiCapo RD (1984) Hereditary haemorrhagic telangiectasis: sonographic findings in the liver. *Radiology* **150**: 521

49. Ralls PW, Johnson MB, Radin DR *et al* (1992) Hereditary haemorrhagic telangiectasis: findings in the liver with colour Doppler sonography. *American Journal of Radiology* **159**: 59

50. Ludwig J, Hashimoto E, McGill DB, van Heerden JA (1990) Classification of hepatic venous outflow obstruction: ambiguous terminology of the Budd–Chiari syndrome. *Mayo Clinic Proceedings* **65**: 51–55

51. Hosoki T, Kuroda C, Tokunaga K, Marukawa T, Masuike M, Kozuka T (1989) Hepatic venous outflow obstruction: evaluation with pulsed duplex sonography. *Radiology* **170**: 733–737

52. Lee DH, Ko YT, Yoon Y *et al* (1994) Sonography and colour Doppler imaging of Budd-Chiari syndrome of membranous obstruction of the inferior vena cava. *Journal of Ultrasound in Medicine* **13**: 159

53. Sakugawa H, Higashionna A, Oyakawa T *et al* (1992) Ultrasound study in the diagnosis of primary Budd–Chiari syndrome (obstruction of the inferior vena cava). *Gastroenterology Japan* **27**: 69

54. Boyer TD (1990) Portal hypertension and bleeding esophageal varices: portal hypertension. In: Zakim D, Boyer TD (eds). *Hepatology: a Textbook of Liver Disease*, p 592. Philadelphia: WB Saunders

55. Brown BP, Abu-Youssef M, Farner R *et al* (1990) Doppler sonography: a non-invasive method for evaluation of hepatic venocclusive disease. *American Journal of Radiology* **154**: 721

56. Herbetko J, Grigg AP, Buckley AR *et al* (1992) Veno-occlusive liver disease after bone marrow transplantation: findings at duplex sonography. *American Journal of Radiology* **158**: 1001

57. Abu-Yousef MM (1991) Duplex Doppler sonography of the hepatic vein in tricuspid regurgitation. *American Journal of Radiology* **156**: 79–83

58. Dodd GD III, Miller WJ, Baron RL *et al* (1992) Detection of malignant tumours in end-stage cirrhotic livers: efficacy of sonography as a screening technique. *American Journal of Radiology* **159**: 727

59. Taylor KJW, Ramos I, Morse SS *et al* (1987) Focal liver masses: differential diagnosis with pulsed Doppler ultrasound. *Radiology* **164**: 643

60. Tanaka S, Kitamura T, Fujita M *et al* (1990) Colour Doppler flow imaging of liver tumours. *American Journal of Radiology* **154**: 509

61. Suzuki M, Takahashi T, Sato T (1987) Medial regression and its functional significance in tumour-supplying host arteries: a morphometric study of hepatic arteries in human livers with hepatocellular carcinoma. *Cancer* **59**: 444

62. Miller MA, Balfe DM, Middleton WD (1996) Peripheral portal venous blood flow alterations induced by hepatic masses: evaluation with colour and pulsed Doppler sonography. *Journal of Ultrasound in Medicine* **15**: 707–713

63. Marn CS, Bree RL, Silver TM (1991) Ultrasonography of liver: technique and focal and diffuse disease. *Radiology Clinics of North America* **29**: 1151

64. Wang S-S, Chiang J-H, Tsai Y-T *et al* (1990) Focal hepatic fatty infiltration as a cause of pseudotumours: ultrasonographic patterns and clinical differentiation. *Journal of Clinical Ultrasound* **18**: 401

65. Yates CK, Streight RA (1986) Focal fatty infiltration of the liver simulating metastatic disease. *Radiology* **159**: 83

66. Golli M, Mathieu D, Anglade M *et al* (1993) Focal nodular hyperplasia of the liver: value of colour Doppler US in association with MR imaging. *Radiology* **187**: 113

67. Learch TJ, Ralls PW, Johnson MB *et al* (1993) Hepatic focal nodular hyperplasia: findings with colour Doppler sonography. *Journal of Ultrasound in Medicine* **12**: 541

68. Kudo M, Tomita S, Minowa K *et al* (1992) Colour Doppler flow imaging of hepatic focal nodular hyperplasia. *Journal of Ultrasound in Medicine* 11: 553

69. Okuda K, Kojiro M, Okuda H (1993) Neoplasms of the liver: benign tumours of the liver. In: Schiff L, Schiff E (eds) *Diseases of the Liver*, p 1236. Philadelphia: JB Lippincott

70. Dachman AH, Lichtenstein JE, Friedman AC *et al* (1983) Infantile haemangioendothelioma of the liver: a radiologic-pathologic-clinical correlation. *American Journal of Radiology* 140: 1091

71. Kew MC (1990) Tumours of the liver: benign hepatic tumours. In: Zakim D, Boyer TD (eds) *Hepatology: a Textbook of Liver Disease*, p 1232. Philadelphia: WB Saunders

72. Pardes JG, Bryan PJ, Gauderer MWL (1982) Spontaneous regression of infantile haemangioendotheliomatosis of the liver: demonstration by ultrasound. *Journal of Ultrasound in Medicine* 1: 349

73. Boyer TD (1990) Portal hypertension. In: Zakim D, Boyer TD (eds) *Hepatology: a Textbook of Liver Disease*, p 602. Philadelphia: WB Saunders

74. LaFortune M, Patriquin H, Pomier G *et al* (1987) Haemodynamic changes in portal circulation after portosystemic shunts: use of duplex carotid sonography in 43 patients. *American Journal of Radiology* 149: 701

75. Rosch J, Hanafee WN, Snow H (1969) Transjugular portal venography and radiologic portacaval shunt: an experimental study. *Radiology* 92: 1112–1114

76. Chong WK, Malisch TA, Mazer MJ, Lind CD, Worrell JA, Richards WO (1993) Transjugular intrahepatic portosystemic shunt: US assessment with maximum flow velocity. *Radiology* 189: 789–793

77. Feldstein VA, Patel MD, La Berge JM (1996) Transjugular intrahepatic portosystemic shunts: accuracy of Doppler US in determination of patency and detection of stenoses. *Radiology* 201: 141–147

78. Foshager MC, Ferral H, Finlay DE, Castaneda-Zuniga WR, Letourneau JG (1994) Colour Doppler sonography of transjugular intrahepatic portosystemic shunts (TIPS). *American Journal of Radiology* 163: 105–111

79. Longo JM, Bilbao JI, Rousseau HP *et al* (1993) Transjugular intrahepatic portosystemic shunt: evaluation with Doppler sonography. *Radiology* 188: 529–534

80. Surratt RS, Middleton WD, Darcy MD, Melson GL, Brink JA (1993) Morphologic and haemodynamic findings at sonography before and after creation of a transjugular intrahepatic portosystemic shunt. *American Journal of Radiology* 160: 627–630

81. Foshager MC, Finlay DE, Longley DG, Letourneau JG (1994) Duplex and colour Doppler sonography of complications after percutaneous interventional vascular procedures. *Radiographics* 14: 239–253

82. Zemel G, Katzen B, Grubbs G, Moore B, Benenati J, Becker G (1994) Sonographic indicators of unsuccessful transjugular intrahepatic portosystemic shunts. *Radiology* 193(P)(Suppl): 167

83. Dodd GD, Zajko AB, Orons PD, Martin MS, Eichner LS, Santaguida LA (1995) Detection of transjugular intrahepatic portosystemic shunt dysfunction: value of duplex Doppler sonography. *American Journal of Radiology* 164: 1119–1124

84. Mituzani P, Saxon R, Alexander P, Barton R, Koslin D (1993) Duplex ultrasound screening after transjugular intrahepatic portosystemic shunt placement. *Radiology* 189(P)(Suppl): 254

85. Nazarian GK, Ferral H, Castaneda-Zuniga WR *et al* (1994) Development of stenoses in transjugular intrahepatic portosystemic shunts. *Radiology* 192: 231–234

86. Coldwell DM, Ring EJ, Rees CR *et al* (1995) Multicentre investigation of the role of transjugular intrahepatic portosystemic shunt in management of portal hypertension. *Radiology* 196: 335–340

87. US Department of Health and Human Services, Public Health Service (1997) *Annual report of the US Scientific Registry of Transplant Recipients and the Organ Procurement and Transplantation Network, 1988–1996*

88. Neuhaus P, Platz KP (1994) Liver transplantation: newer surgical approaches. *Baillière's Clinical Gastroenterology* 8: 481

89. Houssin D, Boillot AO, Soubrane O *et al* (1993) Controlled liver splitting for transplantation in two recipients: technique, results and perspectives. *British Journal of Surgery* 80: 75

90. Dodd GD III, Memel DS, Zajko AB *et al* (1994) Hepatic artery stenosis and thrombosis in transplant recipients: Doppler diagnosis with resistive index and systolic acceleration time. *Radiology* 192: 657–661

91. Platt JF, Yotzy GG, Bude RO *et al* (1997) Use of Doppler sonography for revealing hepatic artery stenosis in liver transplant recipients. *American Journal of Radiology* 168: 473–476

92. Kok T, Haagsma EB, Klompmaker IJ *et al* (1996) Doppler ultrasound of the hepatic artery and vein performed daily in the first 2 weeks after orthotopic liver transplantation. *Investigative Radiology* 31: 173

93. Hall TR, McDiarmid SV, Grant EG *et al* (1990) False-negative duplex Doppler studies in children with hepatic artery thrombosis after liver transplantation. *American Journal of Radiology* 154: 573–575

94. Propeck PA, Scanlan KA (1992) Reversed or absent hepatic arterial diastolic flow in liver transplants shown by duplex sonography: a poor predictor of subsequent hepatic artery thrombosis. *American Journal of Radiology* 159: 1199

95. Otobe Y, Hashimoto T, Shimizu Y *et al* (1995) Formation of a fatal arterioportal fistula following

needle liver biopsy in a child with a living-related liver transplant: report of a case. *Surgery Today* **25**: 916

96. Jabbour N, Reyes J, Zajko A *et al* (1995) Arterioportal fistula following liver biopsy: three cases occurring in liver transplant recipients. *Digestive Diseases and Science* **40**: 1041

97. Davidson BR, Gibson M, Dick R *et al* (1994) Incidence, risk factors, management, and outcome of portal vein abnormalities of orthotopic liver transplantation. *Transplantation* **57**: 1174

98. Durham JD, LaBerge JM, Kam I *et al* (1994) Portal vein thrombolysis and closure of competitive shunts following liver transplantation. *Journal of Vascular and Interventional Radiology* **5**: 611–616

99. Fujimoto M, Moriyasu F, Someda H *et al* (1995) Evaluation of portal haemodynamics with Doppler ultrasound in living-related donor liver transplantation in children: implications for ligation of spontaneous portosystemic collateral pathways. *Transplant Proceedings* **27**: 1174–1176

100. Salizzoni M, Andorno E, Bossuto E *et al* (1994) Piggyback techniques versus classical technique in orthotopic liver transplantation: a review of 75 cases. *Transplant Proceedings* **26**: 3552

101. Rossi AR, Pozniak MA, Zarvan NP (1993) Upper inferior vena caval anastomotic stenosis in liver transplant recipients: Doppler US diagnosis. *Radiology* **187**: 387

102. Van Thiel DH, Gavaler JS, Wright H *et al* (1993) Liver biopsy: its safety and complications as seen at a liver transplant centre. *Transplantation* **55**: 1087

The kidney

PAUL A. DUBBINS

The kidney is a highly vascular organ, receiving approximately 20% of the cardiac output. Many of the diseases of the kidney have a major vascular component, and systemic diseases such as hypertension are mediated through the vascular control system of the juxtaglomerular apparatus. The kidney would therefore appear to be a fertile field for examination by Doppler. Renal and renovascular disease might be expected to produce changes in the vascular supply, in the microvascular circulation and in venous return.

ANATOMY AND TECHNIQUE

Examination of the *renal arteries* requires a knowledge of vascular anatomy, anatomical relations, anatomical variations and surface anatomy. It also requires an understanding of the effects of geometry on the ability to record a Doppler signal. The right renal artery is an anterolateral branch of the aorta and courses laterally and posteriorly behind the inferior vena cava and then behind the ipsilateral renal vein to the hilum of the kidney (Fig. 8.1). Its anterior relations are predominantly bowel: the duodenum, small bowel and transverse colon. At the hilum of the kidney it divides into anterior and posterior branches, then into interlobular arteries and subsequently the arcuate arteries, which send out striate branches to the cortex (Fig. 8.2). On the left, the renal artery arises as a posterolateral branch of the aorta and courses posteriorly laterally and inferiorly immediately behind the third and fourth parts of the duodenum, subsequently passing behind the transverse and descending colon. Both arteries therefore trace an arc that runs parallel to the arc of the anterior abdominal wall. Geometrically this favours visualization but compromises the Doppler examination; however, visualization is also compromised by bowel which overlies much of ·the course of both renal vessels. Furthermore, 40% of individuals do not conform to this simple anatomical arrangement, with one or more accessory arteries supplying either or both kidneys. These may arise from the aorta immediately adjacent to the main renal artery, but their origin may be from anywhere along the abdominal aorta down to and including the iliac arteries (Fig. 8.3). The polar artery is another common variant, branching early from the main renal artery to pass into either the upper, or more usually the lower, pole without traversing the renal hilum. No single imaging approach can circumvent the difficulties relating to geometry, vessel course and the anterior abdominal relations of gas-filled bowel. Each renal artery must therefore be examined with a flexible technique. Anatomical variations in particular are difficult to image with ultrasound, although supplemental arteries are being identified increasingly with improved equipment resolution and improved sensitivity of colour and power Doppler (Fig. 8.3).

The *renal veins* follow a course parallel to the renal arteries. The right renal vein is the shorter, coursing anteriorly, medially and towards the head in front of the right renal artery. It normally joins the inferior vena cava just cephalad to the right renal artery as it crosses beneath the cava. On the left, the renal vein travels medially and anteriorly, usually superior to the renal artery, passing between the aorta and the superior mesenteric artery, where it may occasionally be compressed by the 'nutcracker effect' between the two vessels. This may cause dilatation of the more proximal portion of the vein but this is not of any clinical significance (Fig. 8.4). The right renal vein usually has no major tributaries but on the left the adrenal, lumbar and gonadal veins usually join the renal vein; of these, only the gonadal vein is regularly imaged on ultrasound as it

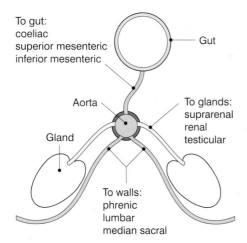

To gut:
coeliac
superior mesenteric
inferior mesenteric

Gut

Aorta

To glands:
suprarenal
renal
testicular

Gland

To walls:
phrenic
lumbar
median sacral

Fig. 8.1 Anatomy of the renal vessels demonstrating their posterolateral course.

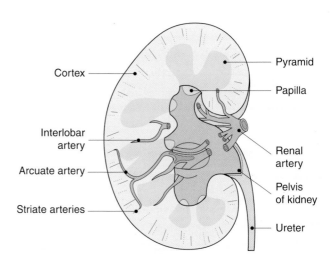

Cortex

Pyramid

Papilla

Interlobar
artery

Arcuate artery

Renal
artery

Pelvis
of kidney

Striate arteries

Ureter

Fig. 8.2 Intrarenal vascular anatomy.

(a)

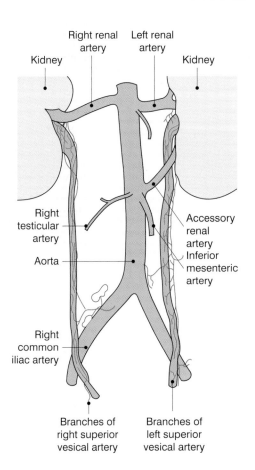

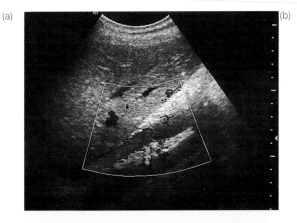
(b)

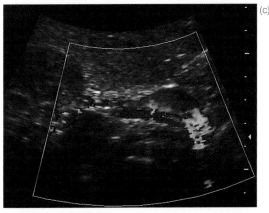
(c)

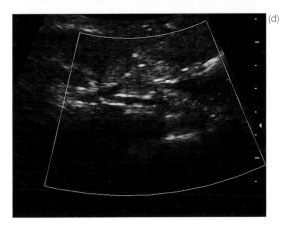
(d)

Fig. 8.3 (a) Origin of the renal arteries including an accessory renal artery supplying the lower pole on the left.
(b) Two right renal arteries. Oblique scan through the aorta and inferior vena cava demonstrating the origin of the two renal arteries from the right lateral wall of the aorta.
(c) Transverse scan demonstrating the larger of the two renal arteries (in red) beneath the corresponding renal vein (in blue) coursing towards the hilum of the right kidney.
(d) Similar transverse image of the accessory renal artery, which is much smaller than the more superior renal artery, but also beneath the corresponding renal vein coursing towards the hilum of the kidney.

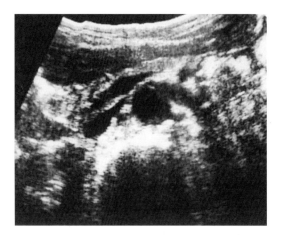

Fig. 8.4 Transverse scan through the upper aorta demonstrating the left renal artery arising from the posterior and lateral aspect of the aorta. The left renal vein arches over the anterior surface of the aorta between the aorta and the superior mesenteric artery and joins the inferior vena cava.

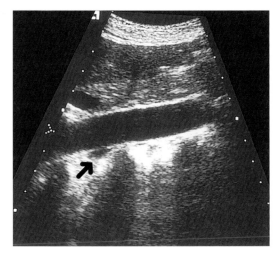

Fig. 8.5 Longitudinal scan through the aorta in a patient with a retro-aortic renal vein, which is represented by the small oval structure posterior to the aorta (arrow).

enters the inferior aspect of the vein near the aorta. Multiple renal veins are common, occurring in approximately one third of the population – the most common of these being an accessory left renal vein traversing to the right behind the aorta – a retro-aortic vein (Fig. 8.5).

Technique – patient positioning and scan orientation

With the patient supine, the aorta is localized with a longitudinal scan just to the left of the midline. The probe is rotated through 90° and the superior mesenteric artery identified (Fig. 8.4). Approximately 1 cm below the origin of the superior mesenteric artery, the right renal artery can be identified arising from the anterolateral surface of the aorta. Occasionally the left renal artery can also be demonstrated at its origin from the posterolateral or lateral surface of the aorta. Both renal veins and their junction with the inferior vena cava can usually be demonstrated in this plane (Figs 8.4 and 8.6). On moving the probe slightly to the right of the midline, the right renal artery is seen to turn posteriorly and laterally. In slim patients it

is occasionally possible to follow the renal artery and vein into the hilum of the kidney by applying compression with the transducer and slightly oblique angulation. Doppler signal recording is best performed at the origin of the artery, by slight displacement of the probe to the right of the midline and angulation to the left to identify the course of the first short segment of the left renal artery (Fig. 8.7). Reversing the angulation to the right approximately 20° from the perpendicular allows signal recording from the posterior and lateral coursing right renal artery[1].

The patient is then turned into the left posterior oblique position. Scanning just posterior to the right mid-axillary line in the longitudinal plane and angling towards the major vessels, both aorta and inferior vena cava can be identified lying parallel to one another (Fig. 8.8). In this plane the section cuts through both the right and left renal arteries and the origins of both can usually be identified (Fig. 8.9). Alteration of the patient position to the right posterior oblique position will identify the junction of the renal veins with the inferior vena cava (Fig. 8.10).

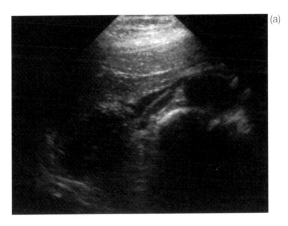

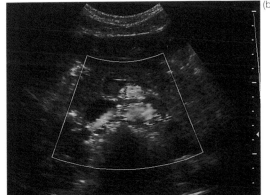

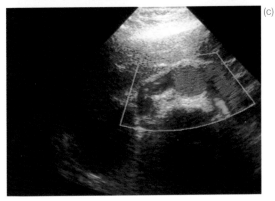

Fig. 8.6 (a) Transverse scans through the aorta demonstrating the origin of the right renal artery from the right anterolateral surface of the aorta coursing posteriorly to the inferior vena cava. (b) Colour flow Doppler evaluation of the right renal artery (in blue) coursing to the right and posteriorly from its origin from the right anterolateral surface of the aorta. (c) Transverse scans through the upper aorta demonstrating the left renal artery (in blue) coursing laterally and posteriorly away from the aorta. The corresponding left renal vein is demonstrated (in red) anteriorly and laterally to the aorta.

Doppler signal recording is possible in this plane from both renal arteries (Fig. 8.11), although occasionally, particularly in heavy or overweight patients, the left renal artery signal is poorly recorded, either because of its depth and difficulties with pulse repetition frequency, or simply because of attenuation of the beam. Scanning from the right flank and angling the probe anteriorly to align the sonographic plane with the coronal plane of the kidney allows the vessels at the renal hilum and within the kidney to be sampled. These can be observed with colour Doppler radiating from the hilum (Fig. 8.12).

The right lobe of the liver acts as an acoustic window to the right renal artery. On the left there is no such acoustic window and visualization of the left renal artery from origin to hilum is extremely difficult. This may be facilitated by compression, or by using the coronal approach to the kidney and following the course of the renal artery retrogradely towards its origin, although in this author's experience the left renal artery is rarely seen in its entirety. The origin may be seen in transverse plane, scanning from the anterior approach and angling slightly to the left (Figs 8.4 and 8.6c), or it may be seen with the patient in the left posterior oblique position as described above. The more distal portion of the main renal artery may be demonstrated just proximal to the hilum by the coronal approach, but the mid-portion of the left renal artery is only rarely seen except in slim patients. By contrast much of the left renal vein is demonstrated with the patient in the supine position; its more anterior and superior location, together with larger diameter, allowing visualization using the left lobe of the liver as an acoustic window (Fig. 8.13).

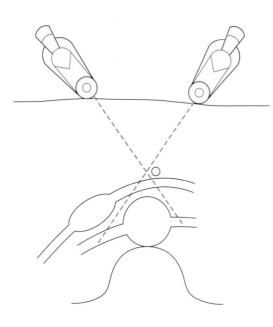

Fig. 8.7 Representation of the approach to Doppler evaluation of the renal arteries from the anterior approach.

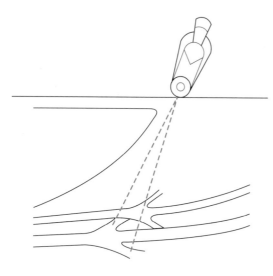

Fig. 8.8 Representation of the approach to the renal arteries scanning from the right flank.

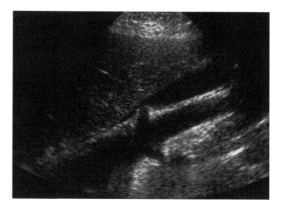

Fig. 8.9 Oblique view through the aorta scanning from the right flank, demonstrating the origin of both renal arteries and the adjacent inferior vena cava. From Dubbins[33], with permission.

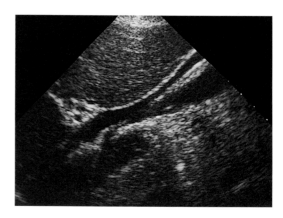

Fig. 8.10 Oblique scanning from the right flank, demonstrating the aorta and inferior vena cava, the origin of the right renal artery and the junction of the right renal vein with the inferior vena cava. From Dubbins[33], with permission.

The intrarenal vessels

Demonstration of the anatomical location and course of the intrarenal vessels is almost exclusively restricted to colour Doppler, although pulsations can be seen on real-time at the site of the interlobar vessels, and occasionally at the bright reflectors at the corticomedullary margin which represent the arcuate vessels. The arteries are each accompanied by a vein; they divide into branches to the upper and lower poles and to the anterior and posterior parenchyma (Fig.

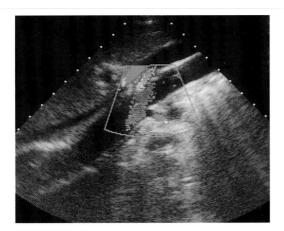

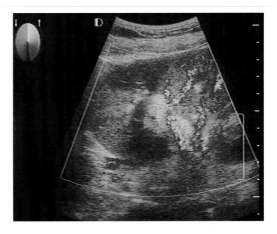

Fig. 8.11 Colour flow Doppler examination of the origin of the renal arteries scanning from the right flank. The right renal artery is demonstrated (in red) between the aorta and inferior vena cava and the left renal artery (in blue) coursing to the left.

Fig. 8.12 Colour flow Doppler image demonstrating blood flow at the hilum and within the kidney. Note there is absent flow to the upper pole in this patient with focal pyelonephritis.

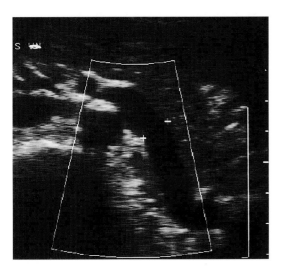

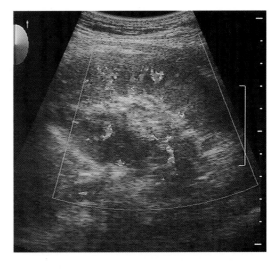

Fig. 8.13 Transverse scan of the left renal vein coursing from the hilum of the kidney anteromedially and then between the superior mesenteric artery, where it is compressed before it joins the inferior vena cava to the right of the aorta. This compression is called the nutcracker phenomenon.

Fig. 8.14 Colour flow Doppler evaluation of the normal kidney, demonstrating parenchymal flow.

8.14). The interlobar vessels course into the renal parenchyma on either side of the renal papillae, giving tiny (invisible) branches to the medulla before arching over the surface of the medulla as the arcuate arteries, giving off multiple small striate branches which extend out towards the cortex. With more modern and sensitive machines, the capsular artery can occasionally be demonstrated at the margin of the kidney, curving around the surface.

It is important to recognize that in the evaluation of the kidneys there are factors other than the Doppler study which contribute to the diagnosis. Both kidneys should be examined carefully with respect to size, echogenicity and smoothness of outline, together with an assessment of the corticomedullary differentiation. The adrenal areas should also be carefully examined to exclude any obvious mass. The time taken to perform a complete vascular examination of the kidney is wasted if the initial examination has missed a renal mass, an adrenal tumour, or a small or absent kidney.

Technique – Doppler examination

Throughout the course of examination of the renal artery, colour Doppler is frequently switched on to confirm the nature and direction of flow. The optimum pulse repetition frequency is selected to detect moderate flow velocities, although it may need to be modified to detect high velocities if a stenosis with aliasing of the colour signal is present. For spectral Doppler, the sample volume is placed on the selected vessel shown on the colour display. Recording spectral Doppler is better performed in duplex rather than triplex mode, since the processing required for triplex imaging reduces

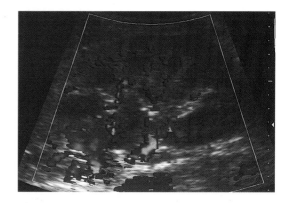

Fig. 8.16 Colour flow Doppler of the normal kidney. Zoom mode has been employed and the colour box opened widely to demonstrate the global renal perfusion but the pixel 'fill in' is diminished because of compromise of the frame rate.

both the frame rate and the pulse repetition frequency, compromising further the discrimination of high-velocity signals at depth.

Colour Doppler is invaluable in the assessment of intrarenal vessels. With the system set to detect low or moderate velocities, flow can be identified in almost all patients in the vessels at the renal hilum, particularly if the angle of incidence is optimized to achieve angles of less than 60° relative to the course of the vessel. Angling the probe medially from the right or left flank will allow assessment of the intrarenal vessels. Peripheral, smaller vessels are usually better demonstrated with power Doppler, although in this situation the directional information is lost

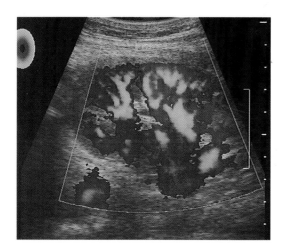

Fig. 8.15 Colour power Doppler of the normal kidney, demonstrating flow within small vessels but the lack of directional information.

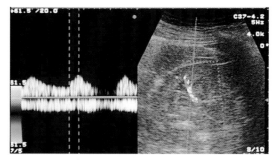

Fig. 8.17 Colour box reduced in size to demonstrate single intrarenal vessel prior to sampling for spectral Doppler.

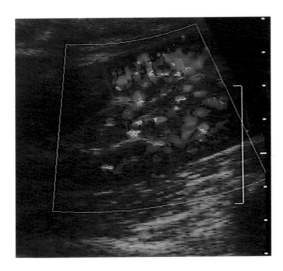

Fig. 8.18 Colour blush within the normal kidney following the injection of intravenous contrast (Levovist).

prior to spectral sampling (Fig. 8.17). It is frequently of value to activate the zoom function on the machine prior to interrogation with colour Doppler, as this allows for greater sensitivity of colour signal recording within the intrarenal vessels. Using this technique, the hilar and interlobular vessels are demonstrated in all patients, although arcuate and striate arteries are only seen in slimmer patients. In the case of the arcuate vessels, this is partly due to their course, which is usually at right angles to the incident beam. Advances in technology have widened the group in whom the entire renovascular pattern can be identified. The use of ultrasound contrast material further enhances visualization of parenchymal vessels (Fig. 8.18)[2].

(Fig. 8.15). The development of systems with directional power Doppler and with greater colour Doppler sensitivity will improve vessel discrimination.

Evaluation of global blood flow requires that the colour box be opened to its fullest extent in order to visualize relative blood flow distribution (Fig. 8.16). This is also important in the evaluation of renal tumours so that flow in the lesion can be compared with that in normal adjacent renal tissue. However, this compromises temporal resolution with lower frame rates and pulse repetition frequency; the size of the colour box should therefore be minimized

Characteristics of the Doppler spectrum

The typical spectra from the renal arteries are shown in Fig. 8.19. There is a rapid systolic upstroke, which is occasionally followed by a secondary slower rise to peak systole (although this is more frequently seen with advancing age, hypertension, etc.). There is subsequently a gradual diastolic decay but with persistent forward flow in diastole.

Renal vein spectra are often different for right and left veins (Fig. 8.20). The right renal vein is short and often therefore mirrors the pulsatility of the inferior vena cava, while the left, particularly if it is sampled to the left of

(a)
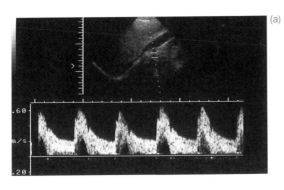

(b)
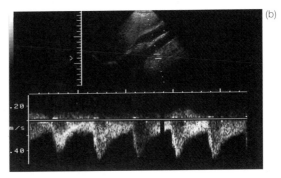

Fig. 8.19 (a) Normal Doppler spectrum from the right renal artery. (b) Corresponding normal Doppler spectrum from the left renal artery using the oblique approach from the right flank.

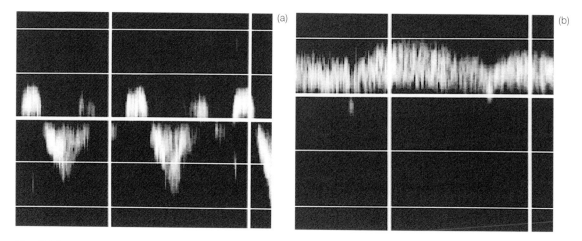

Fig. 8.20 (a) Venous flow within the right renal vein reflecting the pulsatile nature of flow within the inferior vena cava. (b) Damped flow within the left renal vein, presumably modified by the effect of the superior mesenteric artery. From Dubbins[33], with permission

the superior mesenteric artery, may show only slight variability of flow velocities consequent upon cardiac and respiratory activity.

Indices used in the assessment of renal blood flow

A multiplicity of indices is used for evaluation of renal blood flow. The wide range indicates that no single index provides all the information that is necessary for adequate evaluation of renal pathophysiology. The indices used, together with normal values, are shown in Table 8.1, and some examples are shown in Fig. 8.21. Pulsatility and resistance indices in the renal arteries increase with age and in hypertensive patients. This is presumably consequent upon the effect of the juxtaglomerular apparatus

producing vasoconstriction, but also perhaps on the development of hypertensive nephrosclerosis[3-5]. A further cause of variability of Doppler indices relates to differences of opinion as to the optimum site for Doppler sampling. Some authors suggest the renal sinus as the optimum site, while others recommend the interlobar and arcuate artery level[6]. There is significant variety in normal spectral indices but in this author's view this is best minimized by using the same site in order to standardize measurement technique.

DISEASES OF THE MAJOR RENAL VESSELS
General principles

Evaluation of the renal arteries should include an assessment of the aorta, particularly around the origins of the renal arteries, to look for atheromatous plaques. The demonstration of atheromatous plaque within the more distal renal artery by direct visualization is usually rather more difficult, and its presence is inferred from alterations in the Doppler signal. With careful evaluation along the course of the renal artery, it is occasionally possible to demonstrate the irregular beaded appearance associated with fibromuscular

Table 8.1 Normal renal artery Doppler indices.

Index	Range
Pulsatility index (PI)	0.7–1.4
Resistance index (RI)	0.56–0.7
Peak systolic velocity (PSV)	60–140 cm/s^{-1} (<180)
Diastolic/systolic ratio (D/S)	0.26–0.4
Renal artery/aorta ratio (RAR)	<3.5
Time to maximum systole (TMS) (systolic rise time)	42–57 ms
Acceleration index	250–380 cm/s^{-2}

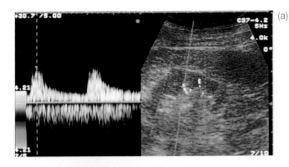

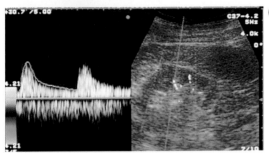

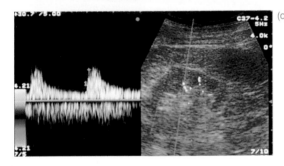

Fig. 8.21 (a) Measurement of the resistance index. (b) Measurement of the pulsatility index. (c) Measurement of the acceleration time or time to maximum systole.

hyperplasia. As at other vessel sites, focal dilatation of the artery may represent a post-stenotic dilatation associated with a proximal stenotic segment.

Renal artery stenosis

The pathology of narrowing of the renal artery is largely divided into stenosis produced by atheroma and that resulting from renal artery fibromuscular hyperplasia. The prevalence of the different types of renal artery disease depends to a very large degree on the age group; fibromuscular dysplasia is predominantly a disease of younger age groups, whereas atheroma becomes more common with increasing age. Atheromatous renal artery stenosis is the cause of the majority of cases of renal artery stenosis. This is particularly the case for those patients presenting with renovascular renal failure, rather than isolated aggressive hypertension. The findings on ultrasound imaging are different in the two conditions.

In cases of atheromatous disease, the stenosis tends to be located near the origin of the artery (Fig. 8.22), although it may occur along the course of the artery. In fibromuscular hyperplasia, the affected segment tends to lie distal to the origin of the vessel. Doppler findings within the main renal artery are variable. For a haemodynamically significant stenosis of more than 50% diameter reduction, there is typically an increase in flow velocity greater than 180 cm s^{-1} associated with spectral broadening (Fig. 8.23); the renal artery/aortic peak systolic ratio (RAR) is increased beyond 3.5. Spectral broadening may be the only sign in stenoses of lesser severity and may predominate in fibromuscular hyperplasia[7]. Colour Doppler findings include narrowing of the luminal diameter and aliasing of the colour signal (Fig. 8.24). The value of

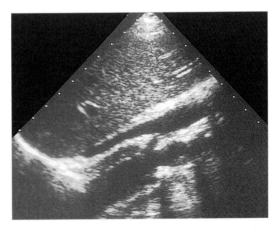

Fig. 8.22 Oblique scans through the aorta, demonstrating the origin of the right renal artery. The infrarenal aorta is atheromatous and there is a plaque of atheroma at the origin of the left renal artery.

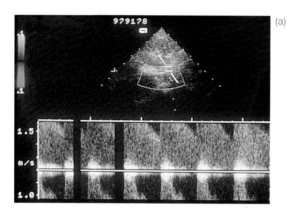 (a)

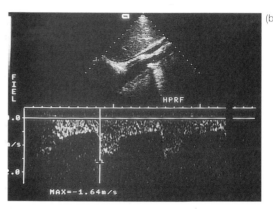 (b)

Fig. 8.23 (a) Renal artery stenosis. There is significant increase in flow velocity within the right renal artery, with spectral broadening and aliasing consistent with marked increased flow velocity and disturbance of flow. (b) Same patient as Fig. 8.22. Flow velocities within the left renal artery only reach 1.64 m s^{-1}. It is difficult in this situation to be confident of a haemodynamically significant stenosis.

using the renal artery/aortic ratio, rather than absolute measurements of velocity, is that it takes into account poor inflow; it is important to remember that these patients are often arteriopaths and consequently may have poor cardiac output[8].

However, initial enthusiasm for the technique of direct evaluation of the main renal arteries for signs of renal stenosis has been markedly tempered by the results of more recent studies. Some of these have indicated that the sensitivity of detection may be as low as 20% in comparison to early claims of sensitivities in excess of 80%[9]. Much of the difficulty relates to the poor imaging of the entire length of the renal artery, and it is possible that the situation may improve with the enhanced visualization of the main renal arteries resulting from the use of effective ultrasound contrast agents.

Findings in the intrarenal vessels

The intrarenal vessels can be imaged in most patients. Haemodynamically significant stenoses will produce significant downstream effects within the intrarenal arteries. These have been described as a 'tardus parvus' pattern, with a low-amplitude signal that has a prolonged systolic acceleration time and which appears delayed in relation to the QRS complex of the ECG. Duplex indices used to characterize this waveform include a systolic acceleration time above 0.07 s, an increase in the acceleration index in excess of 378 cm s^{-2}, a reduced resistance index of less than 0.5 and decreased peak systolic velocities (Fig. 8.25)[10, 11]. In practice these changes will only reliably identify stenoses greater than 70% diameter reduction, lesser degrees of stenosis may not be picked up.

Fig. 8.24 Colour flow Doppler of the origin of the right renal artery in a patient with renal artery stenosis. There is significant disturbance of the flow with a mosaic pattern within the colour signal.

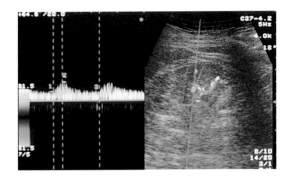

Fig. 8.25 The tardus parvus pattern of renal artery stenosis. Assessment of the intrarenal vessels demonstrates a delay in the time to maximum systole and an increase in the acceleration index.

Furthermore, diffusely diseased arteries will also show these changes, with a significant false-positive rate. Considerable care is necessary in the interpretation of intrarenal waveforms.

Screening for renal artery stenosis

Patients with renovascular hypertension and those with renal failure consequent upon disease of the main renal artery may benefit from a number of possible revascularization techniques such as angioplasty. Duplex ultrasound is one of a number of techniques which have been proposed as possible screening tools. However, direct signs of renal artery stenosis require visualization of the main renal artery; most reports would indicate that this is possible in at best only 70% of cases, and that this is only marginally improved by the use of currently available ultrasound contrast, because the problems of obesity and bowel gas remain. Significant interest has therefore centred around the role of the indirect signs from the intrarenal vessels, since these measurements are simpler and quicker to perform and are possible in more than 90% of patients. There are, however, wide variations of 60–90% in the reported sensitivity of this technique, with some authors reporting even lower values[11, 12].

Most authors would not, therefore, advocate the use of renal Doppler as a screening test for renal artery stenosis. The predominant role appears to be in the evaluation of equivocal angiographic findings and follow-up after angioplasty[13].

Renal artery aneurysm

Renal artery aneurysms are uncommon. Previously on static B-mode imaging, mistaking the dilated left renal vein, produced by the nutcracker effect on the vein by the superior mesenteric artery, led to false diagnoses of renal artery aneurysm. With modern real-time equipment an aneurysm can almost always be identified in continuity with the renal artery. Colour Doppler will demonstrate the flow direction and characteristic venous pulsatility in the case of a prominent vein, or the disordered arterial flow associated with an aneurysm.

Aortic dissection

Ultrasound is of value in assessing dissection of the abdominal aorta. Although this is significantly less common than thoracic aortic dissection, it can occur as a consequence of the extension of a thoracic dissection into the abdominal aorta, or subsequent to interventional procedures performed via the transfemoral route. The aortic flap can be identified on real-time ultrasound, while flow within both the true and false lumen can be documented. Flow may be towards the legs in both channels, or may be reversed in the false lumen (Fig. 8.26). The course of the dissection is often spiral; consequently one renal artery may be supplied by the true lumen of a dissection and the other by the false lumen. Documentation of impaired flow within one or other of the renal arteries, or in the intrarenal vessels, is of significant prognostic value in cases such as this, since it will identify a kidney

181

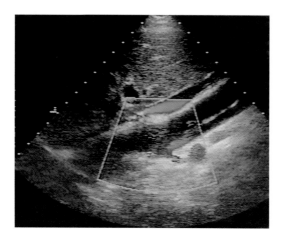

Fig. 8.26 Colour flow Doppler examination of the aorta in a case of aortic dissection. There is reverse flow in the false lumen which modifies flow within the left renal artery. The reverse flow is demonstrated (in blue) underneath the linear echogenic dissection flap. From Dubbins[33], with permission.

at risk of ischaemia. In such cases, revascularization may be considered[14].

Arteriovenous malformation/fistula

In the native kidneys these are almost invariably posttraumatic following penetrating injury. Small arteriovenous fistulae following renal biopsy are usually short lived, although when large they can compromise renal function and renal survival. These are described in the section on renal transplantation (see Chapter 9). Larger arteriovenous fistulae can be encountered following trauma such as knife injuries. In these cases, both the main renal artery and the main renal vein are enlarged, with increased flow velocities, decreased pulsatility and resistance indices within the renal artery, and high flow velocities within the renal vein. The site of the arteriovenous communication is identified by reducing the colour sensitivity, so that only high velocity is detected. In this situation no flow is demonstrated within the normal renal parenchyma but there remains a high-intensity colour signal at the site of the fistula. This is frequently

accompanied by a tissue 'bruit' visible on colour Doppler as a mosaic of colour extending into the renal parenchyma around the fistula (Fig. 8.27)[15].

Atheroembolic disease

Embolism of atheroma within the renal vascular tree is a cause of significant renal dysfunction, producing wedge-shaped infarcts and subsequent scarring. Theoretically colour Doppler, and in particular power Doppler with its increased sensitivity to low-flow states, should be able to provide a global view of renal perfusion (Fig. 8.28). While it is possible with both colour and power Doppler to show focal ischaemia and focal infarcts, both techniques suffer from limitations of inadequate penetration to the posterior kidney. Therefore focal colour-free segments in this area cannot reliably be defined as infarcts, as the features may simply be the result of technical difficulties with colour sensitivities. Ultrasound contrast has been advocated as a tool to resolve some of these difficulties. The blood pool contrast

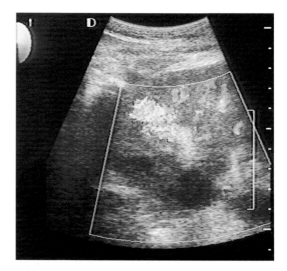

Fig. 8.27 Arteriovenous fistula. Colour flow Doppler demonstrates increased focal flow within the kidney, with a tissue bruit of colour outwith the renal vessels caused by vibration of the adjacent renal substance.

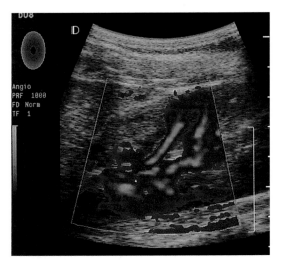

Fig. 8.28 Colour power Doppler evaluation of a patient with focal ischaemia of the kidney. There is normal perfusion in the lower and mid-poles but the anterior surface of the upper pole is avascular.

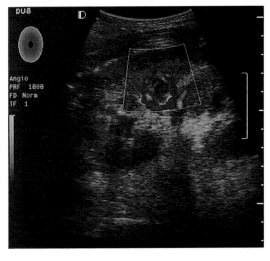

Fig. 8.29 Flash flow of renal vein thrombosis. Poverty of flow to the kidney with only brief demonstration of flow within the central vessels.

agents certainly demonstrate tissue perfusion, even in difficult patients, but gas microbubbles may produce significant sound attenuation, which will degrade the signal from the more deeply situated renal parenchyma with the same potential for perfusion defect artefacts. With newer contrast agents it appears possible to maximize Doppler enhancement while minimizing the shadowing effect[16].

Renal vein thrombosis

This is an uncommon condition in adults; it occurs most commonly in association with the extension of a renal tumour (see below). Rarely, extrinsic compression or haematological conditions which produce an increased tendency to thrombosis may predispose to renal vein thrombosis. In infants, renal vein thrombosis may occur as a complication of dehydration.

Colour Doppler may show no flow in the renal parenchyma, or 'flash flow' where the colour signal is seen only transiently, corresponding to peak systole (Fig. 8.29). Occasionally a 'to and fro' pattern may be seen

with alternating red and blue colour signals visible within the renal arteries. Spectral Doppler may show absent, or reversed, diastolic flow. A 'W' shape to the arterial diastolic flow component, in association with absent venous flow on colour Doppler, is thought to be characteristic of renal vein thrombosis, although other conditions may produce reversed diastolic flow, including acute tubular necrosis and cardiac abnormalities such as aortic incompetence (Fig. 8.30)[17].

Renal infection

The findings in renal infection are extremely variable. Renal infection may be focal or diffuse. Blood flow findings, however, depend not only on the focal or diffuse nature of the condition but also upon the influence of the balance between hyperaemia consequent upon infection, and reduced flow consequent upon renal swelling and capsular stretching. Thus there may be a global or focal increase in blood flow, with a reduction in the Doppler indices; or, more commonly, there may be reduction in

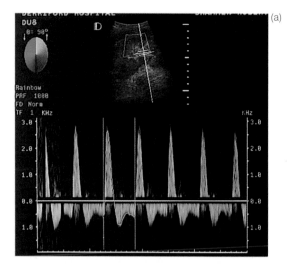

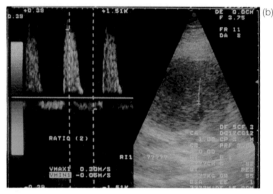

Fig. 8.30 (a) Renal vein thrombosis. Spectral pattern demonstrating the W-shaped flow pattern in diastole characteristic of renal vein thrombosis. (b) Reversed flow in diastole consequent upon aortic incompetence. Image courtesy of Dr D.L. Cochlin.

blood flow and an increase in the Doppler indices. In focal pyelonephritis, this may allow the demonstration of a hypoechoic mass with an associated perfusion defect (Fig. 8.12)[18]. However, even specific findings of this nature rarely influence management, and it is only if renal abscess is demonstrated that a different therapeutic approach would be adopted.

Renal abscess

The development of a renal or perirenal abscess is an uncommon complication of renal infection. The appearances are, however, fairly characteristic, with a renal mass lesion showing central necrosis subsequently developing into an irregular cystic lesion with thick walls. Blood flow is usually increased around the margin of the lesion, producing a 'colour halo', although this is indistinguishable from a necrotic renal tumour. Usually a combination of clinical history and grey-scale features, as well as colour Doppler, will allow the correct diagnosis (Fig. 8.31).

Renal tumour

Angioneogenesis occurs as part of the disordered growth of renal tumours. As a consequence it was felt that both colour Doppler and spectral Doppler might provide a means of assessment of angioneogenesis. However, reports are varied in terms of the success of colour Doppler in distinguishing between malignant and benign pathology of the kidney[19–21]. Comparisons with contrast angiography suggest that the accuracy of the technique is likely to be less than has been hoped, as both benign and malignant tumours can be either hypo- or hypervascular. Angio-

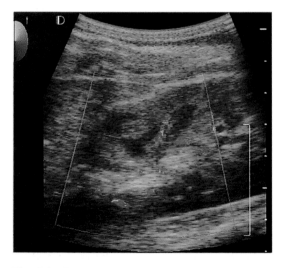

Fig. 8.31 Renal abscess. Colour flow Doppler of the kidney. There is an irregular area within the upper pole of the kidney. There is no flow within the centre of the lesion but circumferential flow.

myolipomata, for example, can be extremely vascular and demonstrate blood pooling while, conversely, transitional cell tumours are characteristically hypovascular[22].

Examination of renal tumours with colour Doppler requires the colour box to be opened to include the whole of the tumour and a small portion of the adjacent normal renal parenchyma, so as to demonstrate the difference in size, distribution and communication of the abnormal blood vessels. High- and low-velocity blood flow patterns have been described, predominantly in the margin of the tumour but also extending within the tumour mass. Clearly, if there is necrosis, or the tumour is hypovascular, this pattern will not be seen (Fig. 8.32). Characteristic colour flow patterns are of large irregular marginal vessels extending into the

centre of the tumour with an abnormal irregular branching pattern (Fig. 8.18). The use of 3-D power Doppler, with and without the use of contrast agents, is being explored in an attempt to characterize blood flow patterns specific for benign and malignant tumours, but this work is still in its infancy. Spectral Doppler may show scattered high-frequency signals both at the margin and within the body of the tumour, presumably representing flow through vessels supplying arteriovenous communications[21]. In very large hypervascular tumours with extensive arteriovenous shunting, blood flow within the main renal artery is abnormal with increased systolic flow velocities and spectral broadening.

Colour Doppler may refine the ability of real-time scanning to evaluate invasion/thrombosis of the renal vein. When thrombus is present the

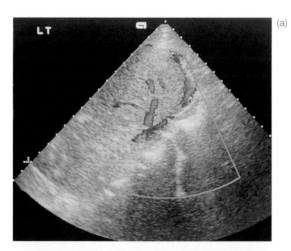

(a)

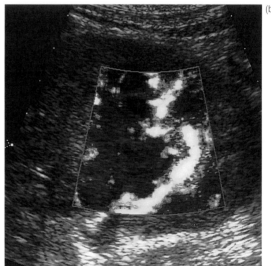

(b)

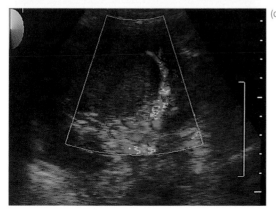

(c)

Fig. 8.32 (a) Large renal tumour demonstrating predominantly circumferential flow but with a few intratumoral vessels. (b) Large central renal tumour demonstrating numerous irregular vessels but with central necrosis. (c) Hypovascular tumour with peripheral flow only. From Dubbins[33], with permission.

185

renal vein is distended and contains low-level echoes (Fig. 8.33). Colour Doppler demonstrates flow around the thrombus or tumour thrombus. It is only rarely possible to identify blood flow within the tumour thrombus itself and thus distinguish between tumour and non-tumour thrombosis. In total occlusion of the renal vein, no colour flow signal is identified and the spectral flow within the renal artery demonstrates a high-resistance flow pattern with absent or reversed flow in diastole (Fig. 8.34).

Obstruction

Although the intravenous urogram and, more recently, computed tomography (CT) are the mainstay of diagnosis of acute obstruction, ultrasound has long had a role in the demonstration of hydronephrosis, particularly in long-standing outflow tract obstruction and ureteric obstruction. Features of obstruction on real-time imaging include dilatation of the calyces and of the renal pelvis; dilated ureters can also be identified posterior to the urinary bladder. In acute obstruction, however, there is often no evidence of calyceal or pelvic dilatation and the kidney may appear structurally normal on ultrasound. In this situation, repeat ultrasound after 8–12 hours will usually demonstrate the development of pelvicalyceal dilatation. However, there are alterations in intrarenal pressure consequent upon the obstruction and these may be detected by the use of Doppler techniques. Thus in acute obstruction an increase in the

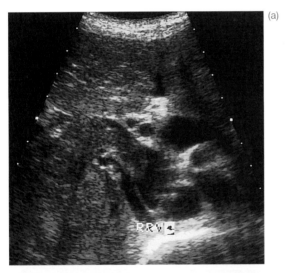
(a)

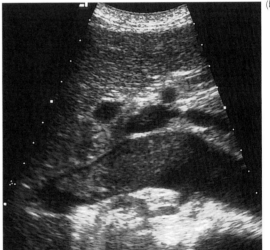
(b)

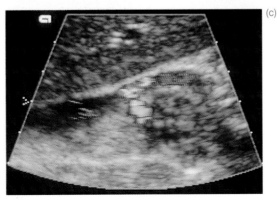
(c)

Fig. 8.33 (a) Transverse scan through the left renal vein. The left renal vein is distended and filled with echogenic material, indicating either extension of tumour into the vein or renal vein thrombosis. (b) Same patient – extension of the echogenic thrombus/tumour into the inferior vena cava. (c) Distortion of the inferior vena cava and encasement of the adjacent right renal artery by tumour extending beneath the inferior vena cava from the adjacent right kidney.

Contrast media

The advent of third-generation ultrasound contrast media now allows the demonstration of blood pool enhancement in the kidney. Currently, the duration of enhancement by commercially available ultrasound contrast media is only short lived, being of the order of 2–3 min after bolus injection; this may possibly be extended by the use of infusion techniques. No clinical role has as yet been established for contrast media in the enhancement of Doppler signals from the kidney, but if the duration of enhancement can be extended (some newer media may allow enhancement in excess of 10 min), and if suitable software is developed for ultrasound machines, then it may be possible to visualize the entire renal vascular supply, measure global and regional volume flow, and also document abnormal areas of perfusion[32].

SUMMARY

Doppler techniques now allow the assessment of intrarenal vessels in most patients (Table 8.2). Currently, however, the role of Doppler in the kidney is limited. It may help to resolve problems with mass lesions, including the differentiation of tumours from pseudotumours such as a hypertrophied column of Bertin. It may allow the assessment of renal obstruction when there is a contraindication to X-ray contrast agents. It may clarify the diagnosis of renal artery stenosis in the case of an equivocal angiogram, and it will allow the identification of significant renal venous disease. The greater sensitivity of modern ultrasound systems combined with improved visualization with echo-enhancing agents may allow visualization and assessment of the entire renal vascular supply in the future.

Table 8.2 Indications for renal Doppler.

Investigation/purpose	Possible cause/indication
1. To confirm renal perfusion	Renal trauma Reduction in renal size, etc.
2. Diagnosis of renal vein thrombosis	Tumour Dehydration (infant) Hypovolaemia Abnormal clotting
3. Renal obstruction	Contrast hypersensitivity Pregnancy
4. Renal tumour vs. pseudotumour	
5. Renal artery stenosis	Equivocal angiogram Follow-up to angioplasty, etc. (Screening)
6. Arteriovenous abnormalities	
7. Aortic aneurysm and aortic dissection	

REFERENCES

1. Dubbins P (1986) Renal artery stenosis – duplex Doppler evaluation. *British Journal of Radiology* **59**: 225–229
2. Taylor GA, Ecklund K, Dunning PS (1996) Renal cortical perfusion in rabbits: visualization with colour amplitude imaging and an experimental microbubble-based US contrast agent. *Radiology* **201**(1): 125–129
3. Keogan MT, Kliewer MA, Hertzberg BS, DeLong DM, Tupler RH, Carroll BA (1996) Renal resistive indexes: variability in Doppler US measurement in a healthy population. *Radiology* **199**(1): 165–169
4. Gill B, Palmer LS, Koenigsberg M, Laor E (1994) Distribution and variability of resistive index values in undilated kidneys in children. *Urology* **44**(6): 897–901

5. Boddi M, Sacchi S, Lammel RM, Mohseni R, Serneri CG (1996) Age-related and vasomotor stimuli-induced changes in renal vascular resistance detected by Doppler ultrasound. *American Journal of Hypertension* 9(5): 461–466

6. Knapp R, Plotzeneder A, Frauscher F et al (1995) Variability of Doppler parameters in the healthy kidney: an anatomic-physiologic correlation. *Journal of Ultrasound in Medicine* 14(6): 427–429

7. Taylor DC, Kezzler MD, Moneta GL et al (1988) Duplex ultrasound scanning in the diagnosis of renal artery stenosis: a prospective evaluation. *Journal of Vascular Surgery* 7: 363–369

8. Strandness DE (1993) The renal arteries. In: *Duplex Scanning in Vascular Disorders*, 2nd edn, pp 197–215. New York: Raven Press

9. Berland LL, Koslin DB, Routh WD, Keller FS (1990) Renal artery stenosis: prospective evaluation of diagnosis with colour duplex US compared with angiography: work in progress. *Radiology* 174: 421–423

10. Handa N, Fukunaga R, Etani H, Yoneda S, Kimura K, Kamada T. (1988) Efficacy of echo Doppler examination for the evaluation of renovascular disease. *Ultrasound in Medicine and Biology* 14: 1–15

11. Stavros AT, Parker SH, Yakes WF et al (1992) Segmental stenosis of the renal artery: pattern recognition of parvus and tardus abnormalities with duplex sonography. *Radiology* 184: 487–492

12. Strunk H, Jaeger U, Teifke A (1995) Intrarenal colour Doppler ultrasound for the exclusion of renal artery stenosis in cases of multiple renal arteries: analysis of the Doppler spectrum and tardus parvus phenomenon. *Ultraschall In Der Medizin* 16: 172–179

13. Baxter GM, Aitcheson F, Sheppard D et al (1996) Colour Doppler ultrasound in renal artery stenosis, intrarenal waveform analysis. *British Journal of Radiology* 69: 810–815

14. Thomas E, Dubbins PA (1990) Duplex ultrasound of the abdominal aorta – a neglected tool in aortic dissection. *Clinical Radiology* 42: 330–334

15. Ozbek SS, Memis A, Killi R, Karaca E, Kabasakal C, Mir S (1995) Image-directed and colour Doppler ultrasonography in the diagnosis of postbiopsy arteriovenous fistulas of native kidneys. *Journal of Clinical Ultrasound* 23(4): 239–242

16. Correas J-M, Kessler D, Worab D, Quay SC (1997) The first phase-shift ultrasound contrast agent: Echogen. In: Goldberg BB (ed.) *Ultrasound Contrast Agents*, pp 101–120. London: Martin Dunitz

17. Tublin ME, Dodd GD (1995) Sonography of renal transplantation. *Radiology Clinics of North America* 33: 447–459

18. Winters WD (1996) Power Doppler sonographic evaluation of acute pyelonephritis in children. *Journal of Ultrasound in Medicine* 15: 91–96

19. Hirai T, Ohishi H, Yamada R et al (1995) Usefulness of colour Doppler imaging in differential diagnosis of multilocular cystic lesions of the kidney. *Journal of Ultrasound in Medicine* 14(10): 771–776

20. Erden I, Beduk Y, Karalezli G, Aytac S, Anafarta K, Sfak M (1993) Characterization of renal masses with colour flow Doppler ultrasonography. *British Journal of Urology* 71(6): 661–663

21. Yamashita Y, Takahashi M, Watanabe O et al (1992) Small renal cell carcinoma: pathologic and radiologic correlation. *Radiology* 184(2): 493–498

22. Horstman WG, McFarland RM, Gorman JD (1995) Colour Doppler sonographic findings in patients with transitional cell carcinoma of the bladder and renal pelvis. *Journal of Ultrasound in Medicine* 14(2): 129–133

23. Platt JF, Rubin JM, Ellis JH (1989) Distinction between obstructive and non-obstructive pyelocaliectasis with duplex Doppler sonography. *American Journal of Radiology* 153: 997–1000

24. Platt JF (1992) Duplex Doppler evaluation of native kidney dysfunction: obstructive and non-obstructive diseases. *American Journal of Radiology* 158: 1035–1042

25. Tublin ME, Dodd GD, Verdile VP (1994) Acute renal colic: diagnosis with duplex Doppler US. *Radiology* 193: 697–701

26. Weston MJ, Dubbins PA (1994) The diagnosis of obstruction: colour Doppler ultrasonography of renal blood flow and ureteric jets. *Current Opinion in Urology* 4: 69–74

27. Renowden SA, Cochlin DL (1992) The effect of intravenous frusemide on the Doppler waveform in normal kidneys. *Journal of Ultrasound in Medicine* 11: 65–68

28. Platt JF, Rubin JM, Ellis JH (1990) Intrarenal arterial Doppler sonography in patients with non-obstructive renal disease: correlation of resistive index with biopsy findings. *American Journal of Radiology* 154: 1223–1227

29. Argalia G, d'Ambrosio F, Mignosi U et al (1995) Doppler echography and colour Doppler echography in the assessment of the vascular functional aspects of medical nephropathies. *Radiologia Medica* 89(4): 464–469

30. Yoon DY, Kim SH, Kim HD et al (1995) Doppler sonography in experimentally induced acute renal failure in rabbits. Resistive index versus serum creatinine levels. *Investigative Radiology* 30(3): 168–172

31. Forsberg F, Goldberg BB (1997) New imaging techniques with ultrasound contrast agents. In: Goldberg BB (ed.) *Ultrasound Contrast Agents*, pp. 177–191. London: Martin Dunitz

32. Cosgrove D (1996) Ultrasound contrast enhancement of tumours. *Clinical Radiology* 51(Suppl. 1): 44–49

33. Dubbins P (1998) *Urogenital Ultrasound: A Text Atlas* London: Martin Dunitz

Doppler ultrasound evaluation of renal transplantation

MYRON A. POZNIAK

Graft and patient survival following renal transplantation has progressively improved[1]. One-year graft survival rates currently approximate at 84% for cadaveric and 93% for living-donor kidney transplants, with 1-year patient survival rates at 94% for cadaveric recipients and 98% for living-related kidney recipients[2]. The improving results are primarily due to refined surgical techniques, better immuno-suppressive agents, advances in human leuko-cyte antigen (HLA) typing for recipient/donor matching, and the creation of coordinated transplant sharing systems[3]. As the number of kidney recipients increases, a corresponding increase in patients presenting for emergency care to non-transplant centres can also be expected. The chances for graft survival can be significantly improved with timely identification of the aetiology of renal transplant dysfunction, allowing prompt medical and/or surgical intervention when necessary.

When screening laboratory test results indicate renal transplant dysfunction, imaging studies are often required to evaluate renal morphology and perfusion. Doppler ultrasound is an ideal tool for this purpose because of its non-invasive nature, ready availability, and ability to detect and distinguish many of the vascular abnormalities that are found with transplant dysfunction. Occasionally, ultrasound can suggest functional problems such as rejection or acute tubular necrosis.

Examination of the transplanted kidney requires careful attention to scan technique and an awareness of the potential problems. The main features of the examination are given in Table 9.1 and the main abnormal findings which may be demonstrated are listed in Table 9.2.

ULTRASOUND ANATOMY OF THE RENAL TRANSPLANT

In most cases, the transplant kidney is positioned extraperitoneally in the right iliac fossa with an end-to-side anastomosis of the renal vasculature to the external iliac artery and vein. The transplanted ureter is implanted directly into the superior surface of the bladder (Fig. 9.1). In approximately 20% of transplants, multiple arterial or venous anastomoses may be required. Because numerous technical variations exist in the way kidneys are transplanted, it is very important that the sonologist and sonographer are familiar with the surgical technique common to their institution and the specific anatomic details of the patient being scanned[4, 5]. With the numerous possible variations, proper documentation and communication of the surgical record is very important in ensuring correct understanding and interpretation of imaging findings and Doppler flow profiles in renal transplantation. Ideally, if the transplant is non-standard a drawing is provided which shows the orientation of the

9

Table 9.1 Renal Transplant Sonographic examination checklist.

1. Review any available prior imaging studies. Review the surgical record, especially with regard to the vasculature.
2. Evaluate the renal collecting system: if dilated, make sure that bladder outflow obstruction is not the underlying cause.
3. Measure the renal length. Record any change.
4. Rule out perinephric fluid collections: record any change in size if previously present.
5. Rule out lymphocoele.
6. Verify uniform parenchymal perfusion by colour Doppler: rule out tardus parvus waveform by examining the interlobar or segmental arterial waveforms for resistance and delayed systolic upstroke.
7. Examine the main renal artery, particularly near its anastomosis (especially if a tardus parvus waveform is observed within the transplanted kidney).
8. Verify renal vein patency.

Table 9.2 Sonographic findings and possible causes.

- Increase in size of transplanted kidney
  Hypertrophy of the kidney
  Allograft rejection
  Postoperative infection
  Renal vein thrombosis

- Reduction in size of transplanted kidney
  Ischemia
  Chronic rejection

- Increased renal arterial flow resistance
  . Compressive effect by transducer, adjacent mass,
     or fluid collection
  Infection
  Advanced stages of rejection
  High-grade obstruction
  Acute tubular necrosis

- Decreased renal arterial flow resistance
  Renal artery stenosis
  Severe aortoiliac atherosclerosis
  Arteriovenous fistula

- Renal collecting system dilatation
  Obstructive hydronephrosis
  Ureteral anastomosis stenosis
  Chronic distention of flaccid denervated system
  Sequela of prior obstructive episode
  Bladder outlet obstruction (neurogenic bladder)

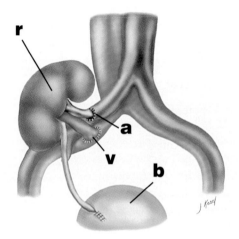

Fig. 9.1 Artist's rendering of a renal transplant (r) located in the right iliac fossa. The transplant renal artery is typically anastomosed to the common iliac artery (a). The transplant renal vein anastomosis is to the common iliac vein (v). The ureter is connected to the urinary bladder (b). Reproduced with permission from McGann and Goldberg[34].

kidney and its vasculature, the number and location of anastomoses, and any other atypical anatomic information.

DOPPLER ULTRASOUND TECHNIQUE

Successful Doppler evaluation of the transplanted kidney can only be accomplished when scan quality is optimal. This requires the use of equipment that provides high Doppler sensitivity. The examiner must optimize the Doppler settings, since improper adjustment can result in slow flow being overlooked and thrombosis being incorrectly diagnosed. Additionally, two important scanning factors that must be taken into account to ensure a successful examination are optimizing the angle of insonation relative to vessel orientation, and minimizing transducer pressure.

Scale setting (pulse repetition frequency)

For the initial scan, the colour and spectral Doppler scales should be set as low as possible.

By doing so, the examiner will be able to localize the vessel in question with colour Doppler and then demonstrate adequate excursion on the spectral Doppler tracing. If aliasing occurs, the examiner can always increase the scale setting until the optimal level for that particular vessel is achieved.

Doppler gain

The gain should be set at the highest level possible without creating noise in the image or tracing.

Filtration level

The Doppler filter reduces noise in both colour and spectral modes. If the filtration level is set too high, it can eradicate the display of very slow flow in a vessel. Initially, filtration should be set at the lowest possible level and only increased incrementally when the low setting does not allow for an effective examination.

Optimizing angle of insonation relative to vessel orientation

To ensure proper perception of flow by colour Doppler, or an accurate display of the spectral velocity, the angle of insonation should be less than 60°. Finding an appropriate angle can be especially problematic when examining transplanted kidneys because their vessels may be extremely tortuous and a committed search for a suitable Doppler window is required[6].

Minimizing transducer pressure

Often the imaging study is limited because intervening adipose tissue increases the distance from the patient's skin to the transplanted kidney or there is gas in the overlying bowel. By applying sufficient pressure, fat or bowel loops can be displaced. Doing so, however, will compromise the Doppler examination as the renal parenchyma is compressed and inflow during diastole is impeded (Fig. 9.2). This results in an elevation of the measured resistive index. Thus, care must be taken not to apply pressure to the kidney, or its vessels, so that any diagnosis made on the basis of the resistive index or velocity measurement is more accurate[7].

COMPLICATIONS OF RENAL TRANSPLANTATION

Functional complications

These include hyperacute rejection, acute rejection, chronic rejection, perioperative ischaemia, acute tubular necrosis, and drug

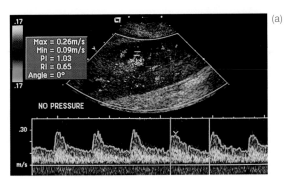
(a)

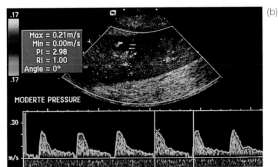
(b)

Fig. 9.2 (a) Renal transplant interlobar artery spectral Doppler tracing acquired with gentle transducer contact. Note the normal waveform and 65% resistive index. (b) When moderate pressure is applied by the transducer the tracing of the same artery now exhibits an elevated resistive index of 100%. Transducer pressure alone is responsible for this alteration in resistance.

toxicity (most commonly immunosuppressive agents)[8,9]. Imaging techniques, including ultrasound with Doppler, are limited in their ability to identify and distinguish these functional complications.

With hyperacute rejection, graft failure occurs rapidly secondary to the presence of preformed anti-donor circulating antibodies. This condition is most often observed in patients undergoing retransplantation. Because renal function is so short-lived, ultrasound has little role in its evaluation.

Acute rejection is a cellular-mediated process, whereby the immune system attacks the foreign renal allograft. It is controlled by the use of steroids, cyclosporine, and other immunosuppressive agents. Occasional elevation in a transplant recipient's immune status (from viral illness or non-compliance with drug therapy) can result in an acceleration of acute rejection to a critical level. The kidney becomes oedematous and swollen, intracapsular pressure rises, eventually resistance to vascular perfusion increases (Fig. 9.3). Although early investigators proposed that resistive index elevation was useful in identifying acute rejection as the cause of kidney transplant dysfunction, subsequent laboratory and clinical studies have shown it to be unreliable. Indeed, it has been found in a canine study that resistive index decreases in the mild to moderate stages of acute rejection. With mild to moderate rejection, the physical effects of increased intrarenal pressure are counteracted by intrarenal hormonal autoregulatory mechanisms. Elevation of resistive index, therefore, does not manifest until the late stages of severe acute rejection[10].

In truth, the resistive index is rarely affected by mild to moderate rejection and when it is, its specificity is low[11]. It is not until acute rejection progressses to severe levels that the resistive index becomes consistently elevated. This, however, can also occur from many other causes such as hydronephrosis, acute tubular necrosis, infection, and compression of the kidney by an adjacent mass or fluid collection. Thus, specificity for the diagnosis of acute rejection by Doppler ultrasound is unacceptably low and renal biopsy is still needed to establish the diagnosis[10-15].

Chronic rejection is primarily an antibody-mediated process, but the pathophysiology is not entirely understood. Doppler indices rarely show any significant alteration in flow profiles with chronic rejection[14].

Perioperative ischaemia can result in transient compromise of renal function, but the

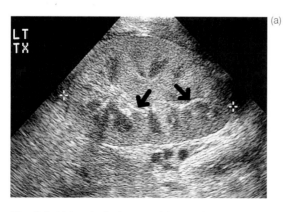 (a)

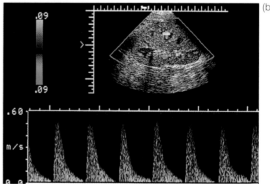 (b)

Fig. 9.3 (a) Longitudinal grey-scale image of a recently transplanted kidney. Note the rounded globular configuration of the kidney. The central hilar space (arrows) is compressed due to oedema and swelling. (b) Spectral Doppler tracing at the interlobar artery level. Resistive index approximates 100%. Biopsy confirmed severe acute rejection.

condition typically resolves within 1–2 weeks of transplantation. The kidney appears oedematous, especially the medullary pyramids, and Doppler studies will show an increase in the resistive index. Although these findings may indicate acute tubular necrosis, they are not considered specific[10, 16] (Fig. 9.4).

Anatomical complications

These include haematomas, seromas, urinomas, abscesses, lymphocoeles, obstructive hydronephrosis, focal masses, arterial and venous stenosis or thrombosis, and intrarenal arteriovenous fistula and pseudoaneurysm[8, 9]. Unlike functional complications, most anatomic complications are readily identified by ultrasound.

Perinephric fluid is a common sequela of renal transplantation and is not considered significant if it is crescentic in shape, or decreases in size over time. Most are *haematomas* or *seromas* which result from oozing from the transplant bed; *urinomas* are relatively uncommon and usually are the result of breakdown at the ureteral anastomosis to the bladder. Doppler examination is of limited value in these cases.

A patient with a rounded, expansile collection with internal debris and associated signs of infection usually has an *abscess*. It is usually difficult to diagnose an abscess by sonography alone and computed tomography (CT) is considered a better imaging study for this purpose. Occasionally colour Doppler may reveal hyperaemia of the tissues surrounding the abscess.

Lymphocoeles usually become apparent about 6–8 weeks postoperatively and are seen as rounded or lobulated collections near the vascular anastomoses. They are the result of surgical disruption of lymphatic channels when the vascular anastomosis to the transplanted kidney is created. An expanding lymphocoele may cause ureteric compression and hydronephrosis. If a lymphocoele becomes large enough, it may compress or kink the renal vascular pedicle. In this situation, Doppler examination may show findings similar to arterial or venous stenosis (Fig. 9.5).

Transient dilatation of the collecting system as a result of anastomotic oedema frequently occurs immediately after renal transplantation, or removal of the ureteral stent. The presence of a

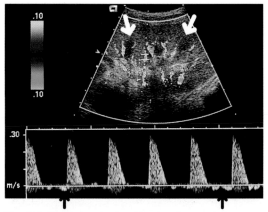

Fig. 9.4 Spectral and colour Doppler ultrasound of a transplant kidney within 24 hours of implantation. This cadaver organ experienced prolonged ischaemic time. Note the prominent hypoechoic medullary pyramids (arrows). The resistive index is elevated to over 100% since reversed flow can be perceived in diastole (arrowheads).

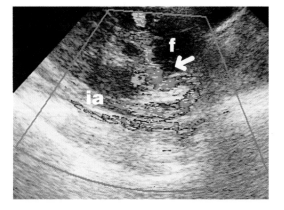

Fig. 9.5 Oblique colour Doppler image of a renal transplant in the iliac fossa. A rounded, lobulated fluid (f) collection is identified inferomedial to the kidney, displacing it cephalad. This large lymphocoele caused a kink in the main renal artery (arrow). External iliac artery is shown (ia). Reproduced with permission from McGann and Goldberg[34].

dilated transplant collecting system does not automatically signify an obstructed system under pressure, as a denervated, flaccid collecting system can become markedly dilated, particularly when the urinary bladder is distended[16]. Platt *et al*[17, 18] proposed use of an elevated resistive index to distinguish obstructive hydronephrosis from chronic dilatation in the renal transplant. Although this measurement may be sensitive, its specificity is very poor because of the many other factors that also affect renal haemodynamics. At this time, the Whitaker test remains the 'gold standard' for diagnosing significant obstruction of the renal transplant collecting system.

Vascular complications

Following renal transplantation, vascular complications are observed in less than 10% of recipients; however, when present, they are associated with a high morbidity and mortality. Complications include renal artery or vein stenosis, compression, kinking, thrombosis, intrarenal arteriovenous fistulae and pseudo-aneurysms. If identified promptly, they can often be successfully repaired prior to transplant failure. Doppler sonography is a very effective, non-invasive screening modality for identifying significant vascular complications[19–21].

Renal transplant artery stenosis

This is most often observed within 1–2 cm of the anastomosis, usually as a result of vessel wall ischaemia due to surgical disruption of the vasa vasorum. Stenosis should be suspected if a tardus parvus waveform and relatively low-resistance flow are noted in the intrarenal branches. A tardus parvus waveform is characterized by a delayed upstroke in systole (>0.07 s), rounding of the systolic peak and obliteration of the early systolic notch. A flow velocity greater than 2 m s^{-1} with associated distal turbulence near the renal artery anastomosis is diagnostic of renal artery stenosis (Fig. 9.6). The examiner should conduct a thorough examination from the renal hilum to the iliac artery in search of a focal stenosis, especially if an intrarenal tardus parvus waveform is noted[22–26] (Fig. 9.7). A vascular kink can cause similar haemodynamic changes and is better identified on colour or power Doppler images.

Approximately 20% of transplanted kidneys require more than one arterial anastomosis due to the presence of accessory arteries. If one of these vessels becomes compromised, then perfusion to the subtended segment of the kidney is decreased. Again, a tardus parvus waveform may be seen, this time limited to the area perfused by the affected artery. If

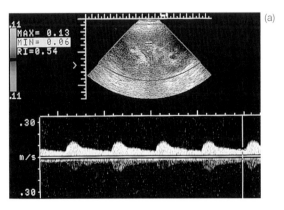
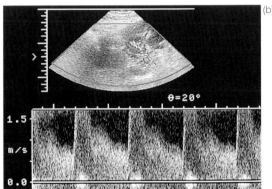

Fig. 9.6 (a) Renal transplant arcuate artery spectral Doppler tracing in a hypertensive recipient with elevated serum creatinine. The intrarenal arterial waveform manifests a slow systolic upstroke, a rounded systolic peak and relatively low resistance. These findings suggest a more proximal stenosis. (b) Spectral Doppler tracing just distal to the anastomosis of the main renal artery to the iliac artery. Note the very high, turbulent flow characteristic of renal artery stenosis.

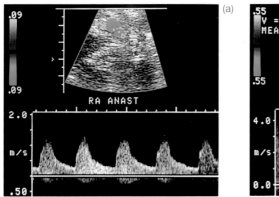 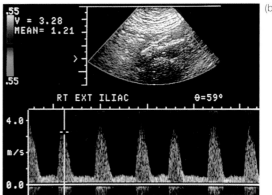

Fig. 9.7 (a) Spectral Doppler tracing of a transplant main renal artery. Tardus parvus changes were present in this waveform but no anastomotic stenosis was perceived. (b) Spectral Doppler tracing of the external iliac artery. A high-velocity jet is identified with velocities of >3 m s⁻¹. This diabetic recipient had an atheromatous lesion in the iliac artery compromising inflow to the renal transplant.

thrombosis of this artery occurs, then the subtended area shows no flow on colour or power Doppler and an arterial tracing will not be identified by spectral Doppler. The area affected will vary depending on the anatomic vascular distribution (Fig. 9.8).

Renal parenchymal scarring secondary to chronic rejection may result in focal stenosis within branch arteries. This should be suspected if there is irregular distribution of flow on colour Doppler through the kidney. Segmental or interlobar renal artery stenosis

can be confirmed by the presence of intrarenal high-velocity flow. Because these lesions are typically multiple and distal, treatment options are limited[27].

Renal vein stenosis

Vein stenosis is an uncommon complication following kidney transplantation, but when present, it is a significant cause of graft dysfunction. Venous stenosis may be seen as a focal narrowing with associated dilatation of the

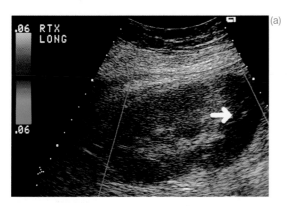 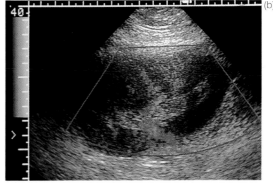

Fig. 9.8 (a) Colour Doppler image of a poorly functioning transplant kidney. The lower pole is hypoechoic (arrow). Little flow is seen throughout the kidney. (b) With power Doppler, flow is identified through the mid- and upper kidney but none is seen in the lower pole. Thrombosis of the lower pole artery was suggested and confirmed angiographically. Ultrasound-guided biopsy of the upper pole confirmed acute rejection.

9

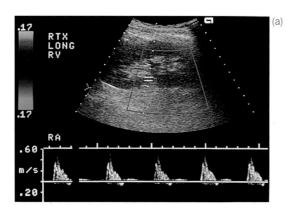

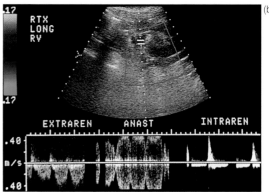

Fig. 9.9 (a) Spectral Doppler tracing at the level of the main renal artery of a poorly functioning transplant kidney. There is very high resistance to arterial inflow. (b) Spectral Doppler tracing obtained at various points long the renal vein. There is slow velocity at the intrarenal component, increasing velocity with some periodicity at the extrarenal component, and a very high velocity with turbulence at the anticipated point of anastomosis. Stenosis of the renal vein was confirmed at venography and treated with angioplasty.

proximal vein. However, to confirm the diagnosis of a significant stenosis, there should be at least a three- to fourfold velocity gradient across the lesion. If the gradient is less than threefold, it is seldom considered clinically significant, even though it may have a dramatic appearance on Doppler examination[28] (Fig. 9.9).

Renal vein thrombosis

This is also a relatively rare posttransplantation complication. It is usually seen within the first week following surgery. It may be the result of technical difficulty with the venous anastomosis, it may be due to preservation injury, or it may occur during an episode of severe acute allograft rejection. Extremely high resistance (resistive index typically greater than 100%) will be seen on the renal arterial waveforms on spectral Doppler. In most cases, the thrombus results in partial rather than complete occlusion of the vein and some renal venous outflow can be detected on spectral Doppler. To prevent a false-negative diagnosis, it is important that the examiner conduct a careful imaging and colour Doppler evaluation of the vein when high arterial resistance is noted[29] (Fig. 9.10).

Intrarenal arteriovenous fistulae and pseudoaneurysms

These are typically the result of renal transplant biopsy. The true incidence of these complications varies from centre to centre depending on biopsy technique. Arteriovenous fistulae manifest as a flash of colour, or 'visible bruit', in the adjacent parenchyma when the

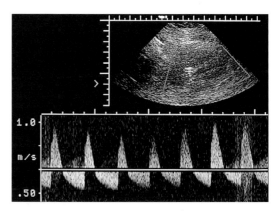

Fig. 9.10 Spectral Doppler tracing of the main renal transplant artery in a recent recipient with a rapidly rising creatinine. The arterial waveform reveals to-and-fro flow with the retrograde component being essentially equal to antegrade flow. The resistive index measures approximately 140%. No flow could be identified by spectral or colour Doppler in the renal veins. Complete thrombosis was confirmed at angiography.

transplanted kidney is examined at normal colour Doppler settings. This phenomenon is caused by vibration of the surrounding tissues secondary to the rapidly flowing blood through the fistula. It is often possible to distinguish the feeding artery and the enlarged draining vein with higher-velocity colour Doppler settings. Spectral Doppler tracings will demonstrate a high-velocity, low-resistance flow within the feeding artery and turbulent, pulsatile flow will be present in the draining segmental vein. If the arteriovenous fistula is large enough, it may be possible to observe pulsatile flow within the main renal vein (Fig. 9.11). Pseudoaneurysms usually appear as a simple cystic structure, or a small collection of paravascular fluid. Colour Doppler, however, immediately reveals that the finding is not a simple cyst. Spectral Doppler tracings show to-and-fro blood flow at the neck of the pseudoaneurysm and a

distorted, turbulent, pulsatile waveform can be observed within the pseudoaneurysm. The vast majority of intrarenal arteriovenous fistulae and pseudoaneurysms resolve spontaneously, but if they increase in size over a period of time, angiographic embolization may be necessary to treat the condition[30, 31].

SUMMARY

In summary, these are very rewarding times in the field of renal transplantation. Advances in kidney procurement and preservation; better matching of donors and recipients; refined surgical techniques; availability of new, more effective immunosuppressive agents; and improved posttransplant monitoring of kidney recipients have contributed to decreased patient morbidity and improved allograft survival. Although Doppler sonography is only able to make a definitive

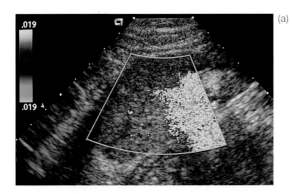
(a)

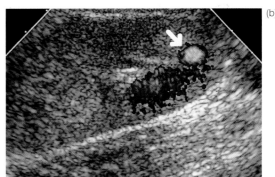
(b)

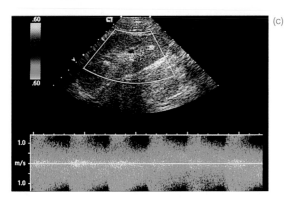
(c)

Fig. 9.11 (a) Colour Doppler image of a renal transplant approximately 2 weeks after biopsy. A burst of colour is seen overlying the lower pole. This flash artefact, due to tissue vibration, suggests an underlying arteriovenous fistula. (b) A power Doppler image with high filtration and pulse repetition frequency reveals the focus of the arteriovenous fistula (arrow). (c) Spectral Doppler tracing obtained at the fistula site reveals a turbulent, high-velocity arterial waveform.

diagnosis in a small percentage of cases, it is extremely useful as a screening tool in the management of renal transplant complica-tions. All of this has allowed transplant patients greater opportunity to return to a more normal lifestyle after surgery[32, 33].

REFERENCES

1. Riehle RA, Steckler R, Naslund EB, Riggio R, Cheigh J, Stubenbord W (1990) Selection criteria for the evaluation of living-related renal donor. *Journal of Urology* **144**: 845–848
2. US Department of Health and Human Services, Public Health Service (1995) *Annual report of the US Scientific Registry of Transplant Recipients and the Organ Procurement and Transplantation Network, 1988–1994*
3. US Department of Health and Human Services, Public Health Service (1996) *Annual report of the US Scientific Registry of Transplant Recipients and the Organ Procurement and Transplantation Network, 1988–1995*
4. Belzer FO (1991) Transplantation of the right kidney: surgical technique revisited. *Surgery* **110**: 113–115
5. Solinger HW, Ploeg RJ, Eckhoff DE *et al* (1993) Two hundred consecutive simultaneous pancreas–kidney transplants with bladder drainage. *Surgery* **114**: 736–743
6. Pozniak MA, Zagzebski J, Scanlan KA (1992) Spectral and colour Doppler artefacts. *RadioGraphics* **12**: 35–44
7. Pozniak MA, Kelcz F, Stratta R, Oberley T (1988) Extraneous factors affecting resistive index. *Investigative Radiology* **23**: 899–904
8. Benoit G, Blanchet P, Moukarzel M *et al* (1994) Surgical complications in kidney transplantation. *Transplant Proceedings* **26**: 287–288
9. Hashimoto Y, Nagano S, Ohsima S *et al* (1996) Surgical complications in kidney transplantation: experience from 1200 transplants performed over 20 years at six hospitals in central Japan. *Transplant Proceedings* **28**: 1465–1467
10. Pozniak MA, Kelcz F, D'Alessandro A *et al* (1992) Sonography of renal transplants: the effect of acute tubular necrosis, cyclosporine nephrotoxicity, and acute rejection on resistive index and renal length. *American Journal of Radiology* **158**: 791–797
11. Genkins SM, Sanfilippo FP, Carroll BA (1989) Duplex Doppler sonography of renal transplants: lack of sensitivity and specificity in establishing pathologic diagnosis. *American Journal of Radiology* **152**: 535–539
12. Kelcz F, Pozniak MA, Pirsch JD *et al* (1990) Pyramidal appearance and resistive index: insensitive and non-specific sonographic indicators of renal transplant rejection. *American Journal of Radiology* **155**: 531–535
13. Perrella RR, Duerincky AJ, Tessler FN *et al* (1990) Evaluation of renal transplant dysfunction by duplex Doppler sonography: a prospective study and review of the literature. *American Journal of Kidney Diseases* **15**: 544–550
14. Akiyama T, Ikegami M, Hara Y *et al* (1996) Haemodynamic study of renal transplant chronic rejection using power Doppler sonography. *Transplant Proceedings* **28**: 1458–1460
15. Saarinen O (1991) Diagnostic value of resistive index of renal transplants in the early postoperative period. *Acta Radiologica* **32**: 166–169
16. Koga S, Tanabe K, Yagisawa TT, Toma H (1996) Urologic complications in renal transplantation. *Transplant Proceedings* **28**: 1472–1473
17. Platt JF, Rubin JM, Ellis JH (1989) Distinction between obstructive and non-obstructive pyelocaliectasis with duplex Doppler sonography. *American Journal of Radiology* **153**: 997–1000
18. Platt JF, Ellis JH, Rubin JM (1991) Renal transplant pyelocaliectasis: role of duplex Doppler US in evaluation. *Radiology* **179**: 425–428
19. Dodd GD, Tublin ME, Shah A *et al* (1991) Imaging of vascular complications associated with renal transplantation. *American Journal of Radiology* **157**: 449–459
20. Pozniak MA, Dodd GD, Kelcz F (1992) Ultrasonographic evaluation of renal transplantation. *Radiology Clinics of North America* **30**: 1053–1066
21. Grenier N, Douws C, Morel D *et al* (1991) Detection of vascular complications in renal allografts with colour Doppler flow imaging. *Radiology* **178**: 217–223
22. Baxter GM, Ireland H, Moss JG *et al* (1995) Colour Doppler ultrasound in renal transplant artery stenosis: which Doppler index? *Clinical Radiology* **50**: 618–622
23. Roberts JP, Ascher NL, Fryd DS *et al* (1989) Transplant renal artery stenosis. *Transplantation* **4**: 580–583
24. Patriquin HB, Lafortune M, Jequier JC *et al* (1992) Stenosis of the renal artery: assessment of slowed systole in the downstream circulation with Doppler sonography. *Radiology* **184**: 479–485
25. Saarinen O, Salmela K, Edgren J (1994) Doppler ultrasound in the diagnosis of renal transplant artery stenosis – value of resistive index. *Acta Radiologica* **35**: 586–589
26. Handa N, Fukunaga R, Etani H *et al* (1988) Efficacy of echo-Doppler examination for the evaluation of renovascular disease. *Ultrasound in Medicine and Biology* **14**: 1–5

27. Stavros AT, Parker SH, Yakes WF *et al* (1992) Segmental stenosis of the renal artery: pattern recognition of tardus and parvus abnormalities with duplex sonography. *Radiology* **184**: 487–492

28. Kribs SW, Rankin RN (1993) Doppler ultrasonography after renal transplantation: value of reversed diastolic flow in diagnosing renal vein obstruction. *Canadian Association of Radiologists' Journal* **44**: 434–438

29. Baxter GM, Morley P, Dall B (1991) Acute renal vein thrombosis in renal allografts: new Doppler ultrasonic findings. *Clinical Radiology* **43**(2): 125–127

30. Middleton WD, Kellman GM, Melson GL *et al* (1989) Postbiopsy renal transplant arteriovenous fistulas: colour Doppler versus US characteristics. *Radiology* **171**: 253–257

31. Hubsch PJS, Mostbeck G, Barton PP *et al* (1990) Evaluation of arteriovenous fistulas and pseudoaneurysms in renal allografts following percutaneous needle biopsy: colour coded Doppler sonography vs duplex Doppler sonography. *Journal of Ultrasound in Medicine* **9**: 95–100

32. Lee HM (1996) Quality of life after renal transplantation. *Transplant Proceedings* **28**: 1171

33. Park IH, Yoo HJ, Han DJ *et al* (1996) Changes in the quality of life before and after renal transplantation and comparison of the quality of life between kidney transplant recipients, dialysis patients, and normal controls. *Transplant Proceedings* **28**: 1937–1938

34. McGann JP, Goldberg B. (1998). *Diagnostic Ultrasound: A Logical Approach*. Philadelphia: Lippincott, Williams & Wilkins.

DOPPLER ULTRASOUND EVALUATION OF RENAL TRANSPLANTATION

Doppler imaging of the prostate

10

FRED T. LEE, Jr.

INDICATIONS

The most important use of colour Doppler imaging of the prostate remains as an aid in cancer detection. This is particularly relevant in patients in whom cancer is suspected based on prostate specific antigen (PSA) elevation without obvious tumour on grey-scale imaging. Other uses for Doppler imaging are largely confined to detection of prostatitis and inflammatory conditions. Controversy continues surrounding diagnosis and treatment of prostate cancer. This is largely attributable to the wide range of biological behaviour found with this disease. Up to 30% of 80-year-old males will have histologic evidence of prostate cancer, yet most will die from other causes. Unfortunately, a more aggressive subset of prostate cancer remains an important cause of mortality among men, with greater than 30 000 deaths a year in the United States.

ANATOMY

The prostate lies immediately anterior to the rectum and inferior to the bladder. Prostatic zonal anatomy has been extensively described by McNeal[1]. In summary, the prostate is composed of three major zonal areas; the peripheral zone, the central zone, and the transition zone (Fig. 10.1). The peripheral zone is the most posterior, and the central zone is a continuation of the peripheral zone cephalad. The transition zone is the most central area of the prostate, and surrounds the urethra as it courses through the prostate. The anterior fibromuscular stroma lines the prostate anteriorly.

Prostate vascular anatomy

The prostate is supplied from two arterial sources: the prostatic arteries and the inferior vesical arteries, both arising from the internal iliac system. The prostatic arteries enter the prostate from an anterolateral location on each side, and give off capsular branches as well as urethral branches. Capsular arteries course along the lateral margin of the prostate, and

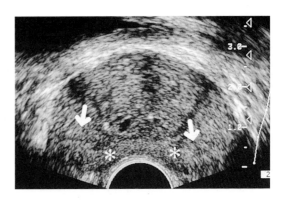

Fig. 10.1 Axial ultrasound of the prostate in a normal patient. Note peripheral zone (asterisks) separated from the more centrally oriented, periurethral transition zone by the surgical capsule (arrows).

give off numerous perforating branches which penetrate the capsule and supply approximately two thirds of the total glandular tissue. The areas of penetration into the capsule are commonly referred to as the neurovascular bundles (Fig. 10.2). The inferior vesical arteries run along the inferior surface of the bladder and also provide urethral branches. In addition to supplying the central portion of the prostate, the inferior vesical arteries also give off branches which supply the bladder base, seminal vesicles and distal ureters (Fig. 10.3)[2, 3]. Both the capsular and urethral branches can be visualized with colour Doppler ultrasound. In the absence of inflammation, neoplasm or hypertrophy, the normal prostate is expected to have low-level periurethral and pericapsular flow, with only a low level of flow in the prostatic parenchyma[4].

EQUIPMENT AND TECHNIQUE

Examination of the prostate by ultrasound requires a high-frequency (5–7.5 MHz) end-fire or biplane transrectal transducer. For the purposes of this chapter, conventional colour Doppler and power Doppler are considered simultaneously. For most general applications, an end-fire transducer is favoured due

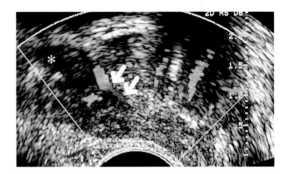

Fig. 10.3 Sagittal image of the prostate at the level of the seminal vesicle (asterisk) demonstrates periurethral flow (arrows) originating from the inferior vesicle artery.

to the ease of switching between axial (coronal) and longitudinal imaging planes, as well as the more favourable angle for transrectal prostatic biopsies. For specialized applications such as prostatic volumetry, brachytherapy and cryosurgery, a true biplane transducer is necessary.

No specific patient preparation is required, although some centres will give the patient a pre-examination enema and have them empty their bladder. The patient is generally placed in the left lateral decubitus position, and the knees brought up to the chest. A digital rectal examination is recommended prior to probe insertion, to rule out any obstructing pathology and also to allow the examiner to evaluate the prostate by digital examination. The probe is covered with a condom into which coupling gel has been placed, and the probe lubricated and gently inserted into the rectal canal.

Examination of the prostate by grey-scale imaging is first performed, and the length, width and height of the gland measured. The prostatic volume is calculated based on the formula for a prolate ellipsoid (length × width × height × 0.523); this allows correlation of the measured PSA with a predicted PSA based on gland volume. Normal prostatic tissue produces approximately 0.3 ng cc^{-1} of PSA, whereas cancerous tissue produces

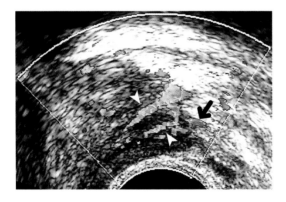

Fig. 10.2 Axial image of the left neurovascular bundle. Note left neurovascular bundle (arrow) with perforating branches penetrating into the prostate (arrowheads).

approximately 3.0 ng cc^{-1} of tumour. Normal levels for polyclonal assays are typically defined as <4.0 ng/ml^{-1}; unfortunately, up to 20% of prostatic cancers present in patients with 'normal' levels of PSA. A 'predicted' PSA can be generated based on the patient's gland volume × 0.2 for polyclonal assays (or gland volume × 0.1 for monoclonal assays). A level of measured PSA that exceeds predicted PSA increases the suspicion of cancer and increases the positive predictive value of prostatic biopsy[5].

Most prostate cancers (70%) arise in the peripheral zone, with a minority originating in the central (10–15%) and transition (10–15%) zones. Because of this, it is very important that the sonographer carefully examines the peripheral zone for signs of tumour. Virtually all prostate cancers will be hypoechoic in relation to normal peripheral zone tissues (Fig. 10.4), although a minority of cribriform carcinomas can demonstrate punctate calcifications. Tumours in the peripheral zone have ready access to sites of anatomic weakness, including the neurovascular bundles, ejaculatory ducts and apex of the gland. This results in more aggressive clinical behaviour of peripheral zone tumours when compared to other locations.

Transition zone tumours tend to behave in a clinically more benign manner because they are distant from sites of anatomic weakness, and

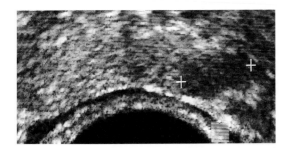

Fig. 10.4 Prostate cancer. Axial image of the prostate at the mid-gland. Hypoechoic tumour (crosses) originates in the left neurovascular bundle area.

thus need to grow quite large before spreading outside of the gland. The main problem with the diagnosis of transition zone tumours is the heterogeneous echotexture of the normal transition zone. Because normal transition zone tissue can be hypoechoic, hyperechoic, or contain calcifications or cysts, it is extremely difficult to diagnose subtle changes in echogenicity that may be associated with neoplasia. Therefore, colour Doppler can play a crucial role in the diagnosis of transition zone tumours by identifying areas of abnormal flow.

COLOUR DOPPLER OF PROSTATE CANCER

Knowledge of the excess PSA for a particular gland is most important from an ultrasound standpoint when an obvious peripheral zone tumour is not found in the face of an elevated measured PSA. As previously mentioned, transition zone tumours are difficult to visualize by grey-scale criteria due to the homogeneous nature of normal transition zone tissue. Once it is established that the patient is at high risk for prostate cancer by PSA criteria, and no peripheral zone cancer has been found, a careful examination of the transition zone should be undertaken. It is in the search for transition zone tumours that colour Doppler ultrasound has proven to be most useful. Prostate cancer is generally hypervascular when compared to normal prostatic tissue, and this is manifested as increased colour-encoding at sensitive instrument settings (Fig. 10.5). These can be targeted for biopsy with increased positive biopsy rates compared to blinded sextant biopsies. Spectral Doppler plays a limited role in the specific diagnosis of prostate cancer. Tumours tend to have low-resistance (high-diastolic) flow, although the exact role and specificity of this finding has yet to be fully elucidated.

The use of colour Doppler in the diagnosis of peripheral zone tumours is more controversial. Several authors have found increased

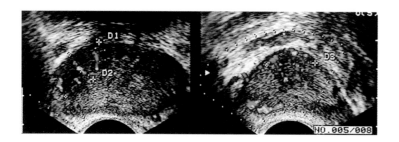

Fig. 10.5 Transition zone prostate cancer (biopsy proven). Axial (left) and sagittal (right) images demonstrate a hypervascular tumour in the transition zone (calipers).

colour Doppler flow to have no significant correlation with the presence or absence of tumour at histology. In addition, there has been no colour Doppler method which consistently discriminates tumour from focal prostatitis in areas of increased flow. Others have found biopsy of sites of increased flow useful in the face of an increased measured PSA (greater than predicted) and no other obvious sites of tumour[6]. This has been found to be particularly useful in black males, where the positive predictive value for biopsy of a focal area of increased colour-encoding has been found to be twice that of white males (32.2% vs. 13.5% respectively)[7]. Most authors now feel that colour Doppler is more of a complementary

test to grey-scale ultrasound, PSA and gland volume rather than a single factor on which to base biopsy decisions (Fig. 10.6).

COLOUR DOPPLER OF PROSTATIC INFLAMMATORY DISEASE

Prostatitis is a difficult condition to diagnose and treat. There are several aetiologies of prostatitis, ranging from bacterial to non-bacterial causes. In the case of bacterial prostatitis, the offending organism is usually *Escherichia coli* or other urinary tract pathogens.

Grey-scale findings of acute prostatitis include a hypoechoic rim around the prostate or periurethral areas, and low-level echogenic

(a)

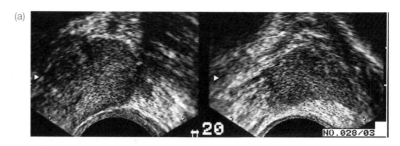

(b)

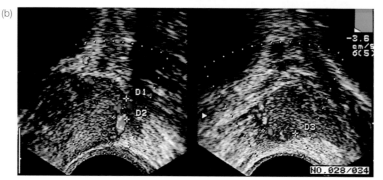

Fig. 10.6 Peripheral zone prostate cancer. (a) and (b) Axial and sagittal grey-scale images demonstrate a subtle hypoechoic area in the left neurovascular bundle (calipers). Biopsy through this area was positive for adenocarcinoma, Gleason score 6. (c) and (d) Axial and sagittal colour Doppler images at corresponding locations demonstrate increased colour flow in areas involved by tumour.

areas within the prostate[8]. Colour Doppler is useful in cases of diffuse bacterial prostatitis. The severity of the inflammatory reaction is mirrored by focal or diffuse increase in the colour signal in the prostatic parenchyma[9]. When focally increased colour signals are seen in cases of prostatitis, there is no reliable non-invasive method to differentiate inflammation from tumour[9]. However, cases of grossly increased flow spread diffusely throughout the gland should be considered prostatitis in the appropriate clinical setting (Fig. 10.7). When the inflammatory process continues to suppuration, a prostatic abscess can develop. On ultrasound, this is seen as a cavity filled with low-level echoes from debris (Fig. 10.8)[10]. Colour Doppler may detect increased flow around the rim of the cavity, although this finding is not necessary to make the diagnosis. Cases of bacterial prostatitis are treated by antibiotics, whereas prostatic abscess requires transrectal catheter or transurethral drainage with unroofing of the abscess cavity.

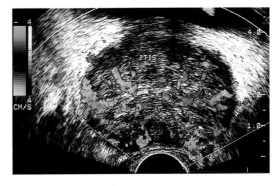

Fig. 10.7 Prostatitis. Colour Doppler image of diffuse prostatitis demonstrates grossly increased flow throughout the gland.

CONCLUSIONS

Doppler ultrasound of the prostate contributes significantly to the diagnostic value of sonography in the assessment of prostatic disease. Colour and power Doppler identify areas of abnormal blood flow, which can then be examined more closely with grey-scale imaging, or biopsied under ultrasound guidance.

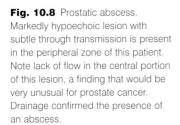

Fig. 10.8 Prostatic abscess. Markedly hypoechoic lesion with subtle through transmission is present in the peripheral zone of this patient. Note lack of flow in the central portion of this lesion, a finding that would be very unusual for prostate cancer. Drainage confirmed the presence of an abscess.

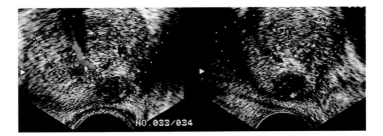

REFERENCES

1. McNeal JE (1968) Regional morphology and pathology of the prostate. *American Journal of Clinical Pathology* 49: 347–357
2. Flocks RH (1937) The arterial distribution within the prostate gland: its role in transurethral prostatic resection. *Journal of Urology* 37: 524–548
3. Clegg EJ (1955) The arterial supply of the human prostate and seminal vesicles. *Journal of Anatomy* 89: 209–217
4. Neumaier CE, Martinoli C, Derchi LE, Silvestri E, Rosenberg I (1995) Normal prostate gland:

examination with colour Doppler US. *Radiology* 196: 453–457
5. Lee F, Littrup PJ, Loft-Christensen L *et al* (1992) Predicted prostate specific antigen results using transrectal ultrasound gland volume: differentiation of benign prostatic hyperplasia and prostate cancer. *Cancer* 70: 211–220
6. DeCarvalho VS, Soto JA, Guidone PL, Kuligowska E (1995) Role of colour Doppler in improving the detection of cancer in the isoechoic prostate gland (abstract). *Radiology* 197(P): 365

7. Littrup PJ, Klein RM, Sparschu RA *et al* (1995) Colour Doppler of the prostate: histologic and racial correlations (abstract). *Radiology* **197**(P): 365

8. Griffiths GJ, Crooks AJR, Roberts EE *et al* (1984) Ultrasonic appearances associated with prostatic inflammation: a preliminary study. *Clinincal Radiology* **35**: 343–345

9. Patel U, Rickards D (1994) The diagnostic value of colour Doppler flow in the peripheral zone of the prostate, with histological correlation. *British Journal of Urology* **74**: 590–595

10. Lee FT Jr., Lee F, Solomon MH *et al* (1986) Ultrasonic demonstration of prostatic abscess. *Journal of Ultrasound in Medicine* **5**: 101

Doppler imaging of the penis

11

MYRON A. POZNIAK and FRED T. LEE, Jr.

Duplex sonography with colour Doppler is rapidly becoming the initial modality of choice for evaluating the penis, because of ease of performance, versatility, minimally invasive nature, reproducibility, and relative availability and low cost[1-5]. Colour Doppler allows the examiner to delineate vascular anatomy, display dynamic variations in blood flow, measure arterial velocity and infer venous drainage[1,2]. By combining Doppler with grey-scale imaging, both anatomical and physiological abnormalities can be assessed during the flaccid and erect states[2-4].

INDICATIONS

The primary application of penile Doppler imaging is to assess the penile vasculature in patients with suspected vasculogenic impotence. While impotence may be the result of psychogenic, neurogenic or hormonal factors, vascular disease is one of the leading causes of erectile dysfunction[4,6]. The initial report of Doppler sonography combined with pharmacological induction of erection to evaluate vasculogenic impotence was by Lue *et al*[7] in the mid-1980s. Today, with advances in Doppler technology, the haemodynamic information available greatly enhances our ability to determine if a patient's impotence is due to a vascular aetiology, such as arterial insuffi-

ciency, venous incompetence, or a combination of the two[2,4,7-19].

Doppler imaging may help to identify arterial or venous injury following acute penile trauma[3,20,21]. In addition, Doppler, and grey-scale ultrasound, may be used to evaluate patients with Peyronie's disease, an idiopathic process which produces fibrous plaques in the penile tunica albuginea[3,22,23], specifically to determine if these plaques cause any significant vascular compromise[24].

PENILE ANATOMY

The penis contains three longitudinal, erectile bodies[1,2]. Two corpora cavernosa are located in the dorsal two thirds of the penile shaft, and a single corpus spongiosum is located in the ventral one third of the shaft. The corpora cavernosa are enclosed by the tunica albuginea, a thick fascial layer. The septum that divides the corpora cavernosa contains fenestrations that create multiple connecting anastomotic channels between the sinusoidal spaces, allowing for free communication across the midline. The dorsal arteries, veins and nerves are situated centrally along the penile dorsum, superficial to the tunica albuginea and deep to Buck's fascia. The urethra is contained within the corpus spongiosum.

Arterial anatomy

The *internal pudendal artery* and its branches are the primary source of arterial supply to the penis[1, 2]. The first three branches are the superficial perineal artery, the bulbar artery and a small urethral artery. The *perineal artery* is a large and constant branch that, in 80% of cases, has an internal and external branch. The *bulbar artery*, which supplies the proximal penile shaft, is usually easily identified during angiography because it is associated with a bulbar parenchymal blush in the early arterial phase. The *urethral artery*, which is of small diameter, arises anterior to the bulbar artery. From this point, the internal pudendal artery continues as the common penile artery. The left and right *common penile arteries* enter the base of the penis and branch into a dorsal artery and a cavernosal artery. The *dorsal artery* extends along the dorsal aspect of the penile shaft towards the glans and terminates at the level of the arterial corona of the glans; it supplies blood primarily to the skin, subcutaneous tissues and glans. Collateral vessels from the dorsal artery often communicate with the cavernosal artery. The *cavernosal* or *deep*

penile artery enters the tunica albuginea proximally and extends the length of the corpus cavernosum. The cavernosal arteries and their helicine branches are the primary source of blood flow to the erectile tissue of the penis. Just as the cavernosal artery supplies blood to the corpus cavernosum, the *spongiosal artery* supplies the corpus spongiosum (Fig. 11.1).

Venous anatomy

Venous drainage of the penile erectile tissue (i.e. the sinusoidal spaces) primarily occurs through *emissary (efferent) veins* which drain the corpus cavernosum, penetrate the tunica albuginea, and empty into the circumflex veins[1, 2]; these then drain into the deep dorsal venous system of the penis. The emissary veins may also drain directly into the *deep dorsal vein*. The *superficial dorsal vein* drains the distal portion of the corpora cavernosa, as well as the skin and glans. The deep and the superficial dorsal veins can be routinely visualized by colour Doppler imaging in the midline of the penile shaft. The most proximal portions of the corpora cavernosa are drained

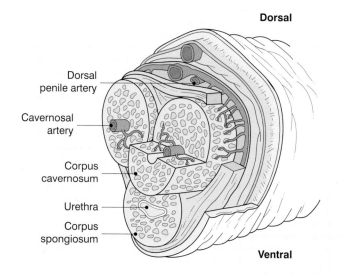

Dorsal

Dorsal penile artery

Cavernosal artery

Corpus cavernosum

Urethra

Corpus spongiosum

Ventral

Fig. 11.1 Normal anatomy. The cavernosal arteries are centrally located in each corpus cavernosus. The urethra courses through the corpus spongiosum. The dorsal penile artery supplies the glans and does not play a direct role in erectile function.

by the cavernosal veins directly into the periprostatic plexus.

Erectile physiology

When the penis is flaccid, its smooth muscle is in a tonic state, the cavernous sinusoids are collapsed, and the cavernous venules are open[4]. The emissary veins drain the sinusoidal spaces and blood circulates into the dorsal veins. During this state, there is high resistance to blood flow into the penis. Erection starts when an autonomic neurogenic impulse relaxes the cavernosal arterioles and sinusoidal spaces[2]. As erection occurs, there is a marked increase in the volume of arterial inflow into the penis as the cavernous arteries dilate. This is accompanied by relaxation of the smooth muscle of the corpora cavernosa, with expansion and elongation of the cavernous sinusoids as they fill with blood. Compression of the cavernous venules between the dilated cavernous sinusoids and the unyielding peripheral tunica albuginea decreases venous outflow. This veno-occlusive mechanism (which depends on neurological stimuli, a sufficient supply of arterial blood, and normal function of the tunica albuginea) maintains sinusoidal distension and rigid erection[1, 2].

Five stages of erectile physiology have been defined by Lue: latent, tumescent, full erection, rigid erection and detumescent[25]. During the latent phase the diameters of the cavernosal arteries are at their greatest and there is maximum inflow of blood with minimal resistance. During tumescence, the sinusoidal cavities of the corpora cavernosa distend with blood. With full erection, blood flow decreases as do the diameters of the cavernosal arteries. With a rigid erection, blood inflow (and outflow) ceases and the diameters of the cavernosal arteries are at their narrowest. Detumescence occurs when the trabeculae and arteries contract in response to a release of norepinephrine (noradrenaline). During the five stages of erection, different arterial diameters and waveform patterns may be seen on Doppler examination.

ULTRASOUND TECHNIQUE

Various techniques for the sonographic examination of the penis have been described, with the changes primarily due to advances in ultrasound technology[1-4, 7, 10, 26]. A linear transducer operating at 7 MHz or higher frequency should be employed. If electronic steering of the Doppler beam is unavailable, a mechanical stand-off wedge may be employed to optimize the Doppler angle of interrogation. Slow-flow sensitivity must be optimized. Filters are set at their lowest levels and the Doppler gain is set just below the noise threshold; the pulse repetition frequency is set to the lowest velocity setting possible. All of these settings can then be adjusted if higher than expected velocity distorts the Doppler display.

The evaluation should be performed in a quiet, private setting with the room comfortably warm and darkened, so that the patient is relaxed and not embarrassed. The scan is performed with the patient lying supine and the penis in the anatomic position (lying superiorly against the anterior abdominal wall). During the examination, the patient may be asked to help keep the penis immobilized by gently holding the corona just under the glans penis and then stretching the shaft along the anterior abdominal wall. Scanning is usually performed on the ventral surface of the penis[1, 3], but the probe can be placed on the dorsal or lateral surfaces if necessary[2, 3]. There should be minimal penile compression with the transducer (Fig. 11.2).

Imaging is performed in both the longitudinal and transverse planes from the base of the penis to the glans, to visualize anatomic details of the corpora cavernosa, cavernosal arteries and surrounding structures, and also to demonstrate any abnormalities such as fibrosis, scarring, plaques, calcification, haematoma or

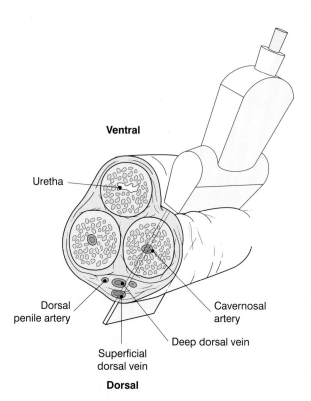

Ventral

Uretha

Dorsal
penile artery

Superficial
dorsal vein

Dorsal

Cavernosal
artery

Deep dorsal vein

Fig. 11.2 Ultrasound technique. A linear transducer is placed in a longitudinal plane along the ventral surface of the penis. Since the cavernosal arteries run parallel to the transducer, electronic steering of the Doppler beam is necessary to interrogate at an appropriate angle.

tumour. The diameter of the arteries and blood flow velocities are measured. Colour Doppler enables the examiner better to correct the angle of insonation, so that peak velocities can be measured more accurately. In addition, with colour Doppler, blood flow direction can be assessed and the presence of any communications between the cavernosal, dorsal and spongiosal arteries can be detected.

PHARMACOLOGICAL INDUCEMENT OF ERECTION

A vasodilating agent is injected into the corpus cavernosum near the base of the penis to induce erection. A number of different agents are available, including papaverine, phentolamine and prostaglandin E1 (PGE1). A standard protocol has not been established and a variety of techniques for using these agents has been reported, either singularly or in various combinations. Reported protocols include 15–60 mg papaverine alone; 30 mg papaverine combined with 1 mg phentolamine; 0.25 ml of a triple mixture of 75 mg papaverine, 2.5 mg phentolamine and 25 μg/4.25 ml PGE1; a 0.2 ml total volume of 6 mg papaverine, 0.2 mg phentolamine, and 2 μg PGE1; and 12.5 mg papaverine combined with 10 μg of alprostadil[1–4, 27].

Some patients may have a poor response to the initial injection of the vasodilating agent and be unable to achieve satisfactory erection. In these cases, manual self-stimulation has been reported to significantly improve erection in many patients[28]. For some patients, a second or third injection may be required before an adequate response is attained[3, 4]. This, however, may run the risk of priapism, a painful complication of over-medication.

Just as there are differences in the use of vasodilating agents, there is no collective consensus as to how soon, how frequently and how long after injection sonographic measurements should be performed. However, it is now generally recognized that waiting until 5 min after injection, as had previously been the practice, can result in falsely low peak systolic velocity findings in the cavernosal arteries, since normal maximum peak systolic velocities can occur in less than 5 min following injection[3]. In addition, premature termination of postinjection measurements (i.e. after 5–10 min) can result in false-positive diagnoses of arterial insufficiency, or venous incompetence, because of temporal variations in the response to vasodilating agents[2]. Early termination may also result in a false-negative diagnosis of venous incompetence. Suggested protocols are summarized in Table 11.1.

DOPPLER EVALUATION AFTER VASODILATOR INJECTION

Doppler evaluation following the injection of a vasodilating agent is performed so that the penile anatomic vasculature can be visualized and haemodynamic parameters measured. There is considerable debate, however, as to which haemodynamic parameters are significant and what constitutes normal and abnormal values. Connolly *et al*[4] have suggested that the most important diagnostic indicators are arterial diameter, peak flow velocity and blood flow acceleration.

To obtain accurate readings, it is important that the examiner is familiar with the physiology of arterial inflow to the cavernosal arteries after pharmacological injection. Particular attention must be paid to the Doppler angle, which should be approximately 60°, or less, to the cavernosal artery[1, 3]. Measurements are most reliable and most easily reproduced when taken at the base of the penis, where the penile vessels angle posteriorly toward the perineum. The arterial diameter and waveform of each cavernosal artery is individually assessed. Peak systolic and end-diastolic velocities are measured and recorded. The examiner should also carefully search for anatomic penile arterial variants that may contribute to vasculogenic impotence. An asymmetric response of the cavernosal arteries during erection or a lack of arterial dilatation may suggest the presence of a significant vascular lesion[29].

Normal Doppler findings

Prior to injection, during the flaccid state, the systolic waveform is dampened and a monophasic flow with minimal diastolic component is present. Following pharmacological inducement of erection, the normal progression of haemodynamic events and the associated Doppler waveform patterns of the cavernosal artery can be classified into different haemodynamic stages[30]. The appearance of the spectral waveform must be correlated with the

Table 11.1 Recommended time protocols for sonographic evaluation of pharmacologically induced erection.

Investigators	Suggested protocols
Hattery *et al*[1]	At 5, 10, 15 and 20 min following injection, with delayed measurements occasionally obtained after 20 min if degree of tumescence or rigidity is increasing
Fitzgerald *et al*[2]	Immediately after injection and at 5 min intervals for 20–30 min or until waveform progression ceases
Herbener *et al*[3]	Immediately after injection and at 1–2 min intervals until there is a plateau of velocity or until velocities peak and then decrease, with examination normally not exceeding 20 min
Herbener *et al*[3]	At 3–5 min intervals until maximum cavernosal artery diameter and peak systolic velocity measurements are obtained
Connolly *et al*[4]	At 3–5 min intervals throughout latent, tumescent and full stages of erection for up to 30 min in order to detect patients who show delayed but eventually normal response to injection

status of the erection, i.e. flaccid, latent, tumescent, full and rigid.

During the initial latent state, there is a sudden increase in both systolic and diastolic blood flow in the cavernosal artery, and a rounded systolic peak is observed. The flow of blood is unidirectional during systole and diastole, with a pronounced forward diastolic component present. This spectral waveform reflects the low resistance to flow within the sinusoidal spaces. Minimal tumescence normally accompanies this stage (Fig. 11.3). Following that, there is an increase in blood flow to the corpora cavernosa, causing the intracavernosal pressure to increase. As intracavernosal pressure rises, a dichrotic notch appears at end-systole and diastolic flow diminishes. When intracavernosal and diastolic pressures are the same, diastolic flow ceases and there is only systolic blood flow. The systolic envelope narrows and systolic velocity may fluctuate. Increasing tumescence normally occurs during this stage (Fig. 11.4).

During full erection, intracavernosal pressure becomes greater than the arterial pressure during diastole because of the veno-occlusive mechanism, flow reversal may be seen during diastole and the systolic waveform narrows. During this stage, maximal systolic velocity

occurs in many patients and strong pulsations are normally seen[4]. In the rigid phase of erection, intracavernosal pressure may equal or exceed arterial systolic pressure, causing additional narrowing of the systolic envelope and, normally, a decrease in systolic velocity. Both systolic and diastolic flow may cease completely as the pressure in the corporal bodies approaches systolic blood pressure (Fig. 11.5)[4].

Cavernosal artery diameter

Obtaining cavernosal arterial diameters can be time-consuming, and the accuracy of the

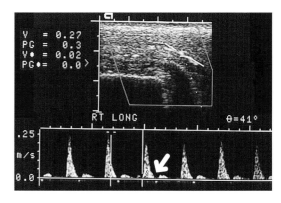

Fig. 11.4 Spectral Doppler tracing in the early tumescent phase. Systolic waveform is narrowed into a sharp spike. Diastolic velocity decreases and a dichrotic notch is present in early diastole (arrow).

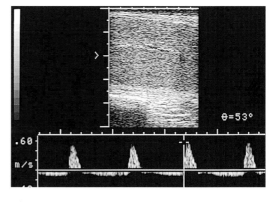

Fig. 11.5 Spectral Doppler tracing at full rigid erection. The systolic peak is narrowed. Note the reversal of flow throughout diastole.

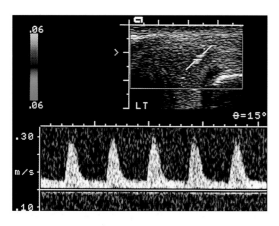

Fig. 11.3 Spectral Doppler tracing during the initial latent phase of the erectile process. Brisk flow is seen in systole, approximating 30 cms^{-1}. At this stage after pharmacologic enhancement, diastolic flow continues in the antegrade direction.

measurement is very dependent on the abilities of the examiner. Considerable controversy exists as to the value of obtaining measurements of the cavernosal artery diameter following pharmacological induction of erection. Some investigators have reported a poor correlation between the degree of increase in cavernosal artery diameter and arteriographic confirmation of arterial integrity. They found that the changes in diameter were not significant enough to be indicative or diagnostic of arterial disease[5, 13, 17, 29, 31, 32].

Other authors use cavernosal arterial diameters as a parameter in determining arterial integrity of the penis. Various percentages of increase in vessel diameter after injection have been reported as indicators of normal vessel compliance (Table 11.2). It is argued that as blood flow in the cavernosal artery is a function of velocity and cross-sectional area of the vessels, the ability of the artery to dilate after pharmacological injection is an important reflection of vessel compliance[1]. Although it is recognized that the degree of change in diameter following injection may not correlate well with other physiological or haemodynamic parameters, Connolly *et al*[4] contend that because increased blood flow during erection is accompanied by an increase in the diameter of the cavernosal arteries, patients with arterial disease will have minimal or no vessel dilatation following injection because of inadequate vessel compliance or blood flow. Thus, they recommend use of the diameter and suggest that the measurement be taken approximately

5 min after injection, since the greatest increase in arterial diameter is observed during the early–latent–stage of erection when blood inflow is at its maximum.

Arterial variants

A high percentage of patients suspected of having arteriogenic causes for their impotence have been found to have abnormal penile arterial anatomy[5, 31, 35, 36]. This includes branching of the cavernous arteries and collaterals from dorsal and urethral arteries. Communications along the cavernosal, dorsal and spongiosal arteries are often found along the shaft of the penis, with those between the dorsal and cavernosal arteries (dorsal-cavernosal perforators) reported in 90% of men[36]. These communications may significantly effect penile blood flow during erection[4, 37]. Spongiosal-cavernosal communications, or 'shunt' vessels, which course from the corpus spongiosum into the corpus cavernosum are another common variant[31, 37]. Although these anatomic variations do not necessarily indicate arterial insufficiency, they may cause inaccurate interpretation if they are not taken into account; for example, lower peak blood flow velocities may be found in patients with a full erectile response if arterial communications are present[31, 38]. Careful scanning of the entire penis from the crura to the glans with colour Doppler is essential in distinguishing these anomalies (Fig. 11.6).

VASCULOGENIC IMPOTENCE

Arterial insufficiency

Measurement of peak systolic velocity in the cavernosal arteries after pharmacological injection is considered one of the most important parameters when evaluating patients whose impotence may be due to arterial disease such as focal stenosis, occlusion or collateral flow between arteries (Fig. 11.7)[1].

Table 11.2 Criteria for indication of normal vessel compliance.

Investigators	Increase in vessel diameter (%)
Lee et al[33]	70
Lue et al[7]	75
Krysiewicz and Mellinger[13]; James[34]	60–75
Collins and Lewandowski[12]	60–100

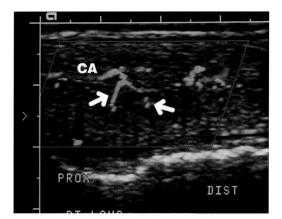

Fig. 11.6 Longitudinal colour Doppler image. There is discontinuity of the cavernosal artery (CA) over a short segment, with collateralization (arrows) to the spongiosal artery.

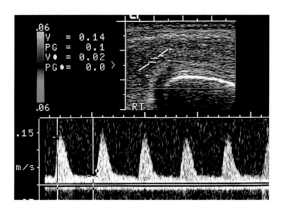

Fig. 11.7 Spectral Doppler tracing in a patient with arterial insufficiency. Despite appropriate pharmaceutical dose, erectile response was suboptimal. Peak systolic velocity in the cavernosal artery is only 14 cm s[-1]. This is well below the accepted range of normal.

What constitutes normal and abnormal values for arterial insufficiency varies, however. Reported peak systolic velocity values indicative of normal arterial function are summarized in Table 11.3; and reported abnormal values indicative of arterial disease as the cause of vasculogenic impotence are summarized in Table 11.4.

In addition to peak systolic velocity values in each cavernosal artery, a comparison of the

values can help in the diagnosis of arterial disease. Asymmetric velocities are considered abnormal if the difference between right and left cavernosal arteries is greater than 10 cm s[-1] [3, 29]; or greater than 10–15 cm s[-1] by Hattery and associates[1]. Underlying arterial disease should be considered in the artery with the lower peak systolic velocity value[34].

Other indicators used to increase the sensitivity of detecting potential arterial disease include reversal of blood flow during systole, a penile blood flow index, and blood flow (or cavernosal artery) acceleration. During rigid erection, reversal of diastolic blood flow is considered a normal finding; however, reversal of arterial blood flow direction during systole is always considered abnormal and may indicate an underlying vascular abnormality[1, 3]. Systolic flow reversal after pharmacological inducement of erection has been observed in patients with significant proximal penile or cavernosal artery stenosis and occlusion, with filling of the distal cavernosal artery secondary to collateral flow.

Lopez *et al*[40] have described a penile blood flow index, which is calculated by adding the percentage increases in the diameters of the right and left cavernosal arteries to the peak flow velocities of both arteries. If the total

Table 11.3 Criteria for normal peak systolic velocity in cavernosal arteries following pharmacologic inducement of erection.

Investigators	Peak systolic velocity (cms[-1])
Lue *et al*[7]; Paushter[32]	≥25
Porst[39]	25–30 or greater
Hattery *et al*[1]; Connolly *et al*[4]; Lee *et al*[33]	≥30
Schwartz *et al*[30]	Mean 39[a]
Herbener *et al*[3]; Benson and Vickers[29]	≥40

[a]Mean peak systolic velocity values are the combined calculated average of the right and left cavernosal arteries.

Table 11.4 Criteria for abnormal peak systolic velocity in cavernosal arteries following pharmacologic inducement of erection.

Investigators	Peak systolic velocity (cm s⁻¹)
Fitzgerald et al[2]; Quam et al[5]; Lue et al[7]; Paushter[32]; James[34]	Mean <25[a]
Hattery et al[1]	<25 abnormal, while 25–30 indeterminate with clinical correlation recommended
Benson and Vickers[29]	<30 considered significant, while 30–40 regarded borderline to mild

[a]Mean peak systolic velocity values are the combined calculated average of the right and left cavernosal arteries.

value is less than 285, vasculogenic impotence is considered likely to be of an arterial nature; this was 97% sensitive and 77% specific in diagnosing impotence due to arterial disease.

Another Doppler index for identifying arterial disease has been referred to both as cavernosal artery acceleration and blood flow acceleration. This index is calculated by dividing the peak systolic velocity by the systolic rise time (cm s⁻²). The systolic rise time is the time from the start of the systolic curve to its maximum value. Proximal arterial disease would be expected to dampen velocity waveforms and prolong the systolic rise time[4]. In a study comprising 30 patients, Valji and Bookstein[14] reported the index more predictive of arterial insufficiency than cavernosal arterial peak systolic velocity by itself. Oates et al[41] found that a systolic rise time of 110 m s⁻¹ or greater had a predictive value of 92% for arteriogenic impotence. Mellinger et al[42] reported that blood flow acceleration seemed to correlate well with subjective evaluation of erections.

Venous insufficiency

Venous incompetence, or failure of the veno-occlusive mechanisms, may be the primary cause of vasculogenic impotence in some patients[2]. Because primary venous leakage is a potentially treatable cause of erectile dysfunction, Doppler examination of the penile venous system may be helpful in identifying these patients who may benefit from additional, more invasive, studies[1, 43]. Patients with normal arterial parameters (e.g. peak systolic velocity >25 cm s⁻¹) but weak erections will very likely have some degree of venous leakage[4]. If the peak systolic velocity is less than 25 cm s⁻¹, however, the veno-occlusive mechanism will not be fully engaged and persistent end-diastolic flow can be expected.

A correlation has been shown between diastolic blood flow velocity within the cavernosal arteries and the presence of venous leakage. With a normal erectile response, there should be minimal, if any, diastolic flow detected within the cavernosal arteries 15–20 min after injection. As previously noted, there will be a decrease and eventually an absence or reversal of diastolic flow in a normal spectral Doppler waveform during rigid erection. If there is veno-occlusive dysfunction, however, this decrease or reversal of diastolic flow may not occur[5, 34, 43]. A persistently elevated diastolic flow in the cavernosal arteries is highly indicative of venous leakage out of the corporal tissue, even after maximum peak systolic velocity has been attained (Fig. 11.8). However, just as there are differences of opinion regarding normal and abnormal peak systolic velocity values, various criteria exist as to what constitutes abnormal diastolic velocity (Table 11.5).

Trauma

Following penile trauma, Doppler ultrasound is useful for identifying the presence of injury

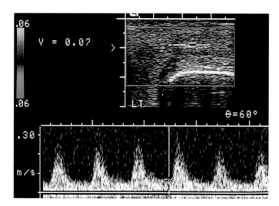

Fig. 11.8 Spectral Doppler tracing of venous insufficiency. Relative high-velocity forward flow (7 cm s^{-1}) persists during diastole.

to the penile vasculature. Imaging can be performed quickly in the emergency setting, or for evaluation of posttraumatic erectile dysfunction[3, 20]. For patients who experience posttraumatic impotence, Broderick *et al*[46] found that a systolic velocity of less than 25 cm s^{-1} and asymmetric velocities of greater than 10 cm s^{-1} were helpful parameters in distinguishing disruption of arterial integrity as a possible cause. In addition, colour Doppler can be used to identify cavernosal artery-corpus cavernosal fistula, an unusual complication of penile trauma in which the patient experiences a prolonged, painful erection (high-flow priapism)[3, 21, 47]. This condition results when the cavernosal artery is lacerated and there is unrestricted blood flow to the cavernosal spaces, creating an arteriosinusoidal or arteriovenous fistula (Fig. 11.9).

Table 11.5 Criteria for abnormal mean arterial end-diastolic velocity.

Investigators	End-diastolic velocity (cm s^{-1})
Herbener *et al*[3]; James[34]	> 3
Quam *et al*[5]; Benson and Vickers[29]; Paushter[32]; Fitzgerald *et al*[44]	>5
Hattery *et al*[1]	>5–8
Montorsi *et al*[45]	>10

Peyronie's disease

Peyronie's disease is an idiopathic disorder of the connective tissue in which fibrous plaques form in the tunica albuginea with induration of the corpora cavernosa of the penis or a fibrous cavernositis. The disease causes a downward bowing of the penis and affected patients typically present with curvature of the penis with erection, or complain of pain during erection[3, 22]. Doppler examination of the penile vasculature is of value in determining if any vascular abnormalities exist because of the fibrous

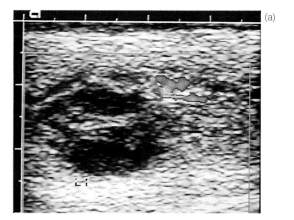

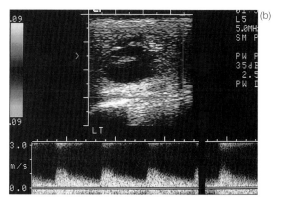

Fig. 11.9 (a) Oblique image of the mid-penis. This patient suffered a traumatic sports injury and presented to the emergency room with a painful priapism. There is an irregular septated fluid collection in the mid-penis. Colour Doppler shows prominent flow in the cavernosal artery immediately adjacent to the haematoma. (b) Spectral Doppler tracing of the cavernosal artery in proximity to the haematoma reveals high-velocity (approx. 1.5 m s^{-1}) turbulent flow. Angiography confirmed an arteriosinusoidal fistula.

plaques[22, 23]. Doppler ultrasound is helpful in detecting the presence of veno-occlusive dysfunction (considered the primary vascular cause of impotence associated with Peyronie's disease) and arterial insufficiency[24].

Other imaging procedures

Doppler ultrasound combined with pharmacological inducement of erection has replaced the use of the penile/brachial pressure index and pudendal arteriography at many institutions for the initial evaluation of patients with suspected vasculogenic impotence[4]. Although arteriography is considered the 'gold standard' for assessing the arteries of the penis, unlike Doppler ultrasound it provides primarily anatomical rather than functional information. If Doppler examination indicates the presence of a surgically correctable lesion, however, many investigators believe a confirmatory arteriogram should be performed before surgery is undertaken.

Colour Doppler ultrasound has also proven helpful in evaluating patients with suspected venous incompetence. However, for patients in whom venous surgery is being considered to correct their condition, dynamic infusion cavernosography is necessary since it provides a more complete preoperative picture of the penile vasculature[1-3]. At many institutions, both cavernosography and cavernosometry are used to determine the presence of veno-occlusive dysfunction and quantify the degree of venous leakage.

REFERENCES

1. Hattery RR, King BF, Lewis RW, James EM, McKusick MA (1991) Vasculogenic impotence: duplex and colour Doppler imaging. *Radiology Clinics of North America* 29: 629–645
2. Fitzgerald SW, Erickson SJ, Foley WD, Lipchik EO, Lawson TL (1992) Colour Doppler sonography in the evaluation of erectile dysfunction. *RadioGraphics* 12: 3–17
3. Herbener TE, Seftel AD, Nehro A, Goldstein I (1994) Penile ultrasound. *Seminars in Urology* 12: 320–332
4. Connolly JA, Borirakchanyavat S, Lue TF (1996) Ultrasound evaluation of the penis for assessment of impotence. *Journal of Clinical Ultrasound* 24: 481–486
5. Quam JP, King BF, James EM *et al* (1989) Duplex and colour Doppler sonographic evaluation of vasculogenic impotence. *American Journal of Radiology* 153: 1141–1147
6. Krane RJ, Goldstein I, Saenz de Tejada I (1989) Medical progress: impotence. *New England Journal of Medicine* 321: 1648–1659
7. Lue TF, Hricak H, Marich KW, Tanagho EA (1985) Vasculogenic impotence evaluated by high-resolution ultrasonography and pulsed Doppler spectrum analysis. *Radiology* 155: 777–781
8. Gall H, Bahren W, Scherb W, Stief C, Thon W (1988) Diagnostic accuracy of Doppler ultrasound technique of the penile arteries in correlation to selective arteriography. *Cardiovascular Interventional Radiology* 11: 225–229
9. Lue T, Tanagho E (1987) Physiology of erection and pharmacological management of impotence. *Journal of Urology* 137: 829–836
10. Mueller SC, Lue TF (1988) Evaluation of vasculogenic impotence. *Urology Clinics of North America* 15: 65–76
11. Desai KM, Gingell JC, Skidmore R *et al* (1987) Application of computerized penile arterial waveform analysis in the diagnosis of arteriogenic impotence: an initial study in potent and impotent men. *British Journal of Urology* 60: 450–466
12. Collins JP, Lewandowski BJ (1987) Experience with intracorporal injection of papaverine and duplex ultrasound scanning for assessment of arteriogenic impotence. *British Journal of Urology* 59: 84–88
13. Krysiewicz S, Mellinger BC (1989) The role of imaging in the diagnostic evaluation of impotence. *American Journal of Radiology* 153: 1133–1139
14. Valji K, Bookstein JJ (1993) Diagnosis of arteriogenic impotence: efficacy of duplex ultrasonography as a screening tool. *American Journal of Radiology* 160: 65–69
15. Aboseif SR, Lue TF (1988) Hemodynamics of penile erection. *Urology Clinics of North America* 15: 1–7
16. Bookstein JJ, Valji K, Parsons L *et al* (1987) Pharmacoarteriography in the evaluation of impotence. *Journal of Urology* 137: 333–337

17. Rajfer J, Canan V, Dorey FJ et al (1990) Correlation between penile angiography and duplex scanning of cavernous arteries in impotent men. *Journal of Urology* **143**: 1128–1130

18. Rosen MP, Schwartz AN, Levine FJ et al (1991) Radiologic assessment of impotence angiography, sonography, cavernosography and cinetrigraphy. *American Journal of Radiology* **157**: 923–931

19. Shabsigh R, Fishman IJ, Scott FB (1988) Evaluation of erectile impotence. *Urology* **32**: 83–90

20. Armenakas NA, McAninch JW, Lue TF, Dixon CM, Hricak H (1993) Posttraumatic impotence: magnetic resonance imaging and duplex ultrasound in diagnosis and management. *Journal of Urology* **149**: 1272–1275

21. Harding JR, Hollander JB, Bendick PJ (1993) Chronic priapism secondary to a traumatic arteriovenous fistula of the corpus cavernosum. *Journal of Urology* **150**: 1504–1506

22. Lopez JA, Jarrow JP (1991) Duplex ultrasound findings in men with Peyronie's disease. *Urological Radiology* **12**: 199–202

23. Amin Z, Patel U, Friedman EF, Vale JA, Kirby R, Lees WR (1993) Colour Doppler and duplex ultrasound assessment of Peyronie's disease in impotent men. *British Journal of Radiology* **66**: 398–402

24. Levine LA, Coogan CL (1996) Penile vascular assessment using colour duplex sonography in men with Peyronie's disease. *Journal of Urology* **155**: 1270–1273

25. Lue TF (1992) Physiology of penile erection and pathophysiology of impotence. In: Walsh PC, Retik AB, Stamey TA, Vaughan ED (eds) *Campbell's Urology*, 6th edn, pp 707–728. Philadelphia: WB Saunders

26. King BF, Hattery RR, James EM et al (1990) Duplex sonography in the evaluation of impotence: current techniques. *Seminars in Interventional Radiology* **7**: 215–221

27. Meuelman EJ, Bemelmans BH, Doesburg WH et al (1992) Penile pharmacological duplex ultrasonography: a dose–effect study comparing papaverine, papaverine/phentolamine, and prostaglandin E$_1$. *Journal of Urology* **148**: 63–66

28. Donatucci CF, Lue TF (1992) The combined intracavernous injection and stimulation test: diagnostic accuracy. *Journal of Urology* **148**: 61–62

29. Benson CB, Vickers MA (1989) Sexual impotence caused by vascular disease: diagnosis with duplex sonography. *American Journal of Radiology* **153**: 1149–1153

30. Schwartz AN, Wang KY, Mack LA et al (1989) Evaluation of normal erectile function with colour flow Doppler sonography. *American Journal of Radiology* **153**: 1155–1160

31. Jarrow JP, Pugh VW, Routh WD, Dyer RB (1993) Comparison of penile duplex ultrasonography to pudendal arteriography: variant penile arterial anatomy affects interpretation of duplex ultrasonography. *Investigational Radiology* **28**: 806–810

32. Paushter DM (1989) Role of duplex sonography in the evaluation of sexual impotence. *American Journal of Radiology* **153**: 1161–1163

33. Lee B, Suresh CS, Randrup ER et al (1993) Standardization of penile blood flow parameters in normal men using intracavernous prostaglandin E1 and visual sexual stimulation. *Journal of Urology* **149**: 49–52

34. James EM (1991) *Penile Ultrasound. Syllabus special course: Ultrasound 1991*, pp 259–266. Presented at the 77th Scientific Assembly and Annual Meeting of the Radiologic Society of North America, Chicago

35. Breza J, Aboseif SR, Orvis BR et al (1989). Detailed anatomy of penile neurovascular structures: surgical significance. *Journal of Urology* **141**: 437–443

36. Bahren W, Gall H, Scherb W, Stiff C, Thon W (1988) Arterial anatomy and arteriographic diagnosis of arteriogenic impotence. *Cardiovascular Interventional Radiology* **11**: 195–210

37. Mancini M, Bartolini M, Maggi M, Innocenti P, Forti G (1996) The presence of arterial anatomical variations can affect the results of duplex sonographic evaluation of penile vessels in impotent patients. *Journal of Urology* **155**: 1919–1923

38. Hattery RR, King BF, James EM et al (1991) Vasculogenic impotence: duplex and colour Doppler imaging. *American Journal of Radiology* **156**: 189–195

39. Porst H (1993) Duplex ultrasound of the penis: value of a new diagnostic procedure based on over 1,000 patients [German]. *Urologe–Ausgabe A* **32**: 242–249

40. Lopez JA, Espeland MA, Jarrow JP (1991) Interpretation and quantification of penile blood flow studies using duplex ultrasonography. *Journal of Urology* **146**: 1271–1275

41. Oates CP, Pickard RS, Powell PH, Murphy LN, Whittingham TA (1995) The use of duplex ultrasound in the assessment of arterial supply to the penis in vasculogenic impotence. *Journal of Urology* **153**: 354–357

42. Mellinger BC, Fried JJ, Vaughen ED (1990) Papaverine-induced penile blood flow acceleration in impotent men measured by duplex scanning. *Journal of Urology* **144**: 897–899

43. Vickers MA, Benson CB, Richie JP (1990) High-resolution ultrasonography and pulsed wave Doppler for detection of co-porovenous incompetence in erectile dysfunction. *Journal of Urology* **143**: 1125–1127

44. Fitzgerald SW, Erickson SJ, Foley WD et al (1991) Colour Doppler sonography in the evaluation of erectile dysfunction: patterns of temporal response to papaverine. *American Journal of Radiology* **157**: 331–335

45. Montorsi F, Bergamaschi F, Guazzoni G *et al* (1993) Doppler colour echography in the diagnosis of impotence. *Minerva Chirurgica* **48**: 99–102

46. Broderick GA, McGahan JP, White RD *et al* (1990) Colour Doppler US: assessment of posttraumatic impotence. *Radiology* **177**(Suppl): 130–134

47. Hakim LS, Kulaksizoglu H, Mulligan R, Greenfield A, Goldstein I (1996) Evolved concepts in the diagnosis and treatment of arterial high-flow priapism. *Journal of Urology* **155**: 541–548

The scrotum

MYRON A. POZNIAK

Sonographic examination of the scrotum was first introduced in the mid-1970s. Today, ultrasound has superseded other imaging technologies in evaluating the scrotum because of advances in high-frequency transducers, an increase in Doppler sensitivity, and the development of power Doppler technology. The addition of haemodynamic information to the imaging findings frequently reinforces and, occasionally, confirms the diagnosis[1-7]. Thus, a thorough ultrasound evaluation of the scrotum must include colour Doppler imaging of the testes and epididymides.

INDICATIONS

Conditions that commonly warrant ultrasound examination include scrotal pain, inflammatory processes, suspicion of spermatic cord torsion, palpable testicular mass, differentiation of a testicular mass from a spermatic cord or epididymal mass, suspicion of a non-palpable neoplasm, trauma, varicocoele, cryptorchidism and infertility.

TESTICULAR ANATOMY

The normal adult testis is an egg-shaped gland which is approximately 3–5 cm in length and 2–4 cm in width and thickness[8]. The testis is covered by the tunica vaginalis, a fascial structure composed of an outer parietal layer and an inner visceral layer which envelops the entire gland, except along the posterior border where the vessels and nerves enter. The potential space between the parietal and visceral layers normally contains a small amount of lubricating fluid, but larger extratesticular collections can occur here forming hydrocoeles.

Deep to the tunica vaginalis is the tunica albuginea, a thin, dense, inelastic fibrous capsule with the tunica vasculosa lying just under it, through which the branches of the testicular artery pass into the gland (Fig. 12.1)[8, 9].

Numerous thin septations (septulae) arise from the visceral layer of the tunica vaginalis and create 250–400 cone-shaped lobules containing seminiferous tubules[10-12]. These tortuous tubules course towards the centre of the testis (the mediastinum) and join to form larger, straight ducts known as tubuli recti, which join with each other to form a plexus in the mediastinum called the rete testis, which then drain as 10–15 efferent ductules into the head of the epididymis.

The epididymis is a tortuous tubular structure that runs along the posterolateral aspect of the testis; it has a head, body and tail. The head is located next to the upper pole of the testis and receives the efferent ductules. The body and tail are composed primarily of the ductus epididymis, which is formed by the

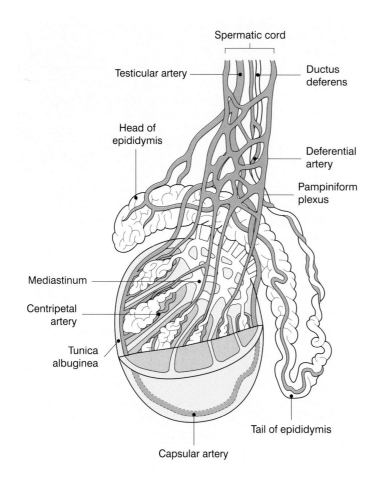

Spermatic cord

Testicular artery

Ductus
deferens

Head of
epididymis

Deferential
artery

Pampiniform
plexus

Mediastinum

Centripetal
artery

Tunica
albuginea

Tail of epididymis

Capsular artery

Fig. 12.1 The testicular artery supplies flow to the epididymis and the testicle. Along the course of the testicular artery within the spermatic cord it is surrounded by the pampiniform plexus of veins. The capsular artery, a branch of the testicular artery, courses just underneath the tunica albuginea. The transtesticular artery may be seen to course along the mediastinum. Centripetal arteries with the recurrent rami supply the testicular parenchyma.

convergence of the efferent ductules. The vas deferens leaves the epididymis from the tail and runs up the spermatic cord.

Testicular arterial anatomy

The testicular arteries originate from the aorta just below the renal arteries; they travel through the ipsilateral inguinal canal in the spermatic cord, accompanied by the cremasteric and deferential arteries, which supply the soft tissues of the scrotum, epididymis and vas deferens. The testicular artery runs down through the mediastinum on the posterior aspect of the testis, giving off capsular branches to each side of the gland. These ramify in the tunica vasculosa and give rise to centripetal

arteries, which run centrally back along the septulae into the parenchyma of the testis towards the mediastinum. Some of their branches course back towards the surface as recurrent rami (Fig. 12.2). In about 50% of testes, small branches are seen passing directly from the testicular artery into the parenchyma; these are known as transmediastinal arteries (Fig. 12.3).

Testicular venous anatomy

Testicular venous outflow is normally through the mediastinum to the pampiniform plexus in the epididymis and spermatic cord and eventually to the testicular veins. The pampiniform plexus is a web-like collection of veins

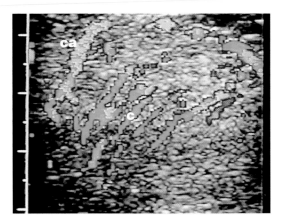

Fig. 12.2 A portion of the capsular artery (ca) can be seen coursing just deep to the tunica albuginea. Several centripetal arteries (c) with their recurrent rami can be seen coursing through the testicular parenchyma.

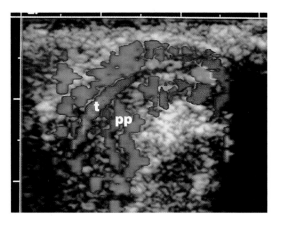

Fig. 12.4 The pampiniform plexus of veins (pp) is a web-like collection of veins surrounding the testicular artery (t) in its course through the spermatic cord.

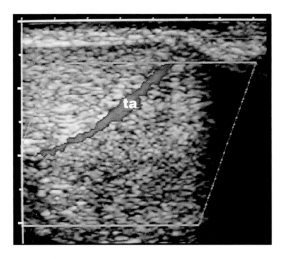

Fig. 12.3 A transtesticular artery (ta) is usually seen obliquely coursing through the testicle along the mediastinum. It is a branch of the testicular artery.

surrounding the testicular artery (Fig. 12.4). One of its functions is to serve as a heat-exchange mechanism, pulling warmth away from the testicular artery. This helps maintain spermatogenesis at a lower, optimum temperature. On the left side, the testicular vein usually drains into the left renal vein; on the right side, drainage is typically directly into the inferior vena cava. These veins normally have valves

that prevent retrograde flow of venous blood to the scrotum, but if they become incompetent a varicocoele will develop[13].

TECHNIQUE

Prior to the ultrasound examination, the testes should be examined with a gloved hand, especially if the sonographic study is being conducted to evaluate a palpable mass. The examination is performed with the patient in the supine position, and a towel is placed under the scrotum for support. If the testis is extremely tender, the patient can be asked to hold it as this facilitates examining patients who may otherwise automatically draw away from the ultrasound transducer because of severe pain. If a small mass is particularly tender, the patient is asked to hold it between his thumb and forefinger, and the ultrasound transducer is then gently placed upon it. Some men may have a vigorous cremasteric response during the examination resulting in the testis being drawn upward and puckering of the scrotum. To avoid shadowing from trapped air, copious amounts of gel need to be worked into these scrotal skin folds. Imaging with the patient standing upright, or while performing a

Valsalva manoeuvre, is useful for evaluating the testicular venous system, in particular for determining valvular competence in patients with possible varicocoeles.

A high-frequency (7.0 MHz or greater) linear array transducer is used for both grey-scale and Doppler imaging, with direct-contact scanning on the scrotal skin. Sequential images are obtained in both the longitudinal and trans-verse planes for each testis to allow assessment of any differences in size and echogenicity between the two sides; a split screen mode is useful to allow a direct comparison between the two sides. An oblique image of the epididymis and spermatic cord should also be obtained. Additional images are taken of any areas of specific interest.

Doppler technique

Ultrasound examination of the scrotum is not complete without colour Doppler. The proce-dure is a mandatory part of the imaging evalu-ation to confirm the presence (or absence) of uniform, symmetric vascular perfusion of the testicle and epididymis. The settings for colour Doppler scanning must be optimized for low-volume and low-velocity flow[14]. If artefact is excessive at low-flow settings and interferes with the examination, colour noise can be decreased by increasing wall filter and scale settings. Temporal resolution can be improved by minimizing the overall image size and limiting the size of the colour box. Use of appropriate technical parameters should assure demonstration of intratesticular vessels in all normal cases[9]. The use of power Doppler can be helpful in very low-flow conditions, such as with paediatric patients, and has replaced nuclear scintigraphy in many cases[11, 12, 15, 16]. The arterial waveforms and velocity measure-ments can be quantified using spectral Doppler[14].

Doppler sensitivity varies greatly between systems and software levels. The examiner must therefore be familiar with normal flow perception on their equipment. A good 'rule of thumb' is to examine the contralateral side (provided it is normal) to establish a colour-flow baseline which can then be used as the standard by which to judge the abnormal testis or epididymis.

Normal ultrasound findings

A normal ultrasound examination of the scrotum reveals uniform, homogeneous echogenicity throughout both testes. The epididymis is usually isoechoic or slightly hyperechoic compared with the testes; the appearances on both sides should be symmet-rical (Fig. 12.5).

Spectral Doppler tracings of testicular arte-rial flow demonstrate relatively low resistance; this is in contrast to the cremasteric and defer-ential arteries which have relatively high-flow resistance. The normal testicular artery resis-tive indices in adults range from 0.46 to 0.78, with a mean of 0.64[9]. Similar findings are reported in the intratesticular arteries of post-pubescent patients, with resistive indices ranging from 0.48 to 0.75 (mean 0.62)[14]. Supratesticular arteries to the vas deferens or cremaster muscle, on the other hand, have

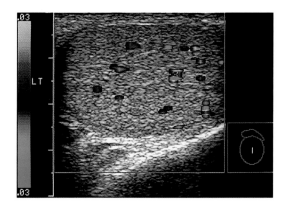

Fig. 12.5 Longitudinal colour Doppler view of a normal testis and epididymis. Note the uniform distribution of relatively low-level colour.

higher impedance with low diastolic flow and resistive indices ranging from 0.63 and 1.0, with a mean of 0.84[1, 9, 14].

Pulsed Doppler is relatively insensitive in detecting arterial flow in prepubescent patients[14, 17, 18]. In contrast, power Doppler showed arterial flow in 92% of testes in prepubescent patients, while colour Doppler demonstrated flow in 83% of cases[4]. In postpubescent patients, both Doppler imaging techniques demonstrated flow in 100% of cases.

INFLAMMATORY DISEASE

Acute epididymo-orchitis is the most common cause of scrotal pain in men over the age of 20 years, accounting for up to 80% of acute scrotal pain, but it is frequently indistinguishable, clinically, from spermatic cord torsion. Patients usually present with an acutely painful, tender, swollen scrotum, with associated erythema, urinary tract symptoms, fever and leukocytosis. Sometimes, however, the signs and symptoms may be less distinct, making clinical differentiation between infection and torsion extremely difficult.

The cause of the inflammatory process varies with the patient's age[19]. In adult patients less than 35 years of age, *Chlamydia* and *Neisseria* are the most common causative organisms and cytomegalovirus is the most common cause in immunocompromised patients. In most normal paediatric patients, a bacterial pathogen is not isolated and the inflammation is presumed to be viral in nature, but paediatric patients who have an underlying urogenital congenital anomaly are prone to infection from Gram-negative bacteria.

The sonographic appearance of epididymo-orchitis varies depending on the chronicity of the condition. In the early, acute stage, the epididymis will be enlarged and either hypo- or hyperechoic[5, 12, 20]. Oedema and swelling of the testis result in an enlarged, ill-defined, hypoechoic image; the wall of the scrotum is thick-

ened. A hydrocoele may be present and may contain some debris. With the onset of tissue breakdown, haemorrhage, and microabscess formation, the appearances become more complex and variable. Scarring and necrosis associated with chronic orchitis result in either a small hypoechoic, or hyperechoic testis.

The sensitivity of grey-scale sonography for detecting epididymo-orchitis has been reported to be about 80%[20]. A study by Ralls *et al*[7] demonstrated 91% sensitivity and 100% specificity for the diagnosis of scrotal inflammatory disease by colour Doppler sonography. Other authors have also reported a sensitivity close to 100%[9, 21]. The diagnosis of inflammation can be made with confidence when hyperaemia with an increased number and convergence of discernible vessels is seen in association with an enlarged, painful, hypoechoic epididymis and/or testis (Fig. 12.6)[1, 2, 5, 20, 21]. Inflammatory hyperaemia vessels typically show a low-resistance flow pattern on spectral Doppler[1], although spectral analysis is rarely necessary to confirm the diagnosis.

Brown *et al*[22] have proposed quantitative guidelines to improve the accuracy of Doppler assessment of acute unilateral epididymitis and/or orchitis. These use peak systolic velocities and ratios of these calculated by using

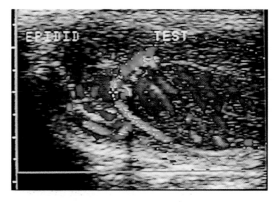

Fig. 12.6 Longitudinal colour Doppler image of the epididymis and testis in a patient with bacterial epididymal orchitis. Note the marked hyperaemia of both the testis and epididymis.

values from the right and left sides. In their study, peak systolic velocities were significantly higher in the patients than in control subjects: a peak systolic velocity of 15 cm s^{-1} resulted in a diagnostic accuracy of 93% for epididymitis and 90% for orchitis. Epididymal peak systolic ratios of 1.7, or testicular ratios of 1.9, were reported diagnostic of acute inflammation, substantially improving diagnostic accuracy.

In cases of severe epididymitis, periepididymal swelling may obstruct testicular venous outflow, leading to testicular ischaemia or infarction. An enlarged, heterogeneous testicle with reduced or absent colour flow and a contiguous abnormal epididymis will be seen on grey-scale images[14]. Hyperaemia of the epididymis helps to differentiate testicular ischaemia following inflammation from that caused by torsion. A high-resistance waveform, along with decreased or reversed diastolic flow, may be seen on the spectral Doppler tracing[23].

Occasionally, testicular or epididymal inflammation results in abscess formation (Fig. 12.7), which normally appears as an enlarged testicle with a fluid-filled mass of mixed echogenicity. It may be difficult to distinguish from a testicular neoplasm, as both can present as complex cystic/solid masses. Older abscesses may have radiating echogenic septa separating hypoechoic spaces[24]. Increased blood flow around the abscess cavity and no internal flow is seen on colour Doppler[1, 20]. Surgical exploration may be necessary to rule out the presence of a tumour and to possibly drain the abscess. Occasionally, testicular inflammation may be focal, even rounded, with areas of decreased echogenicity and swelling. Hyperaemia concentrated in the abnormal area should help differentiate inflammation from neoplasm (Fig. 12.8).

SPERMATIC CORD TORSION

The diagnosis of spermatic cord torsion must be established quickly to allow for prompt surgical correction, since obstruction of blood flow may result in the loss of testicular viability within a few hours of onset of symptoms. Clinical history and physical findings,

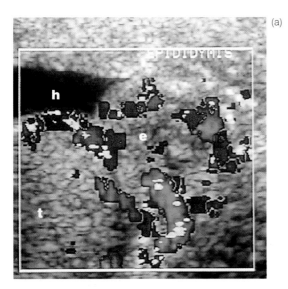 (a)

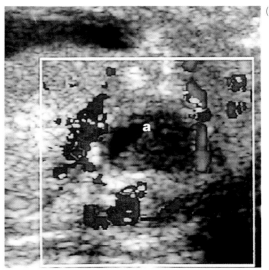 (b)

Fig. 12.7 (a) Transverse image of a patient with acute end epididymitis. Note the hyperaemia of the epididymis (e) as compared to the underlying testicle (t). There is a small hydrocoele (h). (b) Transverse view of the epididymis 10 days later. The patient had a poor response to a course of antibiotics. An irregular fluid and debris collection is now noted within the epididymis with surround hyperaemia. The inflammatory process had evolved into an abscess (a).

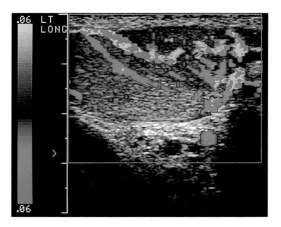

Fig. 12.8 Longitudinal colour view of the testicle. The clinical presentation of this patient was that of an inflammatory process. A focal hypoechoic area at the lower pole shows obvious hyperaemia when compared to the normal upper pole. The diagnosis was focal orchitis.

however, overlap with those of inflammatory disease to such a degree that even an experienced urologist may not be able to differentiate the two conditions. Symptoms and signs include sudden pain in the scrotum, lower abdomen or inguinal area (frequently accompanied by nausea, vomiting and low-grade fever), a tender testicle with a transverse lie, and a swollen, erythematous hemiscrotum[14].

By itself, grey-scale sonography has a low

sensitivity and specificity when evaluating patients with suspected torsion. Findings will depend on the length of time the torsion has been present[1, 2, 5, 21, 25, 26]. During the first few hours, testicular appearance will be normal but after about 4–6 hours, as the veins are obstructed, there is vascular engorgement and the testis becomes enlarged and oedematous, with a hypoechoic appearance[7]. After 24 hours, vascular congestion, haemorrhage and infarction will cause the testis to appear heterogeneous (Fig. 12.9). The epididymis may also be enlarged and hypoechoic because of decreased blood supply.

The addition of colour Doppler increases sensitivity in adults to 90–100% with a high specificity[1, 21, 27]. Unlike grey-scale images, colour Doppler is almost always abnormal even during the early stages of torsion[14]. Instrument settings should be optimised on the *normal* side to detect low-velocity flow before ascertaining that there is decreased blood flow on the *symptomatic* side (Fig. 12.10). If arterial flow cannot be detected in the symptomatic testicle but can in the contralateral testicle, the diagnosis of torsion can be effectively established[14]. The characteristic indication of ischaemia is a completely avascular testicle. In

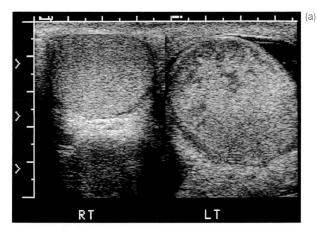

(a)

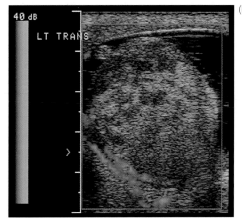

(b)

Fig. 12.9 (a) Transverse view of the mid-testis bilaterally. Note the enlarged left testicle with an irregular heterogeneous echotexture. (b) Power Doppler transverse image of the left testicle shows some scrotal wall flow and perhaps some capsular flow but no flow is perceived within the testicular parenchyma. At surgery this was a grossly necrotic torsed testicle.

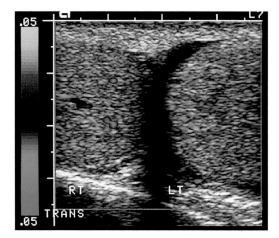

Fig. 12.10 Transverse colour Doppler view of both mid-testes. The Doppler settings are optimized to low flow. Clear asymmetry of colour is perceived with no flow seen on the left while flow is easily perceived on the right. The left testicle was found to be torsed at surgery.

the late stages of torsion, colour Doppler may reveal an increase in peritesticular blood flow because of inflammation in the surrounding soft tissues of the scrotum[1-3, 5, 28].

Evaluation of the small testicles of prepubescent patients, however, can be very difficult because of low-velocity blood flow[14, 27]. In addition, if the patient has intermittent episodes of torsion, or if the torsion resolves spontaneously, blood flow may appear normal on colour Doppler since absence of flow is demonstrated only if torsion is present at the time of sonographic examination. Thus, differentiating between normal and symptomatic testicles may be hard to accomplish in children.

If the testis does spontaneously untwist prior to the ultrasound examination, colour Doppler imaging may show diffuse, reactive hyperaemia. Although this finding may appear similar to that of epididymo-orchitis, spontaneous resolution of acute scrotal pain and increased blood flow are highly indicative of resolution[2, 3, 12, 21]. Colour Doppler ultrasound can also be used to monitor non-surgical detorsion of the testicle as the testis is manually

rotated; if this manoeuvre is successful, blood flow is re-established to the testicle and can be detected on Doppler (Fig. 12.11).

This non-surgical approach, however, is only considered a temporizing measure, it is *not* a substitute for surgical intervention, which is still necessary to correct the underlying anatomic deformity that increases the likelihood of torsion. Hand-held continuous wave Doppler has no role in the evaluation of testicular torsion because of its inability to provide range-gated information, and normal or increased blood flow within the scrotal wall may lead the examiner to incorrectly conclude that intratesticular flow is preserved.

Finally, although testicular torsion may be accurately diagnosed by sonography, this does not guarantee successful surgical salvage; salvage rates depend on the duration of ischaemia.

TESTICULAR NEOPLASMS

Patients with testicular neoplasms usually present with a palpable testicular nodule. For palpable testicular or scrotal masses, ultrasound of the scrotum is widely considered the imaging modality of choice. Most palpable extratesticular masses are benign, whereas intratesticular masses are considered malignant

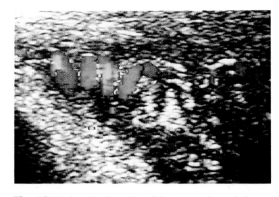

Fig. 12.11 Longitudinal view of the spermatic cord. A twist of the testicular artery is seen to the level of the mid-cord. Monitoring of the cord and testicle with colour Doppler can confirm successful detorsion.

until proven otherwise. Ultrasound can differentiate solid and cystic masses and confirm their extra- or intratesticular location. The main benefit of ultrasound is to identify those masses which may require additional assessment and possible surgical intervention.

On grey-scale images, testicular neoplasms usually appear as a discrete mass whose echo pattern differs from that of the normal testis. Most neoplasms have hypoechoic components[29–32], although heterogeneity of echotexture is frequently observed (particularly with large seminomas and non-seminomatous germ cell tumours). Sonographic differentiation of seminomas, embryonal cell carcinomas, teratomas and choriocarcinomas can be difficult, especially since 40–60% of testicular neoplasms have mixed histologic elements.

Seminomas are the most common single-cell type testicular tumour in adult males (40–50%)[33]. The 'classic' ultrasound appearance of seminomas has been described as a well-defined, uniformly hypoechoic lesion, with no evidence of calcification, haemorrhage, or cystic areas[33]. Modern high-frequency transducers, however, show fine details of the neoplasm's internal structure and seminomas may appear to be less homogeneous than previously described.

The general ultrasound appearance of germ cell tumours is that of an inhomogeneous, small mass with poorly defined margins, anechoic areas due to cystic necrosis, and echogenic foci of haemorrhage[34]. If the tumour invades the tunica, the normal contour of the testicle may be distorted[11].

Teratomas generally appear on ultrasound as extremely inhomogeneous masses with well-defined margins, and areas of various sizes that may be either hyperechoic or hypoechoic[11]. Dense echogenic foci caused by calcification, cartilage, immature bone, fibrosis and non-calcified fibrous tissue can cause acoustic shadowing. Old haemorrhage and necrosis may result in hypoechoic areas. Cysts are a common

characteristic of teratomas and can cause increased thick-walled anechoic areas with through-transmission.

Choriocarcinomas generally appear as small masses on ultrasound but notable haemorrhage may also be seen. Areas containing either solid or cystic components associated with viable tissue, necrosis and haemorrhage may be observed. If calcification is present, a distinct area of increased echogenicity with posterior acoustic shadowing may be present.

Testicular neoplasms have mixed histologic components in 40–60% of cases[35–37], with the most common combination being that of teratoma and embryonal carcinoma (teratocarcinoma). Ultrasound findings of mixed tumours will vary, depending on which cell lines are dominant, and there are no particular ultrasound findings that permit differentiation for possible preoperative planning.

If a testicular mass is suspected of being a tumour, the rest of the scrotum should be examined carefully to exclude any invasion of the tunica albuginea or epididymis by the neoplasm. Enlargement of the epididymis usually indicates epididymo-orchitis or torsion, rather than neoplasm. An extratesticular fluid collection normally indicates inflammation, torsion or trauma, although testicular neoplasms can be associated with hydrocoeles[32]. Because a hypoechoic appearance has also been reported with other testicular conditions (e.g. epididymo-orchitis, trauma, spermatic cord torsion, sarcoid)[29, 32, 38], these additional extratesticular findings help in the differential diagnosis and in the confirmation of neoplasm.

Colour Doppler and spectral Doppler sonography are considered to be of minimal benefit in the evaluation and characterization of adult testicular masses and the diagnosis of testicular neoplasm (Fig. 12.12). This is because masses can be either hypo- or hypervascular. Small lesions tend to be hypovascular while larger lesions may be hypervascular compared with normal testicular parenchyma.

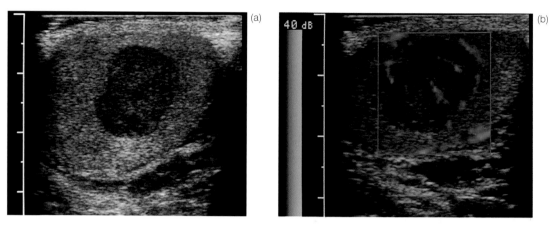

Fig. 12.12 (a) Longitudinal view of the testicle. A large central hypoechoic mass is perceived, suspicious for neoplasm. (b) Power Doppler image shows some flow along the periphery and within the centre of the mass. This was a surgically proven seminoma. Most lesions such as this fail to reveal flow on standard ultrasound equipment, but some of the newer high-resolution units are able to detect subtle flow within these lesions.

An infiltrative neoplasm of the testicle, such as leukaemia or lymphoma, typically presents as an enlarged hypoechoic area on grey-scale imaging[39]. Colour Doppler may demonstrate hyperaemia in the neoplasm with increased flow in areas of leukaemic or lymphomatous involvement, or flow only along the periphery of the lesion (Fig. 12.13), but the appearance is quite similar to inflammation, and clinical or surgical corroboration is required to differentiate these conditions[39].

It has been suggested that colour Doppler imaging may be more useful in evaluating paediatric patients, in whom testicular neoplasms may be difficult to distinguish with grey-scale imaging but tend to be hypervascular on colour Doppler[40].

TRAUMA

Clinical examination of a traumatized, tender testicle can be difficult because of pain and swelling. However, ultrasound evaluation is able to provide information regarding testicular integrity, and the presence of haematoma, haematocoele, fracture or rupture. Colour Doppler sonography provides excellent delineation of blood flow throughout the testis,

differentiating hyperaemic, contused regions from devascularized or ischaemic areas (Figs 12.9 and 12.14).

In the case of testicular rupture, sonographic identification is extremely important because prompt diagnosis and quick surgical intervention is required to successfully correct the condition. If surgery is performed within 72 hours of the trauma, approximately 90% of ruptured testes can be salvaged[41]. If rupture is present, ultra-

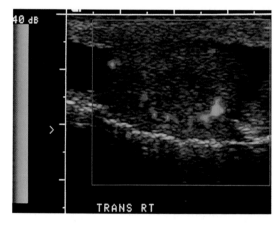

Fig. 12.13 Transverse view of the right testicle in a patient with chronic lymphocytic leukaemia. A subtle rounded area of altered echotexture is perceived within the centre of the testicle. It is much more obvious with the rim of flow on power Doppler. Note the small hydrocoele.

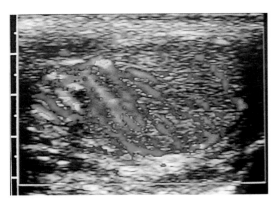

Fig. 12.14 Longitudinal view of a traumatized testicle and epididymis. Note that testicular integrity is maintained but there is marked hyperaemia throughout the epididymis and upper testicle. This injury was treated conservatively and resolved.

sound examination may demonstrate a disrupted hyperechoic tunica albuginea; a heterogeneous testicle with asymmetric, poorly defined margins; thickening of the wall of the scrotum; and a large haematocoele[6, 16, 38]. Perception of blood flow will be diminished or absent on colour or spectral Doppler examination.

Unlike rupture, fractures and small haematomas and haematocoeles do not require surgery if the tunica albuginea has not been interrupted and Doppler imaging shows normal blood flow to the testicle. Sonographic findings associated with a testicular fracture include a linear hypoechoic band crossing the parenchyma of the testicle, a smooth, well-defined testicular outline, an intact tunica albuginea, and often an associated haematocoele. Normal Doppler signals indicate unimpaired blood flow and viable testicular tissue. If Doppler signals are absent, ischaemia is very likely and surgical intervention is called for. Acute haematomas are usually hyperechoic relative to adjacent testicular parenchyma[15, 38]. Older haematomas may have both hyper- and hypoechoic areas, and there may be associated thickening of the scrotal wall. On colour Doppler, haematomas are usually avascular[1-3]. Acute haematocoeles tend to be echogenic, while low-level echoes or separations may be seen in chronic haematocoeles.

VARICOCOELE

Incompetent or absent valves in the testicular veins cause stasis or retrograde blood flow to occur, resulting in dilatation of the pampiniform plexus. This is responsible for the majority of varicocoeles. The characteristic indication of ischaemia is a completely avascular testicle. Varicocoeles occur more commonly on the left; this is attributed to the longer course of the gonadal vein and its direct drainage into the left renal vein. Varicocoeles are important clinically because of their association with infertility.

On ultrasound a varicocoele is seen to consist of dilated, tortuous channels in the epididymis and spermatic cord. Colour Doppler has been shown to be very accurate in detecting varicocoele[13]. Identification of varicocoele by colour Doppler is enhanced by having the patient perform the Valsalva manoeuvre, or by standing up. This increases the abdominal pressure and results in the reversal of blood flow into the pampiniform plexus, thereby causing further distention. When the Valsalva manoeuvre is then released, the direction of blood flow reverts to normal (Fig. 12.15). Whenever a varicocoele is identified, obstruction by a retroperitoneal mass should also be considered as a possible cause, in addition to incompetent or absent valves, and a scan of the upper abdomen performed to assess this possibility.

OTHER IMAGING PROCEDURES

Radio-isotope scanning to evaluate perfusion has essentially been replaced by Doppler sonography. Computed tomography (CT) is primarily used for staging and follow-up of testicular tumours metastatic to the retroperitoneum. Magnetic resonance imaging (MRI), because of its high cost and limited availability, is reserved for problem solving of difficult cases. In general, MRI has not been found to

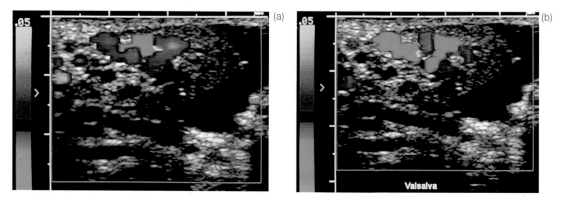

Fig. 12.15 (a) Longitudinal colour Doppler view of the spermatic cord at rest. Note the flow within the large tubular structures indicating a varicocoele. (b) Identical area as in (a) with the patient performing a Valsalva manoeuvre. Note the change of colour within these vessels indicating true flow reversal. In an infertile man, this finding is indicative of incompetent valves within the gonadal vein.

provide significant advantages over ultrasound in the evaluation of the scrotum[42–46].

Prior to the availability of sonography, scintigraphy was the standard diagnostic modality for evaluating testicular arterial perfusion[10, 47, 48]. However, studies comparing Doppler sonography and scintigraphy have shown that the sensitivity of the imaging techniques is similar in detecting testicular flow. In adolescents and adults, the sensitivity has been reported to be 86–100% for colour Doppler, 67–100% for pulsed Doppler, and 80–100% for scintigraphy[1, 5, 21, 28, 47, 49]. In paediatric patients, the sensitivity of colour Doppler has been reported to be 82–100% and 84–100% for scintigraphy[25, 27, 48, 50, 51].

Although scintigraphy continues to be a dependable means of imaging testicular blood flow, it lacks sonography's ability to provide anatomic information, as well as perfusion status, and it exposes the patient to radiation. Therefore, as suggested by Siegel[14], nuclear scintigraphy should be reserved for those situations when the sensitivity of colour Doppler for low-velocity, low-volume testicular arterial flow is not satisfactory and there are questions regarding the findings (e.g. in the small testicles of prepubescent patients) or when the examiner has limited proficiency with colour Doppler evaluation.

Recently, the use of echo-enhancing agents has been studied for improving imaging of small testicles with low-velocity and low-volume flow. In an animal study by Brown et al[52], the authors examined induced testicular torsion with grey-scale imaging, colour Doppler, power Doppler and spectral Doppler analysis. Injection of contrast media did not enhance grey-scale images but visualization of all vessels in both normal and rotated testicles was significantly improved with both colour and power Doppler. Asymmetry of blood flow was more obvious. The authors concluded that diagnosis of testicular ischaemia could be made with more confidence using an intravenous ultrasound contrast agent because of improved demonstration of altered perfusion patterns.

Similar findings were reported by Coley et al[53] in an animal study comparing unenhanced and contrast-enhanced Doppler analysis of acute testicular torsion. The findings from these studies indicate that use of contrast ultrasonography will likely reduce, and possibly eliminate, the need for scintigraphy in currently difficult-to-visualize testicles.

CONCLUSIONS

The scrotal contents are ideally situated for examination by ultrasound. They are small and superficial, allowing high-frequency transducers to be used for examinations. High-resolution images of the testes and associated structures are obtained and Doppler allows information on blood flow to be assessed; careful assessment of the findings will allow many problems to be clarified and managed without the need for further imaging.

REFERENCES

1. Horstman WG, Middleton WD, Melson GL, Siegel BA (1991) Colour Doppler US of the scrotum. *RadioGraphics* 11: 941–957
2. Learner RM, Mevorach RA, Hulbert WC, Rabinowitz R (1990) Colour Doppler US in the evaluation of acute scrotal disease. *Radiology* 176: 355–358
3. Luker GD, Siegel MJ (1994) Colour Doppler sonography of the scrotum in children. *American Journal of Radiology* 163: 649–655
4. Luker GD, Siegel MJ (1996) Scrotal US in pediatric patients: comparison of power and standard colour Doppler US. *Radiology* 198: 381–385
5. Middleton WD, Siegel BA, Melson GL *et al* (1990) Acute scrotal disorders: prospective comparison of colour Doppler US and testicular scintigraphy. *Radiology* 177: 177–181
6. Patriquin HB (1993) Leukemic infiltration of the testis. In: Siegel BA, Proto AV (eds) *Paediatric Disease, 4th series. Test and Syllabus*, pp 667–688. Reston, VA: American College of Radiology
7. Ralls PW, Larsen D, Johnson MB, Lee KP (1991) Colour Doppler sonography of the scrotum. Seminars in Ultrasound, Computed Tomography and Magnetic Resonance 112: 109–114
8. Bannister LH, Dyson M (1995) Reproductive system. In: Williams PL, Bannister LH, Berry MM *et al* (eds) *Gray's Anatomy*, 38th edn, pp 1848–1856. New York: Churchill Livingstone
9. Middleton WD, Thorne DA, Melson GC (1989) Colour Doppler ultrasound of the normal testis. *American Journal of Radiology* 152: 293–297
10. Holder LE, Martire JR, Holmes ER, Wagner HN (1977) Testicular radionuclide angiography and static imaging: anatomy, scintigraphic interpretation, and clinical indications. *Radiology* 125: 739–752
11. Krone KD, Carroll BA (1985) Scrotal ultrasound. *Radiology Clinics of North America* 23: 121–139
12. Middleton WD (1991) Scrotal sonography in 1991. *Ultrasound Quarterly* 9: 61–87
13. Petros JA, Andriole GL, Middleton WD, Picus DA (1991) Correlation of testicular colour Doppler ultrasonography, physical examination and venography in the detection of varicoceles in men with infertility. *Journal of Urology* 145: 785–788
14. Siegel MJ (1997) The acute scrotum. *Radiology Clinics of North America* 35: 959–976
15. Benson CB, Doubilet PM, Richie JP (1989) Sonography of the male genital tract. *American Journal of Radiography* 153: 705–713
16. Siegel MJ (1995) Male pelvis. In: Siegel MJ (ed.) *Paediatric Sonography*, 2nd edn, pp 479–512. New York: Raven Press
17. Jequier S, Patriquin H, Filiatrault D *et al* (1993) Duplex Doppler sonographic examination of the testis in prepubertal boys. *Journal of Ultrasound in Medicine* 12: 317–322
18. Paltiel HJ, Rupich RC, Babcock DS (1994) Maturational changes in arterial impedance of the normal testis in boys: Doppler sonographic study. *American Journal of Radiology* 163: 1189–1193
19. Hermansen MC, Chusid MJ, Sty JR (1980) Bacterial epididymo-orchitis in children and adolescents. *Clinical Paediatrics* 19: 812–815
20. Horstman WG, Middleton WD, Nelson GL (1991) Scrotal inflammatory disease: colour Doppler US findings. *Radiology* 179: 55–59
21. Burks DD, Markey BJ, Burkhard TK *et al* (1990) Suspected testicular torsion and ischaemia: evaluation with colour Doppler sonography. *Radiology* 175: 815–821
22. Brown JM, Hammers LW, Barton JW *et al* (1995) Quantitative Doppler assessment of acute scrotal inflammation. *Radiology* 197: 427–431
23. Sanders LM, Haber S, Dembner A, Aquino A (1994) Significance of reversal of diastolic flow in the acute scrotum. *Journal of Ultrasound in Medicine* 13: 137–139
24. Mevorach RA, Lerner RM, Dvortesky PM, Rabinowitz R (1986) Testicular abscess: diagnosed by ultrasonography. *Journal of Urology* 136: 1213–1216
25. Meza MP, Amundson GM, Aquilina JW, Reitelman C (1992) Colour flow imaging in children with clinically suspected testicular torsion. *Paediatric Radiology* 22: 370–373
26. Middleton WD, Melson GL (1989) Testicular ischemia: colour Doppler sonographic findings in five patients. *American Journal of Radiology* 152: 1237–1239
27. Patriquin HB, Yazbeck S, Trinh B *et al* (1993) Testicular torsion in infants and children: diagnosis with Doppler sonography. *Radiology* 188: 781–785
28. Leahy PF (1986) Diagnosis of testicular torsion using Doppler ultrasonic examination. *British Journal of Urology* 58: 696–697
29. Leopold GR, Woo VL, Scheible FW, Nachtsheim D, Gosink BB (1979) High-resolution ultrasonography of scrotal pathology. *Radiology* 131: 719–722

30. Sample WF, Gottesman JE, Skinner DG *et al* (1978) Grey-scale ultrasound of the scrotum. *Radiology* **127**: 225–228

31. Miskin M, Buckspan M, Bain J (1977) Ultrasound examination of scrotal masses. *Journal of Urology* **117**: 185–188

32. Arger PH, Mulhern CB, Coleman BG *et al* (1981) Prospective analysis of the value of scrotal ultrasound. *Radiology* **141**: 763–766

33. Muir CS, Nectoux J (1979) Epidemiology of cancer of the testis and penis. *National Cancer Institute Monograms* **53**: 157–164

34. Carroll BA, Gross DM (1983) High-frequency scrotal sonography. *American Journal of Radiology* **140**: 511–515

35. Mostofi FK (1973) Testicular tumours: epidemiologic, aetiologic and pathologic features. *Cancer* **32**: 1186–1201

36. Mostofi FK (1994) Tumours of the testis. *IARC Scientific Publications* **111**: 407–429

37. Kurman RJ, Scardino PT, McIntire KR *et al* (1977) Cellular localization of alpha-fetoprotein and human chorionic gonadotropin in germ cell tumors of the testis using an indirect immunoperoxidase technique (a new approach to classification utilizing tumor markers). *Cancer* **40**: 2136–2151

38. Jeffrey RB, Laing FC, Hricak H, McAninch JW (1983) Sonography of testicular trauma. *American Journal of Radiology* **141**: 993–995

39. Mazzu D, Jeffrey RB, Ralls PW (1995) Lymphoma and leukemia involving the testicles: findings on gray-scale and colour Doppler sonography. *American Journal of Radiology* **164**: 645–647

40. Luker GD, Siegel MJ (1994) Pediatric testicular tumors: evaluation with gray-scale and colour Doppler US. *Radiology* **191**: 561–564

41. Gross M (1969) Rupture of the testicle: the importance of early surgical treatment. *Journal of Urology* **101**: 196–197

42. Baker LL, Hajek PC, Burkhard TK *et al* (1987) Magnetic resonance imaging of the scrotum: normal anatomy. *Radiology* **163**: 89–92

43. Baker LL, Hajek PC, Burkhard TK *et al* (1987) Magnetic resonance imaging of the scrotum: pathologic anatomy. *Radiology* **163**: 93–98

44. Seidenwurm D, Smathers RL, Lo RK *et al* (1987) Testes and scrotum: MRI imaging at 1.5T. *Radiology* **164**: 393–398

45. Thurnher H, Hricak H, Carrol PR *et al* (1988) Imaging of the testis: comparison between MR imaging and US. *Radiology* **167**: 631–636

46. Johnson JO, Mattrey RF, Phillipson J (1990) Differentiation of seminomatous and non-seminomatous testicular tumors with MR imaging. *American Journal of Radiology* **154**: 539–543

47. Chen DC, Holder LE, Kaplan GN (1986) Correlation of radionuclide imaging and diagnostic ultrasound in scrotal diseases. *Journal of Nuclear Medicine* **27**: 1774–1781

48. Mendel JB, Taylor GA, Treves S *et al* (1985) Testicular torsion in children: scintigraphic assessment. *Paediatric Radiology* **15**: 110–115

49. Middleton WD, Siegel BA, Melson GL *et al* (1990) Acute scrotal disorders: prospective comparison of Doppler US and testicular scintigraphy. *Radiology* 177–181

50. Atkinson CO, Patrick LE, Ball TI *et al* (1992) The normal and abnormal scrotum in children: evaluation with colour Doppler sonography. *American Journal of Radiology* **158**: 613–617

51. Hollman AS, Ingram S, Carachi R, Davis C (1993) Colour Doppler imaging of the acute paediatric scrotum. *Paediatric Radiology* **23**: 83–87

52. Brown JM, Taylor KJW, Alderman JL, Quedens-Case C, Greener Y (1997) Contrast-enhanced ultrasonographic visualization of gonadal torsion. *Journal of Ultrasound in Medicine* **16**: 309–316

53. Coley BD, Frush DP, Babcock DS *et al* (1996) Acute testicular torsion: comparison of unenhanced and contrast-enhanced power Doppler US, colour Doppler US, and radionuclide imaging. *Radiology* **199**: 441–446

The female pelvis

PAUL A. DUBBINS

Ultrasound has assumed a central role in the investigation of gynaecological physiology and pathology. The advent of transvaginal probes has further advanced gynaecological applications to the extent that it is now an indispensable tool in the evaluation of the female pelvis. Limitations however remain. Ultrasound predominantly assesses structure, and while physiological changes can be documented by sequential ultrasound examinations such as change in the size and the appearance of an ovarian follicle over time, changes in perfusion of the uterus and ovaries at different phases of the menstrual cycle have been shown also to reflect features of subfertility. Similarly there are marked vascular changes known to take place in pathological conditions. For example, neovascularity is an early and persistent feature of tumour growth and if documentation of angiogenesis by Doppler techniques were achievable, this would be of enormous value in differentiation of benign from malignant tumours.

The indications for Doppler ultrasound in the evaluation of pelvic physiology and pathology in the female are therefore potentially large. However, initial optimism about the potential role of Doppler ultrasound in gynaecology showed a great deal of similarity with the situation in other areas of the body. Many pathologies will produce increased blood flow to the pelvic organs, and hitherto our methods of discriminating between the uncontrolled and irregular angiogenesis of malignant tumour from the angiogenesis associated with benign tumour, or even the hyperaemia of inflammatory conditions, have been insufficiently sophisticated to make a reliable distinction. This chapter presents the current state of knowledge for potential applications of Doppler ultrasound in gynaecological disease, while indicating those areas where the role of Doppler ultrasound is established and considering these in more detail.

ANATOMY

Knowledge of the course of the pelvic vessels is important for the proper performance and interpretation of the Doppler examination. Although the attention is drawn to the examination of the ovarian and uterine arteries, the anatomical relations of the pelvic organs to the iliac arteries and veins is also important. Pathological conditions affecting the major vessels in the pelvis may complicate uterine or ovarian pathology, such as iliac venous thrombosis, or may mimic gynaecological pathology, such as an iliac artery aneurysm.

The iliac arteries and veins course inferiorly and laterally from the aortic bifurcation and venous confluence respectively on the antero-

237

medial surface of the psoas muscle, to become the femoral artery and vein as they emerge beneath the inguinal ligament in the groin. Surface markings for the common and external iliac artery and vein are approximated by a line drawn from the umbilicus to the site of maximum pulsation in the groin. The common and external iliac vein lie medial and posterior to the artery. The vessels often form a lateral anatomical relationship to the ovary (Fig. 13.1). The internal iliac artery arises from the medial aspect of the common iliac artery along with the vein approximately 4 cm from the aortic bifurcation. It gives rise to two branches, an anterior and a posterior trunk. At this point, just distal to the bifurcation, the anterior trunk lies posterior to the ureter and to the ovaries. The anterior trunk has several branches, one of which is the uterine artery which runs medially on the surface of the levator ani muscles, crossing above the ureter and ascending in a tortuous fashion lateral to the uterus, giving off uterine branches. It is accompanied through its course by the uterine vein.

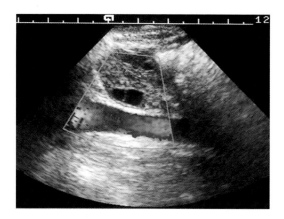

Fig. 13.1 Colour flow Doppler study of the left iliac fossa using compression. The left ovary is demonstrated anterior to the external iliac artery. There is a small amount of intraparenchymal flow within the ovary. The apparent bidirectional flow within the iliac artery is related to the geometry with the proximal iliac artery, indicating flow towards the transducer while the distal artery shows flow away from the transducer.

The ovarian artery is a branch of the renal artery on the left, although on the right it may arise from the aorta. Throughout its course in the abdomen it lies medial and posterior to the ureter, crossing the external iliac artery and vein to enter the true pelvis, where it turns medially in the ovarian suspensory ligament, passing into the broad ligament where its terminal branches supply the ovary and an anastomosis with branches of the uterine artery.

TECHNIQUE

The examination of the pelvic vessels has been significantly altered by the transvaginal technique of evaluation of pelvic anatomy and pathology. The course of the uterine artery is particularly suitable for transvaginal assessment, with ideal geometry for Doppler signal recording (Fig. 13.2). Similarly, however, it is possible to record Doppler signals transabdominally with an empty bladder, when the uterus is normally anteverted, for similar reasons of geometry. When the bladder is full, however, the angle of incidence of the Doppler beam to the uterine arteries is not optimized in spite of good visualization of the body of the uterus (Figs 13.3 and 13.4). The ovarian arteries, running a somewhat transverse course through the pelvis, are more difficult to assess, although greater sensitivity of signal recording is almost invariably achieved with transvaginal scanning.

Demonstration of the uterine and ovarian vessels requires colour flow Doppler for their identification. It is difficult to be prescriptive about colour flow settings but the following generalizations apply:

Filtration

The lowest possible filtration, particularly when investigating pelvic venous disease and conditions affecting 'perfusion' of tissues.

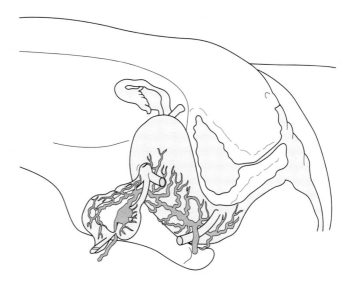

Fig. 13.2 Uterine and ovarian artery distribution. The uterine artery is a branch of the internal iliac artery and ascends on the lateral border of the uterus. It sends branches to the ovary and to the fallopian tube. The ovary is also supplied by the ovarian artery, a branch usually of the renal artery.

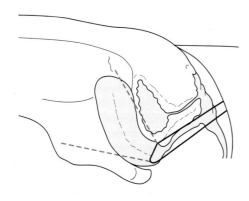

Fig. 13.3 Sagittal sections through the pelvis demonstrating the optimum geometry achieved by a transvaginal scan with an empty bladder.

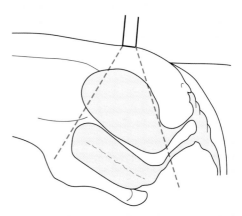

Fig. 13.4 Sagittal planes through the abdomen demonstrating that with a full urinary bladder the geometry for Doppler assessment of blood flow is suboptimal.

Colour/B-mode priority

For the most part small vessels are being investigated and it is less critical to exclude 'colour bleed' outwith the wall of the vessel; high colour priority should therefore be selected.

Persistence

A moderate persistence setting should be selected.

Velocity range

Selection of velocity range depends upon whether arteries or veins are being interrogated. Arterial flow within the uterine and ovarian arteries is usually within the range of 10–50 cm s^{-1} peak systolic velocity, although this may be lower, particularly in post-menopausal ovarian vessels. Flow velocity in pelvic veins is in the region of 1–10 cm s^{-1}. Velocity range settings should be chosen to reflect these predicted velocities.

Motion artefact

Most machines now have specific algorithms to reduce motion artefact and these should be employed.

Spectral Doppler settings

These reflect the colour Doppler settings but the need to use low filtration is particularly important in order to detect slow flow in veins and diastolic flow in arteries.

Angle of insonation

As with all Doppler applications, it is important to optimize the angle of insonation of the Doppler beam on the vessel but this may be compromised by the direction of flow and the limitations that transducer position, both abdominally and intravaginally, provide for variation of this angle. Where possible angles of less than 60° should be employed, although this is less important if velocities are not being measured. Although Doppler indices such as the resistance index (RI) and the pulsatility index (PI) are widely used in gynaecology and are angle independent, these are often supplemented in clinical applications by measurements of peak systolic velocity, which will require stringent attention to angle optimization and correction.

Sample volume

The vessels under study are small and therefore sample volume size should be at a minimum.

Technique for evaluating pathology

It is important when assessing pelvic pathology with Doppler techniques that optimum signal-recording methods are used. Evaluation of vessels is straightforward but in the demonstration of mass lesions, inflammatory processes, etc., careful attention to technique will ensure that the vascular supply is accurately mapped and Doppler spectra precisely recorded.

When a suspected pathological process is identified on real-time ultrasound, it is assessed with colour Doppler. Flexibility of the use of the colour box is important: initially for small- to moderate-sized lesions the whole lesion can be contained within the colour box in order to identify regions of increased vascularity, but this large field of view compromises the frame rate and pulse repetition rate, affecting the detection of high velocities and potentially also pulsatile flow. Therefore a smaller colour box is then selected and individual zones within the lesion are interrogated sequentially. Attention is paid to the size, distribution and communications of the vessels together with the vessels of supply and drainage. Throughout the procedure the machine settings are varied to optimize the system for very high and very low velocities. Sampling with spectral Doppler is performed at multiple sites, as some vessels may demonstrate apparently normal flow patterns, while others will demonstrate abnormal flow patterns and Doppler indices. Failure to record signals in this obsessive way will result in a lower accuracy of the technique.

Ultrasound contrast media will enhance the signal in all uterine and ovarian masses. This has the potential to improve the visualization of a wide variety of pelvic pathology, but it is not yet established whether this will improve the differentiation of different pathologies and no distinct application has been identified[1].

NORMAL APPEARANCES

Colour flow Doppler will demonstrate the uterine arteries coursing along the lateral aspects of the body of the uterus (Fig. 13.5).

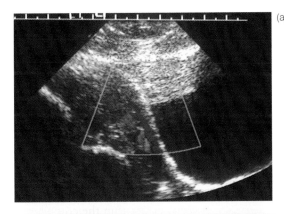

(a)

(b)

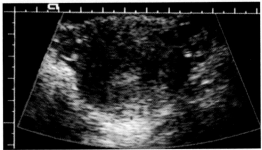

Fig. 13.5 (a) Sagittal transabdominal scan along the left margin of the uterus demonstrating the uterine artery and vein. (b) Transverse scan demonstrating both uterine arteries running along the lateral aspect of the uterus.

The branches of the uterine artery extending towards the ovary and the ovarian artery can be identified in the broad ligament and on the superior aspect of the ovary, respectively. Because of their tortuosity, only short segments of the arteries are usually identified in any particular scan plane (Fig. 13.6).

Pelvic veins

Normal venous structures can be seen within the body of the uterus and in both adnexae coursing towards the ovarian vein and the uterine veins.

Normal Doppler spectra

Normal Doppler spectra vary throughout the menstrual cycle. This variation is particularly

(a) marked in the ovarian artery which demonstrates a low-resistance pattern at the time of the development of the corpus luteum. However, there is wide variation in reported normal values of stromal ovarian and ovarian artery flow. Typically the resistance index in the early follicular phase is in the region of 0.65–0.7, falling to 0.55–0.6 in the late follicular phase and returning to early follicular phase values in the early luteal phase. However, published normal values range between 0.4 and 0.8 and pulsatility index values vary from 0.6 to 2.5. Similar values for ovarian vascular indices have also been recorded in postmenopausal ovaries but the cyclical variation is lost[2]. Thus an individual measurement of ovarian artery impedance is of limited value in assessment of ovarian

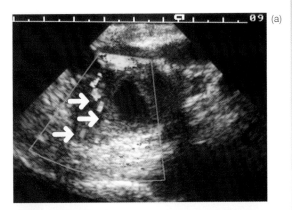

(a)

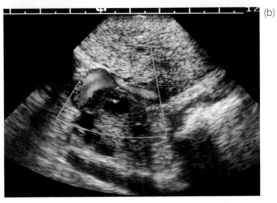

(b)

Fig. 13.6 (a) Left ovary demonstrating uterine and ovarian branches (arrowheads). (b) Blood supply to the fallopian tube and ovary from the uterine artery.

function, although the cyclical change of ovarian flow does correlate with development of the corpus luteum.

Cyclical variation in uterine artery flow is well defined and also appears to correlate with fertility; normal values are given in Table 13.1. It is important to note, however, that mean values for uterine artery flow in post-

menopausal patients are similar to those recorded for the mid-luteal phase in premenopausal patients. Again, therefore, it appears that cyclical variation is more important in the assessment of normal reproductive physiology, rather than using individual values[3, 4]. Normal Doppler spectra are illustrated in Figs 13.7–13.10.

Table 13.1 Variation in Doppler indices in the uterine and ovarian arteries in the menstrual cycle.

	RI OVA[a]	PI OVA[a]	VEL OVA[a] (cm s⁻¹)	PI UTA[a]
Early follicular	0.65–0.7	1.8–2.2	20	1.67 ± 0.22
Late follicular/ovulation	0.55–0.6	1.0–1.3	40	1.89 ± 0.4
Luteal	0.6–0.65	1.3–1.8		2.23 ± 0.67
Non-conception	0.6–0.7	1.8–2.2		3.85 ± 1.1
Postmenopausal	0.6–1.0	1.3–4.0		1.8–3.8

[a]RI = resistance index; PI = pulsatility index; OVA = ovarian artery; VEL = velocity; UTA = uterine artery.

(a)

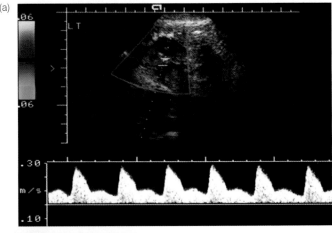

(b)

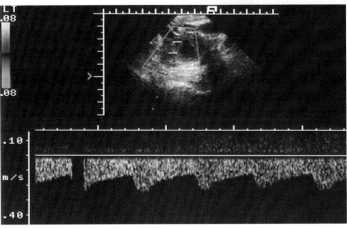

Fig. 13.7 (a) Doppler spectrum of ovarian blood flow within the follicular phase. (b) Low-resistance blood flow at the time of ovulation.

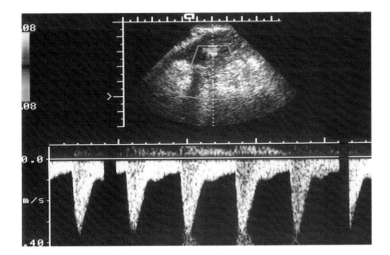

Fig. 13.8 Doppler spectrum of normal uterine artery blood flow in the late follicular phase.

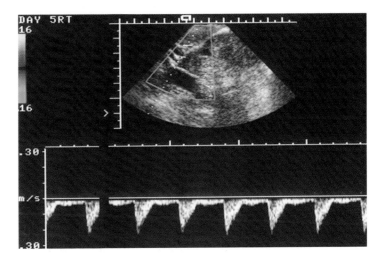

Fig. 13.9 Doppler spectrum of uterine artery blood flow in the luteal phase.

Pelvic venous diameter is extremely variable but pelvic veins are normally less than 5 mm in diameter and flow velocities between 5 and 10 cm s^{-1}. In this author's experience reverse flow on Valsalva is short lived and of low velocity (<2 cm s^{-1}).

ERRORS AND ARTEFACTS[5]

There are a number of factors which will contribute to alterations in flow and which are not related to pelvic pathology. These are common to all vessels and include the following:

Hypertension

Indices will be uniformly slightly increased.

Abnormalities of heart rate and rhythm

Both pulsatility and resistance indices will be decreased in tachycardias and increased in bradycardias. Irregularities such as atrial fibrillation will invalidate the use of any of the Doppler indices.

Sample volume artefacts

Because of the small size of many of the vessels under study, maintenance of the position of the

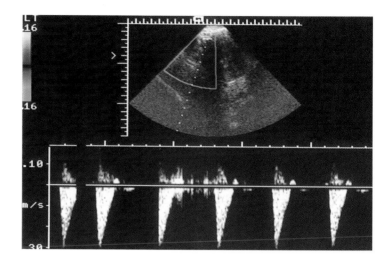

Fig. 13.10 Doppler spectrum of uterine artery blood flow in the postmenopausal uterus.

sample volume within the centre of the vessel is frequently difficult. This has the effect that there may be inaccurate recording of either systolic or diastolic flow velocities, dependent upon vessel movement relative to the sample volume throughout the cardiac cycle. This produces variation in the appearance of the Doppler spectrum and variation in the Doppler indices.

Bowel movement may provide significant imaging artefact, but although this may compromise Doppler signal recording, it is not usually confused for normal or abnormal blood flow patterns.

Bladder distension also has an effect on Doppler spectra, producing a significant increase in the impedance indices compared to the empty bladder[6].

APPLICATIONS

Fertility

The cyclic changes of blood flow characteristics and Doppler indices within the uterine and ovarian arteries suggest a possible application in the diagnosis and management of subfertility. For example, changes in the pulsatility index in the uterine arteries on day 14 correlate with successful pregnancy as well as with

biochemical markers of uterine receptivity, with mean values of uterine artery pulsatility index of less than 2.65 for conception cycles, compared with non-conception cycles of 3.85[7]. These changes can be used to augment morphological information about the uterus and ovaries in the diagnosis and management of subfertility (Fig. 13.11).

The mean pulsatility index in the uterine and ovarian arteries of infertile women in the mid-luteal phase is significantly greater than that in fertile women[8]. However, although there is an increase in blood flow to the ovaries during follicular development, there is no correlation between peak systolic velocity and oocyte quality[9]. It is interesting to note that the changes in flow associated with infertility are seen not only in primary ovarian failure but also in tubal blockage although the causation of this phenomenon is not clear[3].

The periovulatory reductions in pulsatility and resistance index in the ovarian artery are not seen in infertile women. An elevated uterine artery pulsatility index is also seen in patients with polycystic ovarian syndrome, although the ovarian artery pulsatility index is low. A high vascular resistance in the uterine artery and ovarian artery in the luteal phase indicates a poor 'baby take-home rate'.

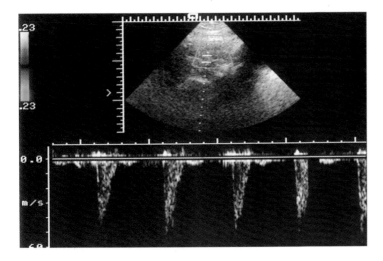

Fig. 13.11 Doppler spectrum of uterine artery blood flow in infertility.

In patients undergoing ovulation induction, the pulsatility and resistance indices are reduced within the ovarian and uterine arteries when induction is successful. If the ovulation induction is ineffective then there are no changes in the indices. Similarly, in ovarian failure, treatment with hormone replacement therapy allows the restoration of normal endometrial flow, which implies improved receptivity for oocyte donation[10].

The small subgroup of infertile patients with a short luteal phase do not have a demonstrable corpus luteum vascularization problem, and these patients do not benefit from colour flow and pulsed Doppler monitoring.

In summary, duplex ultrasound has a significant role to play in the investigation and management of infertility. It is particularly useful in identifying patients for different treatment regimens and represents a more precise technique in the evaluation of uterine receptivity.

Diseases of the uterine body

Fibroids

The vascularity of fibroids is variable. In some patients, blood flow to the uterus yields normal resistance and pulsatility indices with uterine vessels simply being displaced around the fibroids. In other cases, the fibroids may demonstrate marked vascularity with increased number and size of uterine vessels (Figs 13.12–13.14) together with a significant reduction in peripheral resistance to blood flow evidenced by reduction in pulsatility and resistance indices below 0.8 and 2.0, respectively. Indeed Wiener et al[11] indicate that the lowest impedance indices of all the uterine pathologies are recorded in uterine fibroids. There is some evidence that these vascular fibroids respond better to medical suppressive therapy and this may be useful in their management. There is,

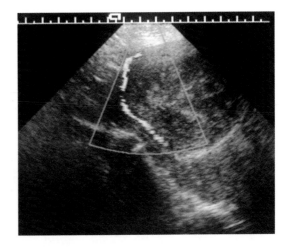

Fig. 13.12 Colour flow Doppler of marginal blood flow in uterine fibroids.

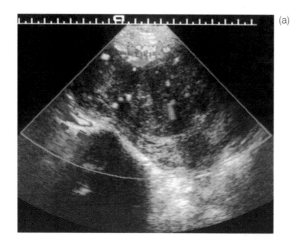

(a)

Fig. 13.13 (a) Irregular blood flow both at the margin and within the uterine fibroids. There was grey-scale evidence of partial necrosis. (b) Doppler spectrum of same patient showing increased systolic and diastolic velocities with reduction in resistance indices indicating uterine hyperaemia with vascular fibroids.

(b)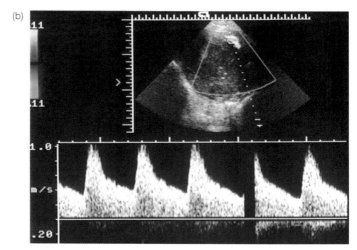

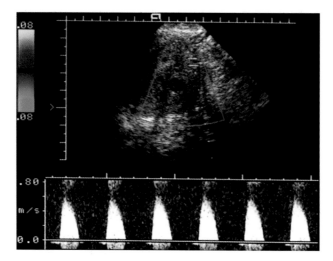

Fig. 13.14 Doppler spectrum of uterine artery flow in postmenopausal uterus with uterine fibroids. No evidence of increase in blood flow velocities, particularly in diastole.

however, no evidence that malignant tumours of the myometrium demonstrate any specific Doppler ultrasound features[12].

Endometrial disease

Endometrial hyperplasia, endometrial polyps and endometrial carcinoma can produce similar appearances on transvaginal ultrasound. There is broadening and inhomogeneity of the thickness of the endometrium. Differentiation of neoplasia from hyperplasia largely depends upon identifying an endometrial thickness greater than 5 mm. While this represents a sensitive method it lacks specificity.

Although flow characteristics within the uterine arteries reflect a reduced resistance to flow in many cases of endometrial cancer, this is not invariably the case, nor is it exclusive to malignancy (Figs 13.15 and 13.16). Nonetheless, in the presence of postmenopausal bleeding and in the absence of uterine fibroids it has been suggested that uterine artery and endometrial Doppler are sensitive in the differentiation of significant pathology from endometrial atrophy. When no pathology of the endometrium is present then resistance

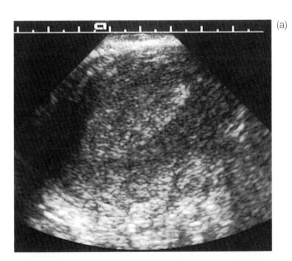
(a)

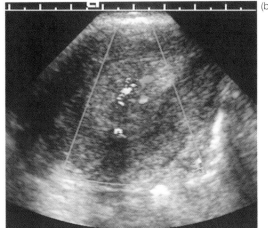
(b)

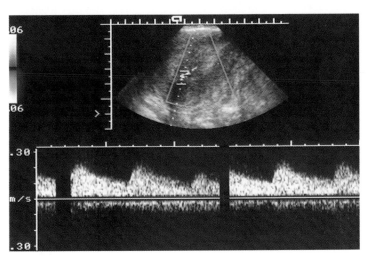
(c)

Fig. 13.15 (a) Transvaginal ultrasound demonstrating endometrial hyperplasia. (b) Same patient. Colour flow Doppler demonstrating endometrial vascularity. (c) Spectral Doppler within the vessels in the endometrium shows resistance indices less than 0.77.

13

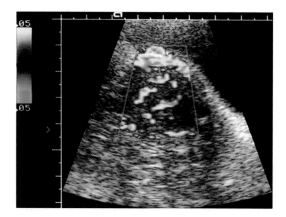

Fig. 13.16 Transabdominal ultrasound of the uterus with abnormal flow demonstrating gross hyperaemia extending to the surface of the uterus in an endometrial carcinoma with extensive myometrial invasion.

index values are 0.85 ± 0.08, whereas if there is pathology present these are 0.77 ± 0.03. Furthermore these authors indicate that, in their experience, malignancy has not been found in patients where the resistance index was recorded as greater than 0.83, perhaps allowing a more conservative approach in this group[11]. Visual assessment of colour Doppler distribution alone has been reported to be only 39% sensitive in the detection of endometrial malignancy[12].

Tamoxifen

Tamoxifen is widely used in the treatment of breast carcinoma and has an oestrogenic effect on the endometrium. This produces significant endometrial thickening and there is an associated increase in the incidence of endometrial carcinoma. There is a concomitant increase in blood flow within the uterine arteries and within the myometrial vessels, which may be demonstrated on colour Doppler and by a decrease in the blood flow indices. However, this is not specific for malignancy and there are no features which will currently allow a specific diagnosis (Fig. 13.17)[13].

Hormone replacement therapy

Hormone replacement therapy produces no significant change in blood flow characteristics to the normal postmenopausal uterus[14]. However, in the presence of uterine fibroids there may be increased blood flow with particular increase in the diastolic component in patients on replacement therapy.

Trophoblastic disease

Hydatidiform mole, invasive mole and choriocarcinoma are rare neoplasms of the endometrium. Thickening and inhomogeneity of the endometrium are characteristic ultrasound features with a varying degree of formation of vesicles within the uterine cavity. Ultrasound imaging is relatively poor at distinguishing the three levels of severity of the disease and, unless there is evidence of distant metastases, it is unreliable at the assessment of degree of invasion. There is a significant increase in myometrial and endometrial blood flow as evidenced by colour Doppler in all of the trophoblastic tumours; this is usually more marked in the more aggressive tumours (Fig. 13.18). Similarly, Doppler indices are altered in trophoblastic disease: a mean peak systolic velocity of 57.5 ± 20.4 (normal 28.3 ± 3. 41) and a resistance index of 0.56 ± 0.19 (normal 0.86 ± 0.05) have been demonstrated, although the resistance index may vary from 0.2 to 0.8. Nonetheless, the extent of intratumoral flow correlates with the prognosis: the higher the resistance index, the lesser the need for prolonged treatment cycles[15, 16]. Furthermore, the return of the Doppler indices to normal values is good evidence of successful surgical or medical treatment.

Ovarian disease

Ovarian cancer

Detection and characterization of ovarian tumours has depended upon the demonstration

(a)

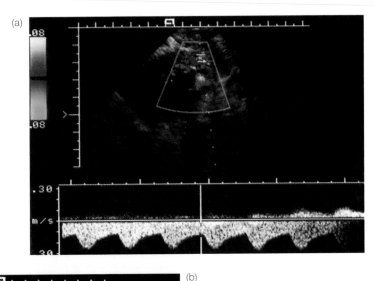

(b)

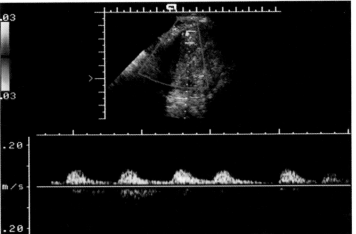

Fig. 13.17 (a) Spectral Doppler of uterine artery demonstrating increased uterine blood flow in patient on tamoxifen. (b) The return of uterine blood flow to normal values after withdrawal of tamoxifen.

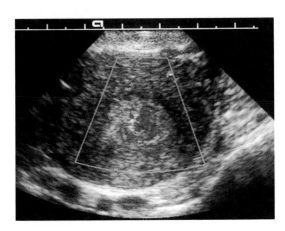

Fig. 13.18 Colour flow Doppler of flow in trophoblast. In this case this was retained products of conception but similar features can be seen in trophoblastic tumours.

of ovarian enlargement and the identification of both cystic and solid masses within the ovary. Criteria for malignancy include the size and complexity of lesions. However, not all malignant lesions demonstrate characteristic ultrasound features. Furthermore, if ultrasound is to have a role in screening for ovarian carcinoma, then features must be sought that would allow the early identification of a potentially malignant lesion prior to the development of frank malignant morphology.

Considerable research work has suggested that malignant tumours demonstrate higher diastolic flow and consequently lower resistance and pulsatility indices than those seen in benign tumours. Similarly, the pattern of colour flow in benign and malignant tumours is reportedly different (Figs 13.19–13.23). However, the reported accuracy of colour flow and spectral Doppler is the subject of wide variability within the literature. Chou et al[17] and Sengoku et al[18] suggest a sensitivity of 100% with a negative predictive value of 100%, while Bromley et al[19] and Brown et al[20] record sensitivities of only 66% and 50%, respectively. The uncertainty about the value of Doppler is perhaps best reflected in the variation of criteria used by different authors to indicate the presence or absence of malignancy. The cut-off values for the resistance index range between 0.4 and 0.6, while others simply use a visual assessment of the colour Doppler pattern. It is important therefore to compare the results of Doppler findings with the reported sensitivity of ovarian morphology alone in predicting malignancy, which is in the region of 91–98%[19, 21].

In isolation, therefore, Doppler does not appear to confer a significant advantage in the diagnosis of malignant disease over ultrasound imaging alone. Studies attempting to combine a morphological score with Doppler features and indices suggest that although diagnostic sensitivities may be unaltered, there may be significant improvement in positive predictive value from 60% to 94%[22]. It is not surprising that the early results have not been borne out by subsequent studies. The process of angioneogenesis is a microscopic one and is at least partly dependent on cell type and morphology[23].

The situation in premenopausal patients is more complex still. The presence of low-resistance flow in a corpus luteum requires that any suspicious lesion be examined in the early proliferative phase of the menstrual cycle to ensure that the neovascularity is not a physiological response (Fig. 13.24).

The current situation is probably best summed up by Carter et al[24], who conclude that colour Doppler has neither the sensitivity nor the specificity to distinguish between benign and malignant disease of the ovary.

At present the role in identifying malignant tumours relies on Doppler indices that were developed for documentation of severity of vascular disease. It is possible that the development of new techniques for the assessment and quantification of Doppler data may enhance this role. For example, in diseases of the breast, demonstration of abnormal vascular anastomoses appears important for the diagnosis of malignancy. In the evaluation of the prostate, colour Doppler, particularly when contrast

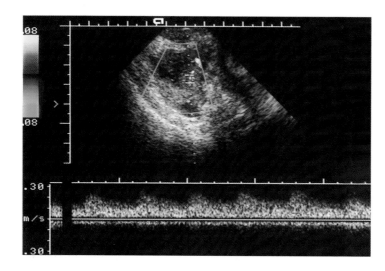

Fig. 13.19 Solid ovarian tumour with colour flow Doppler at the margin and spectral Doppler demonstrating low resistance.

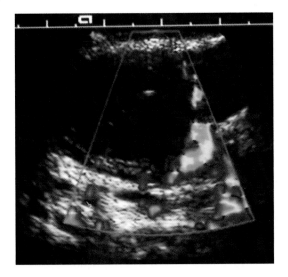

Fig. 13.20 Colour flow Doppler at the margin of an apparently simple cyst but which subsequently proved to have borderline malignancy detectable in the wall.

enhanced, appears to be of value in monitoring the effect of treatment[25].

Screening for ovarian cancer

Although it is clear that transvaginal ultrasound can identify asymptomatic masses postmenopausally, at present there is an assumption rather than proof that this does more than just affect the 'lead time' to the diagnosis of ovarian cancer. Furthermore, the case for cost effectiveness is far from proven. Screening of first-order relatives of those with ovarian cancer may be justified, and in these patients the addition of colour flow and spectral Doppler may contribute to the security of a negative screening result. Doppler may also be of value in the management of patients who

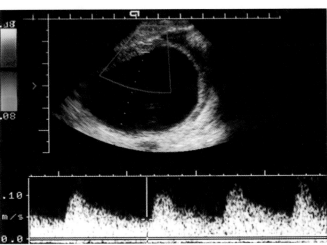

Fig. 13.21 Simple ovarian cyst with spectral Doppler recorded in the cyst wall with relatively low resistance index of 0.64.

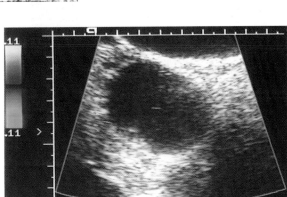

Fig. 13.22 Heterogeneous ovarian mass with cystic and solid elements but little parenchymal flow on colour flow Doppler. This was an ovarian fibroma.

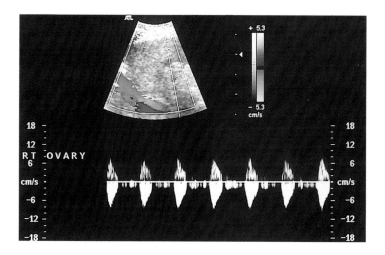

Fig. 13.23 Spectral Doppler of a postmenopausal ovary showing no diastolic flow. Some artefactual flow is demonstrated in both systole and diastole due to the small size of the vessels sampled.

yield masses which appear morphologically benign on transvaginal sonography[26]. There is, however, a diagnostic dilemma when a morphologically normal ovary, or a morphologically benign simple cyst, demonstrates neovascularity. Based on existing studies, about 6% of women screened with ultrasound will have cystic or complex masses. Moreover, in one study an ovarian artery resistance index of <0.4 occurred in 12% of premenopausal patients and 3% of postmenopausal. In this study, only one borderline ovarian tumour and one endometrial malignancy were discovered[27]. The scientific basis for ovarian screening in a low-risk population is therefore unproven and even in patients with a strong family history there is a high false-positive detection rate, particularly in premenopausal patients, using both CA125 and ultrasound. It seems unlikely that Doppler, using current methods of data processing, will further improve on the specificity of the screening technique; it could in fact increase the number of false-positive laparotomies if abnormal colour flow is to be used as another indicator of ovarian abnormality[26].

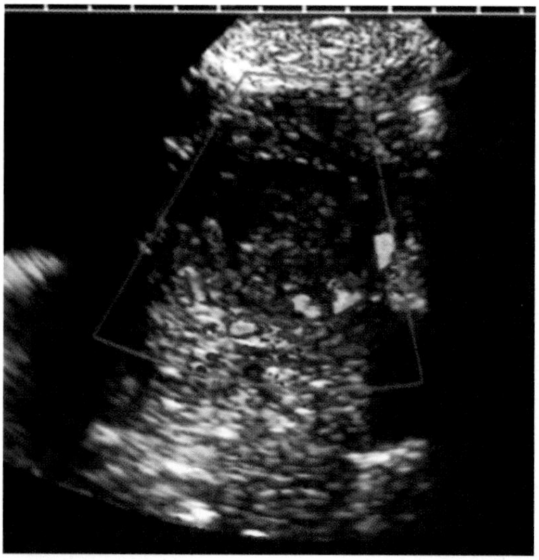

Other adnexal lesions

Inflammatory processes may produce a hyperaemic response, although this is not invariable, and will not allow differentiation of lesions of differing aetiology[28]. *Tubo-ovarian abscess* is the pathology most likely to show evidence of increased Doppler flow with circumferential vessels draped around the cystic component and low resistance indices, often less than 0.5 (Fig. 13.25)[29]. *Endometriomata* demonstrate a wide variety of appearances on colour Doppler, sometimes with circumferential

Fig. 13.24 Colour flow around a complex mass in the ovary of a premenopausal patient. This represented flow in a corpus luteum.

13

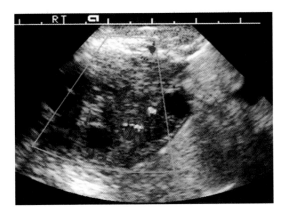

Fig. 13.25 Colour flow Doppler showing adnexal hyperaemia in pelvic inflammatory disease.

vessels, occasionally 'spotty' vessels with resistance indices varying from 0.5 to 0.74[30]. Differential diagnostic features remain dependent upon clinical history and other findings.

Ovarian torsion

Ovarian torsion may produce a variety of appearances on ultrasound including a complex cystic mass, a solid mass, and a solid mass with peripherally placed cysts. The absence of colour signal will not distinguish this from other pathologies, since colour Doppler has been demonstrated both centrally and peripherally in torsion[31]. However, it may allow the distinction of ovaries that are beyond salvage by conservative surgery[32]. If these data are confirmed, then preoperative assessment with colour Doppler could help to determine the nature and extent of surgery. Those patients with demonstrable blood flow within the ovary would be submitted for laparoscopic untorsion, while in those with an absence of flow, open surgery and oophorectomy would be the likely procedure. However, more work is required to confirm these data before such an approach can be recommended in the management of suspected ovarian torsion.

Complications of early pregnancy

The trophoblast is extremely vascular during its development, with two phases of invasion. The vessels contributing to this invasion have thin walls and low peripheral resistance to blood flow. Sampling within the vascular component of the trophoblast will therefore produce characteristic low-impedance signals with resistance indices less than 0.6. Some workers have suggested that this may contribute to the early differentiation of viable from non-viable or complicated pregnancies (Fig. 13.26a). However, the high power output of Doppler, particularly in relation to transvaginal applications, must be considered and, in this author's view, this prohibits its use in most early pregnancy applications. Ectopic pregnancy may be considered an exception to this rule and certain valuable data can be acquired.

Ectopic pregnancy

Ultrasound imaging occupies a central role in the investigation of ectopic pregnancy, with recorded sensitivities of 94% for transvaginal ultrasound[33]. Modern methods of management now suggest that a conservative approach can be adopted in those patients without active trophoblast and that when there is active trophoblast, medical treatment using either systemic or local methotrexate is the preferred first-treatment option. Using colour Doppler as a guide, the vascular trophoblast can be identified within the adnexal region. Sampling the flow within the trophoblast will yield pulsatile flow of low resistance index in the presence of active trophoblast but a resistance index in excess of 0.8 in inactive trophoblast[34]. This may provide a useful guide for conservative, non-operative treatment in these patients (Fig. 13.26b).

Ancillary Doppler findings in ectopic pregnancy are similar to those in a normotopic pregnancy, with flow in uterine vessels and to

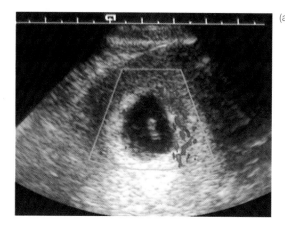

(a)

Fig. 13.26 (a) Normal colour flow pattern in the trophoblast of a normal 7-week intrauterine pregnancy. (This patient subsequently had a termination of the pregnancy.) (b) Vascular trophoblast in the adnexal region. Colour and spectral Doppler demonstrating low-resistance flow, implying active trophoblast and suggesting the need either for administration of methotrexate as medical treatment or operative intervention.

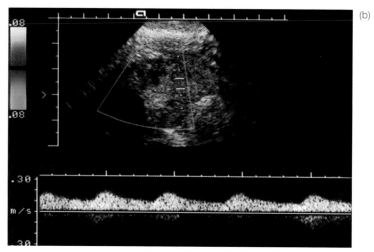

(b)

the corpus luteum displaying comparable impedance indices, although peak velocities within the uterine arteries are reduced. The reported findings do not, however, appear sufficiently specific to allow differential diagnosis[35].

Cervical ectopic pregnancy

Although rare, this form of ectopic pregnancy presents particular difficulties with management. Attempts at evacuation of the uterus are usually unsuccessful, accompanied by heavy bleeding and often necessitating hysterectomy. More recently, direct installation of potassium chloride and subsequently methotrexate into the gestational sac can result in regression of the gestation and either complete resolution,

or a more safely performed uterine evacuation. Colour and duplex Doppler ultrasound have two roles in this situation. First, to identify the position of the uterine arteries joining the uterus, thus confirming the diagnosis of a cervical pregnancy by its position caudal to the uterine arteries. Second, Doppler is used to monitor the regression of the trophoblast by alteration of the pattern of the Doppler signal with time, as this usually mirrors the fall in human chorionic gonadotrophin values.

Other gynaecological tumours

Duplex Doppler ultrasound has no established role in the assessment either of cervical carcinoma or pelvic metastatic disease, including ovarian carcinoma. Certain metastases may show increased vascularity similar to that of primary ovarian tumours, but there are no data to relate vascularity to susceptibility for certain forms of treatment, nor to the likely response to treatment (Fig. 13.27).

Pelvic congestion syndrome

The association between chronic pelvic pain, dyspareunia and pelvic varices has been termed pelvic congestion syndrome. Its aetiology is not clear but some have ascribed it as being due to dilatation of pelvic veins, congestion of the ovaries with resultant ovarian swelling and cyst formation (Fig. 13.28). In its most marked form there may be vulval and leg varices. Some have suggested a psychological component for the condition but it is difficult to assess a particular psychological profile as cause or effect in women with long-term disabling pelvic pain. There is an association between the symptoms and multiple large serpiginous pelvic veins, usually of diameter greater than 4 mm and, in this author's experience, flow velocities within the pelvic veins of less than 5 cm per second. Reverse flow within the pelvic veins during a Valsalva manoeuvre, which exceeds 2 cm s^{-1} peak velocity, appears

to be a prominent feature of the syndrome. Further work is necessary, however, to define this association more clearly.

Other pathologies

Non-gynaecological pathologies can be encountered during pelvic and transvaginal ultrasound examination.

Retroperitoneal mass lesions including lymphadenopathy

The relationship of retroperitoneal masses to the iliac vessels can usually be established without the use of colour flow Doppler.

Iliac artery aneurysm

Common external and internal iliac artery aneurysms can represent a differential diagnostic finding of a pelvic cystic mass. Common and external iliac artery aneurysms are usually easily identified by their relationship to the main arterial trunk, although internal iliac artery aneurysms may require colour flow Doppler for confirmation of their nature. Usually a pulsatile but swirling colour signal can be observed within the true lumen with a variable amount of mural clot.

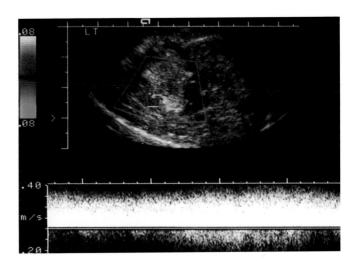

Fig. 13.27 Echogenic ovarian metastasis in patient with primary breast carcinoma demonstrating high-velocity peripheral flow which is normally indicative of shunting.

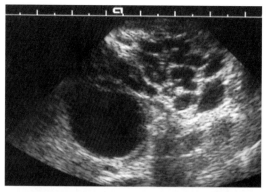

(a)

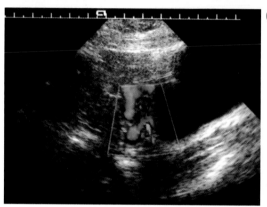

(b)

Fig. 13.28 (a) Large collection of serpiginous vessels in the pelvis adjacent to the right ovary which also contains a cyst. (b) Extension of the distended veins towards the uterine cervix and vaginal vault.

Deep venous thrombosis

Transvaginal ultrasound is not the primary method of diagnosis of deep vein thrombosis but the pelvic extension of clot can be demonstrated by both transabdominal and transvaginal ultrasound, with distension of the iliac veins by intraluminal echogenic clot and either distortion of flow pattern around the clot or complete occlusion.

Bowel masses

Bowel wall thickening is a non-specific feature of bowel pathologies. Similarly, mural hypervascularity is a feature typical of inflammatory bowel pathologies including Crohn's disease, diverticular disease and infective colitides; the degree of vascularity reflects disease activity.

Hysterosalpingo-contrast sonography (HYCOSY)

The use of echo-enhancing agents in the assessment of tubal patency has been shown to be of value in the investigation of infertility. A fine cannula is inserted into the cervical canal under direct vision and between 5 and 10 cc of contrast are injected gently whilst performing a transvaginal scan. This should show the echogenic contrast within the tubes and spill into the peritoneum in similar fashion to that seen with orthodox hysterosalpingography, although the correlation between hysterosalpingography and HYCOSY remains less than 90%. The technique has therefore not fully replaced formal X-ray hysterosalpingograms. The use of colour Doppler in conjunction with ultrasound contrast improves the sensitivity of the technique in the detection of tubal spill[36].

SUMMARY

Colour and duplex Doppler have yet to find well-defined applications in gynaecology. The value in ovarian tumour diagnosis is controversial and in tumours of the endometrium unproven. It may improve diagnostic security in patients with morphologically benign ovarian tumours, but hopes that it would enhance the process of ovarian screening have not been fulfilled. In inflammatory pathology there are no reported features that will allow the distinction between different pathological processes, even torsion of the ovary demonstrating intraovarian flow in many cases.

In the assessment and management of subfertility, Doppler techniques appear to have significant value. Ovarian activity and uterine receptivity can be more accurately monitored than by ultrasound morphology alone. Cyclical changes can be documented and the effects of ovulation induction therapy defined.

In ectopic pregnancy it may have a role in the operative planning process, while in malignant trophoblastic disease it appears to be of value in determining prognosis and in treatment planning.

There is a need for considerable research particularly in the areas of neovascularity and signal processing before Doppler techniques are applicable to common gynaecological conditions, and before this author could advocate its widespread adoption in the investigation of gynaecological conditions.

REFERENCES

1. Suren A, Osmers R, Kulenkampff D, Kuhn W (1994) Visualization of blood flow in small ovarian tumour vessels by transvaginal colour Doppler sonography after echo enhancement with injection of Levovist. *Gynaecologic and Obstetric Investigation* 38: 210–212
2. Sladkevicius P, Valentin L, Marsal K (1995) Transvaginal gray-scale and Doppler ultrasound examinations of the uterus and ovaries in healthy postmenopausal women. *Ultrasound in Obstetrics and Gynecology* 6: 81–90
3. Steer CV, Tan SL, Mason BA, Cambell S (1994) Mid-luteal phase vaginal color Doppler assessment of uterine artery impedance in a subfertile population. *Fertility and Sterility* 61: 53–58
4. Kurjak A, Zalud I (1992) Doppler and color flow imaging. In: Nyberg DA, Hill LM, Bohm-Velez M, Mendelson EB (eds) *Transvaginal Ultrasound*, pp 285–294. St Louis: Mosby Year Book
5. Meire HB (1993) Doppler – artefacts, errors and pitfalls. *Abdominal and General Ultrasound* 5: 83–93
6. Battaglia C, Artini PG, D'Ambrogio G, Galli PA, Genazzini AR (1994) Uterine and ovarian blood flow measurement. Does the full bladder modify the flow resistance? *Acta Obstetrica et Gynecologica Scandinavica* 73: 716–718
7. Steer CV, Tan SL, Dillon D, Mason BA, Campbell S (1995) Vaginal color Doppler assessment of uterine artery impedance correlates with immunohistochemical markers of endometrial receptivity required for the implantation of an embryo. *Fertility and Sterility* 63: 101–108
8. Tinkanen H, Kujansuu E, Laippala P (1994) Vascular resistance in uterine and ovarian arteries: its association with infertility and the prognosis of infertility. *European Journal of Obstetrics, Gynecology and Reproductive Biology* 57: 111–115
9. Balakier H, Stronell RD (1994) Color Doppler assessment of folliculogenesis in *in vitro* fertilization patients. *Fertility and Sterility* 62: 1211–1216
10. Achiron R, Levran D, Sivan E, Lipitz S, Dor J, Maschiach S (1995) Endometrial blood flow response to hormone replacement therapy in women with premature ovarian failure: a transvaginal Doppler study. *Fertility and Sterility* 63: 550–554
11. Wiener Z, Beck D, Rottem S, Brandes LM, Thaler I (1993) Uterine artery flow velocity waveforms and color flow imaging in women with perimenopausal and postmenopausal bleeding. Correlation to endometrial histopathology. *Acta Obstetrica et Gynecologica Scandinavica* 72: 162–166
12. Carter JR, Lau M, Saltzman AK et al (1994) Gray-scale and color flow Doppler characterisation of uterine tumors. *Journal of Ultrasound in Medicine* 13: 835–840
13. Tepper R, Cohen I, Altaras M et al (1994) Doppler flow evaluation of pathologic endometrial conditions in postmenopausal breast cancer patients treated with Tamoxifen. *Journal of Ultrasound in Medicine* 13: 635–640
14. Zalud I, Conway C, Schulman H, Trinca D (1993) Endometrial and myometrial thickness and uterine blood flow in postmenopausal women: the influence of hormonal replacement therapy and age. *Journal of Ultrasound in Medicine* 12: 737–741
15. Carter J, Fowler J, Carlson J et al (1993) Transvaginal color flow Doppler sonography in the assessment of gestational trophoblastic disease. *Journal of Ultrasound in Medicine* 12: 595–599
16. Hsieh FJ, Wu CC, Chen CA, Chen TM, Hsieh CY, Chen HY (1994) Correlation of uterine hemodynamics with chemotherapy response in gestational trophoblastic tumors. *Obstetrics and Gynecology* 83: 1021–1025
17. Chou CY, Chang CH, Yao BL, Kuo HC (1994) Color Doppler ultrasonography and serum CA125 in the differentiation of benign and malignant ovarian tumors. *Journal of Clinical Ultrasound* 22: 491–496
18. Sengoku K, Satoh T, Saitoh S, Abe M, Ishikawa M (1994) Evaluation of transvaginal colour Doppler sonography, transvaginal sonography and CA125 for prediction of ovarian malignancy. *International Journal of Gynaecology and Obstetrics* 46: 39–43
19. Bromley B, Goodman H, Benacerraf BR (1994) Comparison between sonographic morphology and Doppler waveform for the diagnosis of ovarian malignancy. *Obstetrics and Gynecology* 83: 434–437
20. Brown DL, Frates MC, Laing FC et al (1994) Ovarian masses: can benign and malignant lesions be

13

differentiated with color and pulsed Doppler US? *Radiology* **190**: 333–336

21. Stein SM, Laifer-Narin S, Johnson MB *et al* (1995) Differentiation of benign and malignant adnexal masses: relative value of gray-scale, color Doppler, and spectral Doppler sonography. *American Journal of Roentgenology* **164**: 381–386

22. Timor-Tritsch LE, Lerner JP, Monteagudo A, Santos R (1993) Transvaginal ultrasonographic characterisation of ovarian masses by means of color flow-directed Doppler measurements and a morphologic scoring system. *American Journal of Obstetrics and Gynecology* **168**: 909–913

23. Wu CC, Lee CN, Chen TM, Shyu MK, Hsieh CY, Chen HY, Hsieh FJ (1994) Incremental angiogenesis assessed by color Doppler ultrasound in the tumorigenesis of ovarian neoplasms. *Cancer* **73**: 1251–1256

24. Carter JR, Lau M, Fowler JM, Carlson JW, Carson LF, Twiggs LB (1995) Blood flow characteristics of ovarian tumors: implications for ovarian cancer screening. *American Journal of Obstetrics and Gynecology* **172**: 901–907

25. Cosgrove D (1996) Ultrasound contrast enhancement of tumours. *Clinical Radiology* **51** (Suppl. 1): 44–49

26. Muto MG, Cramer DW, Brown DL (1993) Screening for ovarian cancer: the preliminary experience of a familial ovarian cancer center. *Gynecologic Oncology* **51**: 12–20

27. Karlan BY, Raffel LJ, Crvenkovic G *et al* (1993) A multidisciplinary approach to the early detection of ovarian carcinoma: rationale, protocol design, and early results. *American Journal of Obstetrics and Gynecology* **16**: 494–501

28. Quillin SP, Siegel MJ (1994) Transabdominal color Doppler ultrasonography of the painful adolescent ovary. *Journal of Ultrasound in Medicine* **13**: 549–555

29. Tinkanen H, Kujansuu E (1993) Doppler ultrasound findings in tubo-ovarian infectious complex. *Journal of Clinical Ultrasound* **21**: 175–178

30. Aleem F, Pennisi J, Zeitoun K, Predanic M (1995) The role of colour Doppler in diagnosis of endometriomas. *Ultrasound in Obstetrics and Gynecology* **5**: 51–54

31. Stark JE, Siegel MJ (1994) Ovarian torsion in prepubertal and pubertal girls: sonographic findings. *American Journal of Roentgenology* **163**: 1479–1482

32. Willms AB, Schlund JF, Meyer WR (1995) Endovaginal Doppler ultrasound in ovarian torsion: a case series. *Ultrasound in Obstetrics and Gynecology* **5**: 129–132

33. de Crespigny LC (1998) Demonstration of ectopic pregnancy by transvaginal ultrasound. *British Journal of Obstetrics and Gynecology* **95**: 1253–1256

34. Tekay A, Jouppila P (1992) Color Doppler flow as an indicator of trophoblastic activity in tubal pregnancies detected by transvaginal ultrasound. *Obstetrics and Gynecology* **80**: 995–999

35. Jurkovic D, Bourne TH, Jauniaux E, Campbell S, Collins WP (1992) Transvaginal color Doppler study of blood flow in ectopic pregnancies. *Fertility and Sterility* **57**: 68–73

36. Shlief R, Deichert U (1991) Hysterosalpingo-contrast sonography of the uterus and fallopian tubes: results of a clinical trial of a new contrast medium in 120 patients. *Radiology* **178**: 213–215

Clinical applications of Doppler ultrasound in obstetrics

DAVID J. ROWLANDS and PAUL A. DUBBINS

The circulatory changes that occur during pregnancy involve modification of vascular structure within the uterus (spiral arteries), the development of a neocirculation (the placenta and the fetus), and a redistribution of blood flow and alteration in circulating blood volume such that the placenta in the third trimester receives 20% of the total maternal circulation and maternal blood volume increases by a similar value. Certain disease processes and certain complications of pregnancy are at least in part mediated by a microvascular abnormality. Thus, for example, impaired trophoblast migration of the spiral arteries is a major component in pre-eclampsia. As a result there has been considerable interest in the application of Doppler techniques to the detection of complications of pregnancy, detection and characterization of certain fetal abnormalities, as well as an assessment of the value of Doppler in the detection and management of maternal disease.

THE UTEROPLACENTAL CIRCULATION

The uterine artery is a branch of the anterior division of the internal iliac artery, and divides further into four arcuate arteries, each of which divide into more than 25 spiral arteries. There are therefore between 100 and 200 spiral arteries which enter the intervillus space.

During early pregnancy, trophoblast cells invade this space and disrupt the wall of the spiral arteries as part of the process of placental formation. There are two separate waves of invasion. Between implantation and 10 weeks, the trophoblastic invasion is limited to the decidual layer. From about 14 weeks until 22 weeks, the invasion extends as far as the spiral arteries. This invasion of the spiral arteries affects the resistance to blood flow within the spiral arteries and thereby in the arcuate and main uterine arteries[1].

Method of examination

The complexity of the uteroplacental circulation makes accurate identification of the vessel under study difficult with either continuous wave or duplex Doppler ultrasound. Flow velocity waveforms are obtained from the lateral lower quadrants of the uterus, angling the transducer on either side of the uterus towards the cervix. Signals achieved in this way are assumed to be originating from the uterine arteries (see Fig. 13.2)[2, 3]. The uterine arteries are more accurately identified using colour Doppler: the region lateral to the lower uterus is examined and the external iliac artery and the adjacent vein are identified. The uterine artery crosses the external iliac artery on its course from the internal iliac artery to the body of the

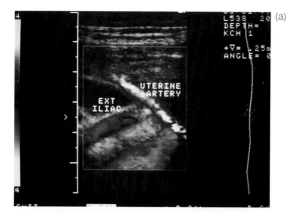

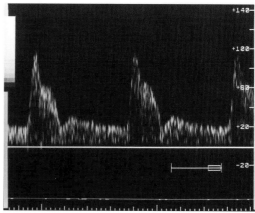

Fig. 14.2 Uterine artery waveform in intrauterine growth retardation demonstrating low diastolic flow and an early diastolic notch.

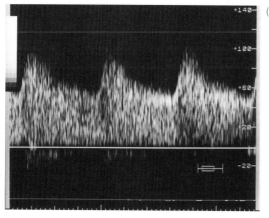

Fig. 14.1 (a) Colour flow Doppler of the uterine artery (red) demonstrating apparent crossover of the external iliac artery (blue). (b) Normal uterine artery flow in the third trimester demonstrating high diastolic flow.

It is possible to calculate several indices to quantify waveform analysis; however, the most commonly used in the uterine artery is the resistance index (RI) (Fig. 14.9a). After 26 weeks of gestation the normal range of resistance index is between 0.45 and 0.58. Decreased end-diastolic flow and consequently raised resistance indices above 0.58 is considered abnormal, as is a notch in early diastole in either uterine artery, suggesting failure of trophoblastic invasion of the spiral arteries (Fig. 14.2)[6,7].

Problems and pitfalls

A comparative histological study of third-trimester placental biopsy at caesarean section[8] has demonstrated that the uterine artery flow impedance reflects impaired trophoblast migration. Nonetheless, there are a number of reasons for caution. Impedance to flow varies throughout the uteroplacental circulation, with the lowest value seen in the arcuate vessels on the placental side of the uterus and the highest value seen in the uterine arteries on the non-placental side of the uterus[9]. The physiological variations and anatomical complexities of the uteroplacental vascular tree make it difficult to

uterus. In this way more accurate identification of the particular vessel being investigated is achieved. It is important to angle the transducer to improve the angle of insonation whilst maintaining vessel identification on colour Doppler. Spectral waveforms are obtained by placing the pulsed Doppler range gate within the vessel at this point (Fig. 14.1a)[4]. The spectral waveform from the normal uteroplacental system is unidirectional, of low pulsatility, and demonstrates frequencies throughout the cardiac cycle (Fig. 14.1b). This is a result of the trophoblastic invasion of the spiral arteries; end-diastolic frequencies increase to a maximum at 24–26 weeks of gestation (see Fig. 14.9)[5].

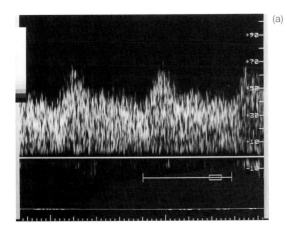
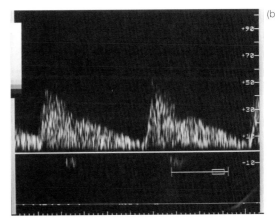

Fig. 14.3 (a) Uterine artery waveform in labour. Blood flow characteristics in the uterine artery between contractions is normal. (b) During a contraction the overall flow velocity within the uterine artery is reduced. However, the diastolic velocity is reduced further than the peak systolic velocity and there is an early systolic notch.

obtain accurate and reproducible measurements using continuous wave Doppler, with inter-observer variations ranging from 3.9 to 17%[10, 11]. In later pregnancy, between 37 and 40 weeks, maternal position may also alter flow patterns, with the umbilical artery resistance being higher in the supine position than in the decubitus[12]. Furthermore, variations in uterine activity (Fig. 14.3), maternal heart rate and exercise also significantly alter the waveform[13, 14]. The examination should therefore be performed with the mother resting and only during a period of uterine inactivity. The effect of exercise is more marked in complicated pregnancies, but there are no data evaluating the effect of exercise to improve sensitivity or specificity of Doppler in predicting fetal outcome. The time of day, or recent eating by the mother, do not appear to have an effect on the uterine artery flow[14, 15]. Most of the antihypertensive drugs appear to have no effect on fetomaternal blood flow[16]. However, nifedipine appears to produce a reduction in umbilical artery resistance, and this has therefore been suggested as a better drug to use during pregnancy[17]. The effect of smoking on blood flow has been somewhat controversial with researchers reporting either no effect, or a significant effect, from smoking a cigarette[18, 19].

However, because of the dispute and the potential for cigarette smoking to alter flow patterns in chronic smokers, these authors advocate that patients should not smoke for at least 1 hour prior to a Doppler study.

Pathology

The association between poor trophoblastic invasion of the spiral arteries with the development of pregnancy-induced hypertension and possibly intrauterine growth retardation led to initial enthusiasm for the use of Doppler as a screening method for pregnancy complications. Screening by continuous wave Doppler is cheap and easy to perform when coupled to an 18-week anomaly scan. However, even in primiparous mothers and using a uterine artery resistance index on the placental side above the 90th centile, only 51% of subsequent pre-eclampsia or small-for-gestational-age infants were detected; the positive predictive value was only 29%[20]. This is typical for results seen in low- and moderate-risk pregnancies. Furthermore, screening can only be useful if there is an intervention available which will improve outcome, and in obstetrics the options are limited. Delivery is not an option in most cases; early results on the use of low-dose aspirin have shown a possible value in preventing early-onset pregnancy-induced hypertension, but further studies are required and it remains to be shown whether Doppler can identify the particular subgroup likely to respond to aspirin treatment.

Coexistent maternal disease

Uterine artery Doppler appears to be of significantly greater utility when there is pre-existing maternal disease. In chronic renal disease, for example, an abnormal artery waveform predicts pre-eclampsia and intrauterine growth retardation with a high degree of accuracy. Only 8% of patients with negative Doppler findings in one study developed complications of pregnancy[21]. By contrast, although the resistance index is increased in the uterine arteries of diabetics with a morphological vasculopathy, there is no relationship with short- or long-term diabetic control and it is not a good predictor of diabetes-related fetal morbidity, presumably because these changes are reflecting the risk of acidosis as a result of hypoxia rather than metabolic acidosis[22, 23]. In patients with pre-existing, essential hypertension, uterine artery Doppler appears to be useful in defining groups of patients who are at risk of developing complications. If the systolic blood pressure is greater than 140 mmHg, then resistance indices in both uterine arteries are increased. If the systolic blood pressure is less than 140 mmHg, three separate groups may be identified: those with (a) bilateral or (b) unilateral abnormalities of the waveform within the uterine arteries; and (c) those with an entirely normal uterine artery flow. The prognosis appears to be related to the degree of abnormality of uterine artery flow. In systemic lupus erythematosus, one study suggests that an abnormal uterine artery Doppler will identify all those pregnancies with an adverse outcome[24].

DOPPLER EXAMINATION OF THE FETOPLACENTAL CIRCULATION (TABLE 14.1)

The placenta rather than the lungs is the organ of gaseous exchange in the fetus. Two umbilical arteries convey deoxygenated blood from the fetus to the placenta, and one umbilical vein returns oxygenated blood to the fetal inferior vena cava. The umbilical arteries take origin from the fetal internal iliac arteries coursing alongside the lateral walls of the bladder in the urachus to the umbilical insertion. The umbilical vein courses posteriorly and cephalad to join the left branch of the portal vein. The oxygenated blood is then shunted through the liver to the inferior vena cava by the ductus venosus. Spectral waveforms from the umbilical artery and vein can usually be easily obtained using continuous wave Doppler ultrasound[25]; a simple Doppler probe is placed on the abdomen and the beam randomly directed into the uterine cavity until the characteristic arterial and venous waveforms are demonstrated (Fig. 14.4). Duplex Doppler allows identification of a loop of cord and the recording of an unambiguous signal from the umbilical vessels. Colour flow Doppler confers few advantages on the evaluation of the umbilical artery, although in patients with oligohydramnios it may be the only way to identify a loop of cord. Furthermore, in twin pregnancies it allows the identification of the individual umbilical arteries.

Ultrasound imaging and colour Doppler allow the optimization of the angle of

Table 14.1 Vessels examined by Doppler.

Maternal	Uterine arteries
	Arcuate arteries
	Placental vessels
Fetal	Umbilical
	Aorta
	Middle cerebral artery
	Carotid
	Renal
	Ductus venosus

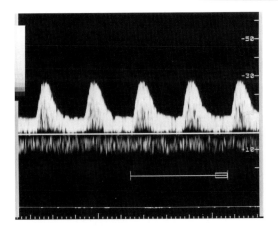

Fig. 14.4 Normal umbilical artery flow in the third trimester. There is variation in the normal pulsatility of the umbilical artery but in this example there is clearly defined continuous end-diastolic flow.

insonation to the umbilical vessels and therefore improve clarity of signal reproduction. However, as the Doppler indices relate systolic to diastolic components of flow, optimal angle of incidence is less important. Volume flow assessment within the fetoplacental circulation was much in vogue in the early 1980s but has not found widespread clinical utility and is not performed in most departments. Sampling of the umbilical artery waveforms can be performed at any point along the vessel. Early suggestions that different signals were achieved at the placental end of the cord compared to the umbilical end have not been confirmed. This

would seem unlikely unless there were pathology of the umbilical vessel itself. Indeed in situations where there is oligohydramnios, and particularly in twin pregnancies with a 'stuck twin', sampling flow from the umbilical arteries within the fetal abdomen as they course alongside the bladder may be the only option to achieve satisfactory Doppler signals (Fig. 14.5).

Normal waveforms from the umbilical artery are unidirectional and demonstrate frequencies throughout the cardiac cycle. Decreased end-diastolic flow (Fig. 14.6) and consequently raised Doppler indices are considered abnormal, and are thought to reflect increased placental resistance caused by damage to placental tertiary villi[26]. In more extreme cases, end-diastolic flow may be absent (Fig. 14.7) or even reversed (Fig. 14.8).

Doppler waveforms within the umbilical artery change with gestational age in a similar fashion to those of the uterine artery. Resistance and pulsatility indices demonstrate a gradual reduction with increase in gestational age. Normal values of the pulsatility index are shown in Fig. 14.9b.

Problems and pitfalls

As end-diastolic values fall, the A/B ratio (peak systole/end diastole) and resistance index tend towards a value of 1. For clinical purposes

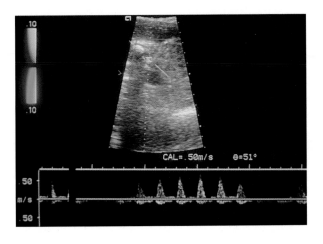

Fig. 14.5 Colour and duplex Doppler of the umbilical artery of a fetus with severe intrauterine growth retardation. There is virtual anhydramnios and the umbilical artery is identified on colour flow as it courses alongside the echo-free fetal bladder within the pelvis. The accompanying spectral Doppler signal demonstrates absent diastolic flow.

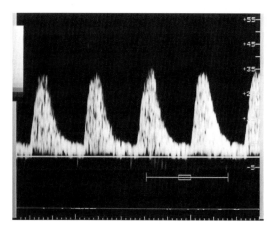

Fig. 14.6 In intrauterine growth retardation there is reduction of end-diastolic flow.

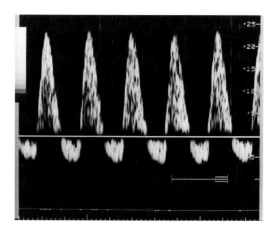

Fig. 14.8 Reversed diastolic flow in the umbilical artery. This implies a fetus at risk of significant morbidity/mortality.

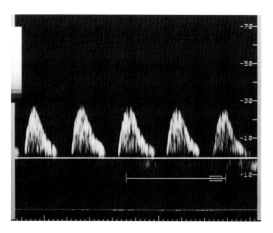

Fig. 14.7 Severe intrauterine growth retardation with absent end-diastolic flow in the umbilical artery.

fetal inactivity and in the absence of fetal breathing; duplex and colour Doppler ultrasound are of value in enabling the waveform to be sampled rapidly and accurately. Measurement of three consecutive cardiac cycles reduces the coefficient of variation of measurements to less than 5%[30].

All Doppler devices have inherent filtration which removes low-frequency noise and vessel wall movement artefact. On most current machines the high-pass filter can be varied, but it is important not to set this higher than 100 Hz and preferably lower than 50 Hz, if a false impression of absent diastolic flow is not to be created.

Pathology and applications (Tables 14.2–14.4)

Intrauterine growth retardation

Reduction in end-diastolic flow velocities within the umbilical artery waveform is thought to occur as a result of reduced tertiary villi formation and therefore could be an indicator of placental dysfunction, intrauterine growth retardation and fetal distress. In spite of the attraction of the hypothesis that Doppler would provide an early indicator of failure of

resistance indices are therefore not sensitive to the quantification of reversed flow, and the pulsatility index is more accurate for situations where there is low, absent or reversed end-diastolic flow. Variations in fetal heart rate[27] and the presence of fetal breathing movement[28] may significantly alter the arterial waveforms, although within the physiological range of 120–160 beats per minute it is not necessary to correct indices for fetal heart rate[29]. Nonetheless, it is important to examine umbilical artery waveforms during a period of

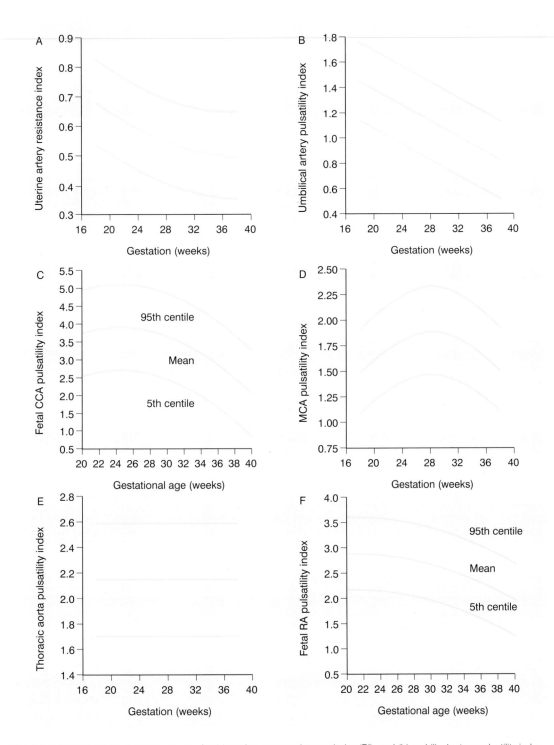

Fig. 14.9 Normal values during pregnancy for (a) uterine artery resistance index (RI), and (b) umbilical artery pulsatility index (PI). Fetal common carotid artery (CCA) PI (c) falls steeply after 32 weeks gestation, mirrored by the middle cerebral artery (MCA) PI (d). Normal values are also shown for the fetal descending thoracic aorta PI (e) and renal artery (RA) PI (f). Reproduced with permission from Pearce[41].

Table 14.2 Indications for Doppler examination in pregnancy.

Uterine artery	Umbilical artery	Middle cerebral artery
? Screening	Intrauterine growth retardation	Intrauterine growth retardation
Pre-existing disease, e.g. renal disease	Post dates	
SLE	Fetal abnormality	
Pre-existing uterine disease		
Trophoblastic disease		

Table 14.3 Features of abnormality.

Uterine artery	Umbilical artery	Middle cerebral artery
Raised indices	Raised indices	Decreased indices
Notch	Absent end-diastolic flow	
	Reversed end-diastolic flow	Ratio of middle cerebral artery to umbilical artery $\leqslant 1$

Table 14.4 Factors contributing to abnormal flow.

Uterine artery	Umbilical artery	Middle cerebral artery
Pre-existing disease	Fetal activity	Direct cerebral compression
Exercise	Breathing	
Uterine activity	Cord compression	
?Antihypertensives	?Cigarettes	
?Cigarettes		

the tertiary villus, it has not proved of value in screening for intrauterine growth retardation. However, in high-risk pregnancies, particularly those in which there is pregnancy-induced hypertension, or which have other clinical or sonographic features to suggest fetal growth retardation, the umbilical artery waveform is a good indicator of fetal compromise. Progressive reduction in the diastolic component of umbilical artery flow mirrors the risk and severity of potential fetal compromise[31, 32]. Furthermore not only may fetuses at increased risk be identified and managed more intensively, but high-risk pregnancies, such as those with established intrauterine growth retardation or pregnancy-induced hypertension, with normal umbilical artery waveforms appear to carry no greater risk of fetal morbidity or fetal loss than a normal pregnancy. The corrected perinatal mortality rate is reduced when the results of umbilical artery Doppler are made available to clinicians, who are then able to act with more appropriate and more timely intervention[33]. The finding of absent or reversed end-diastolic flow in a pregnancy with established intrauterine growth retardation is an indication for the serious consideration of early delivery[34, 35], although there are as yet no precise data indicating the temporal relationship between these end-diastolic flow changes and a subsequent poor outcome.

Post dates pregnancy

The management of a post dates pregnancy is extremely difficult. No single parameter has been established that will confidently predict outcome and, although there has been some enthusiasm for a role for Doppler in the assessment of post dates pregnancy, there is not universal agreement about its value[36]. In these authors' view, therefore, umbilical artery Doppler should be looked upon as one of the factors which contribute to the monitoring of post dates pregnancies, and absence or reversal of diastolic flow is an indication for immediate delivery; an operative delivery may need to be considered. Some authors have advocated the use of the ratio between the Doppler shifts (A/B ratio) in the uterine artery and the fetal middle cerebral artery (UA/MCA ratio) in postterm pregnancy, suggesting that values of <1.05 yield sensitivities of 80% and specificities of 90% in predicting an adverse outcome[37].

Twin pregnancy

In uncomplicated multiple pregnancy, there is the same progressive decrease in placental resistance as is seen in singleton pregnancies, with a consequent fall in indices with increasing gestational age. Doppler appears to be of no value in predicting adverse outcomes in unselected pregnancies[38]. However, in pregnancies with discordant growth patterns, Doppler analysis of the umbilical arteries appears to be a useful adjunct to serial growth measurements, allowing recognition of high-risk twin pregnancies which require more intense surveillance[39].

In twin-to-twin transfusion syndrome, the shared circulation has the result that Doppler waveforms in the umbilical arteries of both twins are similar. Doppler studies of these vessels appear to be of no predictive or management value in this condition, although colour and power Doppler may allow documentation of placental anastomoses and consequent guidance of laser ablation.

Diabetes

Both pre-existing vascular disease and hypertensive disorders of pregnancy are common in mothers with diabetes. In these cases, the value of an abnormal umbilical artery Doppler signal has the same significance in identification of uteroplacental insufficiency as in the non-diabetic population. However, diabetic pregnancies are also at risk of metabolic complications and Doppler flow patterns will not detect these complications, and it is therefore vital that a normal umbilical artery flow does not give either the clinician or the mother false reassurance[22].

Fetal abnormality

Fetuses with autosomal trisomy may also have abnormal placentation with reduced tertiary villi formation[40]. An abnormal umbilical artery waveform should therefore prompt a detailed study of fetal structural anatomy and an assessment of amniotic fluid volume; karyotyping should also be considered[34].

In the presence of a raised alpha-fetoprotein but structurally normal fetus, the appearance of an abnormal uteroplacental Doppler waveform at 20 weeks is associated with a significantly raised perinatal mortality[41], with the commonest contributor to perinatal mortality being placental abruption. Similarly it has been suggested that fetal and placental morphological features should be combined with Doppler to improve prediction of outcome[42].

Preterm pregnancy

Prediction of preterm delivery is a goal that has eluded obstetricians for many years. Early work suggests that a comparison between umbilical artery flow and uterine artery flow, in studies performed between 25 and 36 weeks, will predict an increased risk of preterm delivery if there is an unmatched increase in the resistance index of the uterine artery with normal umbilical artery flow. This is thought to be due to failure of trophoblast migration, but its value in predicting preterm delivery in low-risk pregnancies, or even the management of pregnancies with a previous history of preterm delivery, has not been evaluated[43].

THE FETAL CIRCULATION

The advent of colour Doppler, and more recently power Doppler, has meant that it is now possible to visualize flow within many of the fetal vessels. These include the aorta, inferior vena cava, carotid, intracerebral and renal arteries. Furthermore, it is possible to study cardiac and cardiopulmonary haemodynamics. The detailed study of congenital cardiac abnormalities and the role of Doppler techniques is, however, beyond the scope of this chapter.

There is a redistribution of fetal blood flow in response to hypoxia with a selective increase in blood flow to the brain, heart and adrenal glands at the expense of the viscera. This redistribution reflects the morphological findings in intrauterine growth retardation, with the head continuing to grow at the expense of a relatively smaller abdomen.

Fetal outcome is thought to relate both to the severity and duration of hypoxia, as well as the gestational age at delivery. It is assumed that hypoxia will tend to increase with increasing gestational age in fetuses with growth retardation and that this will lead to a greater redistribution of blood flow.

The descending thoracic aorta

The descending thoracic aorta is selected for study since it allows comparison between the visceral blood supply and cerebral perfusion. The sampling point is distal to the carotid vessels and proximal to the coeliac, mesenteric and renal arteries. The transducer is orientated to the long axis of the fetus and the thoracic aorta is identified. The sample volume is placed just above the diaphragm maintaining an angle of less than 55° and high-pass filter of less than 100 Hz (Fig. 14.10)[44]. The resulting waveform has characteristic features (Fig. 14.11) with

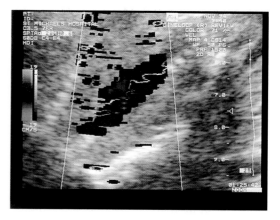

Fig. 14.10 Colour flow Doppler of the descending thoracic aorta and proximal abdominal aorta, demonstrating flow towards the transducer (red), and vena cava, demonstrating flow away from the transducer (blue).

forward flow throughout the cardiac cycle, but the pulsatility and resistance indices are constant throughout gestation (Fig. 14.9e)[45–47]. However, the haemodynamics of the fetal aorta are complex, supplying not only the visceral vessels and the lower limbs but more especially the umbilical arteries. Thus, while fetal hypoxia may produce alterations in the Doppler waveform of the thoracic aorta, much of the information derived from flow redistribution can also be obtained from examining the umbilical

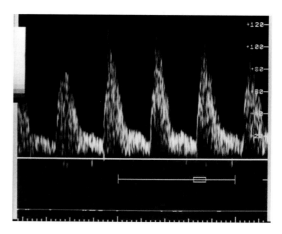

Fig. 14.11 Normal flow in the fetal aorta. The high peak systolic velocity of approximately 100 cm s^{-1} is accompanied by persistent diastolic flow of approximately 20 cm s^{-1}.

artery waveform which is generally easier to obtain.

The fetal cerebral circulation

The common carotid artery can usually be identified on colour Doppler within the neck. It is a relatively straight vessel with a long course and is therefore amenable to pulsed Doppler assessment. The long axis of the vessel is identified and the probe is angled to improve the angle of insonation. The sample volume is placed above the vessel, close to the root of the neck, in order to get a waveform from the common carotid artery and to avoid the external carotid artery.

The middle cerebral artery is the most commonly interrogated of the intracerebral vessels. The skull is scanned as if to perform a biparietal diameter measurement. A colour Doppler examination is then performed in a plane slightly closer to the base of the skull, where the middle cerebral artery will be identified as a vessel coursing towards the probe from the circle of Willis in the Sylvian fissure (Fig. 14.12). Later in gestation the location of the middle cerebral artery can be identified without colour Doppler simply by demonstrating pulsations within the brain substance.

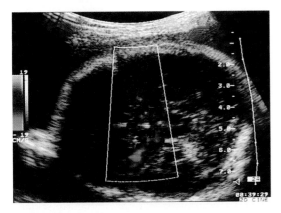

Fig. 14.12 Colour flow Doppler of the middle cerebral artery demonstrating colour-coded flow towards the transducer (in red) and away from the transducer in the contralateral middle cerebral artery (in blue).

Placement of the sample volume either within these pulsations or within the colour signal will allow recording of the Doppler waveforms.

The common carotid artery pulsatility index remains constant until 32 weeks gestation and then falls steeply (14.9c)[45–47] and this is mirrored by changes seen in the middle cerebral artery (Fig. 14.9d)[48].

The renal arteries

The renal arteries are lateral, anterolateral or posterolateral branches of the aorta. Therefore, in order to record Doppler signals from them, the ultrasound beam needs to be angled from the fetal kidney towards the aorta. In practice this is achieved by a coronal scan through the fetal abdomen, angling slightly anteriorly in long axis from the fetal flank. Colour Doppler will then enable visualization of the fetal renal artery running from the aorta to the renal hilum and the sample volume can be placed within the artery to obtain a waveform. The fetal renal artery waveform is difficult to interpret. Early in pregnancy velocities are low with little or no end-diastolic flow, but peak systolic velocity gradually increases with advancing gestational age and, commensurate with this, end-diastolic flow appears (Fig. 14.9f)[49]. It is not clear whether this represents renal maturation and the consequent increase in arteriolar cross-sectional area, or is simply a lack of sensitivity of existing ultrasound equipment for the low velocities and low-volume flow in early pregnancy. However, although renal blood flow will reflect any viscerocephalic redistribution, fetal renal artery Doppler contributes little to the identification of the compromised fetus because the kidneys only receive 3% of the fetal cardiac output and the renal artery velocities are low. This is in stark contrast to the significance of decreased fetal urine production and oligohydramnios as evidence of fetal compromise.

Colour Doppler of the renal vessels may also be used to assess congenital renal abnormalities, such as renal agenesis, where the artery is also absent, although care should be taken as hypoplastic arteries may be difficult to demonstrate on ultrasound, and enlarged adrenal glands may be misidentified as kidney.

Problems and pitfalls

Fetal breathing movements have a marked effect on all fetal Doppler waveforms in addition to the umbilical arteries already discussed, consequently measurements should only be taken during periods of fetal apnoea[50]. Marked fetal movement makes accurate placement of the sample volume and consequent Doppler signal recording difficult. Fetal heart rates within the normal physiological range are not thought to be important.

Care must be taken to avoid fetal head compression with the transducer as the fetal brain is readily compressible. There is a demonstrable rise in pulsatility index and fall in mean blood flow velocity measurement proportional to the transducer pressure applied[51].

Pathology and applications

The preferential supply of blood to the fetal brain is reflected by the high end-diastolic flow in the cerebral circulation. This results in a lower pulsatility index when compared with the descending aorta and renal arteries[52]. Diastolic flow within the intracerebral vessels is maintained in cases of early growth retardation presumably as a neurological protective mechanism and it may therefore be of use in monitoring fetal well-being. The redistribution of blood flow can be quantified by a ratio between the pulsatility index in the cerebral artery and the pulsatility index in the umbilical artery. This ratio is normally 2:1 but tends towards unity as fetal hypoxaemia is reflected in a falling middle cerebral artery pulsatility index and a rising

umbilical artery pulsatility index. It is not clear, however, at what point intervention should be considered. With continued worsening of the hypoxaemia it appears that there is a reversal of adaptation and this seems to be predictive of imminent fetal demise[53]. It is not clear, however, whether prompt surgical intervention will allow neurologically intact babies to be salvaged after the reversal is noted. Data are required to establish whether quantification of redistribution of blood flow can affect management strategy.

Two thirds of small-for-gestational-age fetuses which develop distress in labour can be identified from an abnormal fetal aortic pulsatility index[54], the absence of aortic end-diastolic flow being associated with increased neonatal morbidity and mortality[55]. This is seen most notably as a result of necrotizing enterocolitis, presumably reflecting the redistribution of blood flow and subsequent gut hypoxia and ischaemia.

Redistribution of blood flow and indeed the evaluation of blood flow characteristics in any of the fetal vessels is poor as a population screening tool for intrauterine growth retardation resulting from placental insufficiency[56]. In common with other applications of fetal Doppler, these methods appear to be better suited to the investigation of those fetuses designated as high risk.

Placental abnormalities

The diagnosis of placenta praevia is largely performed by ultrasound imaging. Transabdominal ultrasound has fallen into some disrepute because of reported incidences of low-lying placenta in excess of 40%[57] when scanning is performed before the last trimester; routine screening for placenta praevia in the second trimester is therefore not now widely used. By contrast, when there is antepartum haemorrhage, ultrasound is used to establish the relationship of the placenta to the internal os. This is more commonly now performed using transvaginal ultrasound. The addition of colour Doppler allows the demonstration of the rare but potentially serious vasa praevia. In this situation a vessel, or vessels, can be seen coursing from the margin of the placenta in close proximity to, or covering, the internal os. Similarly, other placental abnormalities can be documented: velamentous insertion of the cord can be identified with colour Doppler and chorio-angioma can be differentiated from a placental haematoma by the demonstration of a rich vascular supply[58].

Postpartum

A small amount of postpartum haemorrhage is a normal feature but where haemorrhage is prolonged, or heavy, the possibility of retained products of conception must be considered. Transvaginal ultrasound will frequently demonstrate abnormalities within the uterine cavity. As a general rule brightly reflective structures are taken to represent retained placental fragments and/or membrane; while echo-poor contents are thought to represent fresh or clotted blood. However, it is frequently difficult to differentiate between retained products of conception and uncomplicated blood clot.

There is a difference in the blood flow characteristics of the uterine artery when there are retained products of conception. Patients with residual trophoblast exhibit a resistance index in the myometrial vessels of 0.35 ± 0.1 whereas those without residual trophoblast have resistance indices in the myometrial vessels of 0.54 ± 0.15. However, the combination of low-impedance flow and intrauterine material is common after abortion and does not necessarily imply retained products of conception. It may simply reflect physiological involution; the temporal course of return to non-pregnant flow characteristics in the uterine vessels has not been documented[59].

TROPHOBLASTIC DISEASE

Transvaginal ultrasound will demonstrate uterine abnormalities in persistent gestational trophoblastic tumour. However, the sensitivity of ultrasound imaging is only 70% but abnormal uterine artery waveforms are seen in 90% of cases with persistent gestational trophoblastic tumour, and raised uterine artery impedance may predict resistance to chemotherapy[60, 61]. However, magnetic resonance imaging (MRI) appears to be more sensitive in the detection of trophoblastic tumour, being more accurate at identifying myometrial invasion and therefore establishing a diagnosis of choriocarcinoma.

MATERNAL HAEMODYNAMICS

Pregnancy is associated with marked changes in maternal haemodynamics. There is an increase in circulating blood volume with a corresponding increase in the cardiac output. This might be expected to have effects on blood flow to a number of the intra-abdominal organs, in addition to the effect that it has on uterine blood flow. Furthermore, it might be hoped that certain conditions, particularly associated with pregnancy and thought to be mediated through an abnormality in maternal physiology, might be reflected in changes in blood flow characteristics detectable by Doppler.

Doppler ultrasound of the maternal kidney in pregnancy

Doppler blood flow characteristics to the maternal kidney appear to alter little during pregnancy. Although certain authors report a slight reduction in the mean resistance index in renal artery examinations, this is not statistically significant. There is no doubt that volume flow is increased in pregnancy but this appears to be mediated largely by vasodilatation of the large supply vessels, although the absolute changes in flow velocity have not been investigated. There is no change in Doppler indices in patients either with essential hypertension, or those with pregnancy-associated hypertension; nor does the renal artery resistance index correlate with the severity of the hypertensive disease, or the status of renal function. However, the outcome of pregnancy is worse in patients with an elevated resistance index in the renal arteries[62].

There is no change in Doppler indices in patients presenting with progressive physiological dilatation of the collecting system of the kidneys during pregnancy. In the past this has been attributed to a combination of a hormonal effect, together with a degree of mechanical obstruction of the ureter by the enlarging uterus. There is no correlation between the degree of dilatation of the collecting system and any change in resistance index in uncomplicated cases, but it may be clinically useful in cases of suspected obstruction in whom Doppler ultrasound may show a significant difference between the affected and unaffected kidney. The obstructed kidney will usually show a resistance index differing by 0.1 or more than that in the unobstructed kidney. In these authors' department, resistance indices are used as a discriminator in deciding which patients with loin pain in association with pregnancy should proceed to an intravenous urogram[63].

Haemodynamic changes in other vessels

There is naturally a decrease in the resistance index in the aorta and common iliac arteries which reflects the increased flow to the uterus that occurs during pregnancy. However, there are also changes in the flow patterns in other vessels consequent upon changes in volume flow. There is, for example, an increase in volume flow through the portal vein and consequently in the hepatic veins. In the hepatic veins this affects not only the volume of flow but also the Doppler waveform where the normal pulsatile flow is lost in most patients. This occurs as early as the first trimester in some patients and therefore does not appear to be related to pressure effects from the enlarging uterus. This is of limited diagnostic significance except that some authors have suggested that changes in hepatic venous flow might be useful in the assessment of diffuse liver disease, including pregnancy-related liver disease. However, there is no correlation between liver disease in pregnancy and changes in hepatic venous flow, whatever the severity[64].

CONCLUSIONS

The role of Doppler in obstetrics has yet to be fully evaluated. The advent of colour Doppler has enabled more precise examination of the uteroplacental and fetoplacental circulations, together with more intricate examination of the fetal vasculature. However, this is an expensive modality and its benefits beyond a research tool have yet to be established. Combined analysis of the uteroplacental and fetoplacental (umbilical) circulation may increase diagnostic accuracy[65]. However, fetomaternal haemodynamics are complex, showing variation in their response to many maternal and fetal physiological and pathological states. It is possible, even likely, that other factors will influence fetal maternal blood flow. Currently Doppler methods appear capable only of detecting gross changes in placentation and gross changes of fetal well-being. For example, umbilical artery waveforms may be normal in a morphologically normal but small placenta. Similarly, chronic hypoxia induces placental changes which are presumably responsible for the altered waveform in umbilical and fetal vessels. However, in experimentally induced acute hypoxia there is no alteration in fetomaternal flow as detected by Doppler techniques[66].

In the same way, the role of uterine artery Doppler in the management of pregnancy is not clear cut. While apparently of value in patients with pre-existing maternal disease, its findings are not sufficiently sensitive or specific, nor does the use of screening Doppler affect perinatal morbidity and outcome[67]. Rather, it appears to be a rather indiscriminate indicator of fetomaternal abnormality. It may be that its use will lie in combination with other investigative parameters, including serum biochemistry.

Doppler ultrasound cannot be recommended as a screening procedure for the identification of pregnancy complications in low-risk pregnancies. Doppler examination of the uterine and umbilical arteries between 18 and 26 weeks gestation in high-risk pregnancies may be predictive of significant pregnancy complications, but at present there is insufficient evidence to suggest that the level of surveillance in the Doppler-negative group can be relaxed. If a relatively safe, cheap and effective treatment for early-onset maternal placental disease becomes established, such as aspirin or one of its analogues, then uteroplacental waveform screening may prove useful in deciding upon early treatment.

Doppler has most potential in the management of high-risk pregnancies consequent upon maternal disease, previously identified placental disease and fetal intrauterine growth retardation. Umbilical artery studies help identify fetuses at risk of hypoxia and acidaemia; when the results are applied clinically they contribute to reduced perinatal mortality rates. Doppler ultrasound of the fetal circulation may identify chronic hypoxia but a clinical role has yet to be established (Tables 14.3 and 14.4). It is likely that the future lies in comparative investigation of the uteroplacental umbilical and one or more fetal vessels. It is important, however, to stress that fetomaternal haemodynamics are not the only indicator of maternal or placental disease, or of fetal well-being. Doppler ultrasound may contribute to, but not replace, other methods of fetal and maternal surveillance.

REFERENCES

1. Pijnenborg R, Dixon G, Robertson WB, Brosens I (1980) Trophoblastic invasion of human decidua from 8 to 18 weeks of pregnancy. *Placenta* 1: 3–19
2. Bewley S, Campbell S, Cooper D (1989) Uteroplacental Doppler flow velocity waveforms in the second-trimester. A complex circulation. *British Journal of Obstetrics and Gynaecology* 96: 1040–1046
3. Schulman H, Winter D, Farmakides G, Coury A, Schneider E, Penny B (1989) Doppler examinations of the umbilical and uterine arteries during pregnancy. *Clinical Obstetrics and Gynaecology* 32: 738–745
4. Bower S, Vyas S, Campbell S, Nicolaides KH (1992) Colour Doppler imaging of the uterine artery in pregnancy: normal ranges of impedance to blood flow, mean velocity and volume flow. *Ultrasound in Obstetrics and Gynecology* 2: 261–265
5. Schulman H, Fleischer A, Farmakides G, Bracero L, Rochelson B, Grunfeld L (1986) Development of uterine artery compliance in pregnancy as detected by Doppler ultrasound. *American Journal of Obstetrics and Gynecology* 155: 1031–1036

6. Fleischer A, Schulman H, Farmakides G, Bracero L, Rochelson B, Koenigsberg M (1986) Uterine artery Doppler velocimetry in pregnant women with hypertension. *American Journal of Obstetrics and Gynecology* 154: 806–813
7. Bower S, Schuchter K, Campbell S (1993) Doppler ultrasound screening as part of routine antenatal screening: prediction of pre-eclampsia and growth retardation. *British Journal of Obstetrics and Gynaecology* 100: 989–994
8. Voigt HJ, Becker V (1992) Doppler flow measurements and histomorphology of the placental bed in uteroplacental insufficiency. *Journal of Perinatal Medicine* 20: 139–147
9. Kofinas AD, Espeland M, Swain M, Penry M, Nelson LH (1989) Correcting umbilical artery flow velocity waveforms for fetal heart rate is unnecessary. *American Journal of Obstetrics and Gynecology* 160: 704–707
10. Rightmire DA, Campbell S (1987) Fetal and maternal Doppler blood flow parameters in postterm pregnancies. *Obstetrics and Gynecology* 69: 891–894

11. Bewley S, Cooper D, Campbell S (1991) Doppler investigation of uteroplacental blood flow resistance in the second trimester: a screening study for pre-eclampsia and intrauterine growth retardation. *British Journal of Obstetrics and Gynaecology* **98**: 871–879

12. Qu LR, Kan A, Masahiro N (1994) Fetal circulation in relation to various maternal body positions. *Chung-Hua Fu Chan Ko Tsa Chih* **29**: 589–591

13. Mulders LG, Jongsma HW, Wijn PF, Hein PR (1988) The uterine artery blood flow velocity waveform: reproducibility and results in normal pregnancy. *Early Human Development* **17**: 55–70

14. Morrow R, Ritchie K (1989) Doppler ultrasound fetal velocimetry and its role in obstetrics. *Clinics in Perinatology* **16**: 771–778

15. Hastie SJ, Howie CA, Whittle MJ, Rubin PC (1988) Daily variability of umbilical and lateral uterine wall artery blood velocity waveform measurements. *British Journal of Obstetrics and Gynaecology* **95**: 571–574

16. Duggan PM, McCowan LM, Stewart AW (1992) Antihypertensive drug effects on placental flow velocity wave forms in pregnant women with severe hypertension. *Australian and New Zealand Journal of Obstetrics and Gynaecology* **32**: 335–338

17. Hirose S, Yamada A, Kasugai T, Ishizuka T, Tomoda Y (1992) The effect of nifedipine and dipyridamole on the Doppler blood flow waveforms of umbilical and uterine arteries in hypertensive pregnant women. *Asia–Oceania Journal of Obstetrics and Gynaecology* **18**: 187–193

18. Castro LC, Allen R, Ogunyemi D, Roll K, Platt LD (1993) Cigarette smoking during pregnancy: acute effects on uterine flow velocity waveform. *Obstetrics and Gynecology* **81**: 551–555

19. Morrow RJ, Ritchie JW, Bull SB (1998) Maternal cigarette smoking: the effects on umbilical and uterine blood flow velocity. *American Journal of Obstetrics and Gynecology* **159**: 1069–1071

20. North RA, Ferrier C, Long D, Townend K, Kincaid-Smith P (1994) Uterine artery flow velocity waveforms in the second trimester for the prediction of pre-eclampsia and fetal growth retardation. *Obstetrics and Gynecology* **83**: 378–386

21. Ferrier C, North RA, Becker G, Cincotta R, Fairley K, Kincaid-Smith P (1994) Uterine artery waveform as a predictor of pregnancy outcome in women with underlying renal disease. *Clinical Nephrology* **42**: 362–368

22. Johnstone FD, Steel JM, Haddad NG, Hoskins PR, Greer IA, Chambers S (1992) Doppler umbilical artery flow velocity waveforms in diabetic pregnancy. *British Journal of Obstetrics and Gynaecology* **99**: 135–140

23. Ben-Ami M, Battino S, Geslevich Y, Shalev E (1995) A random single Doppler study of the umbilical artery in the evaluation of pregnancies complicated by diabetes. *American Journal of Perinatology* **12**: 437–438

24. Kofinas AD, Penry M, Simon NV, Swain M (1992) Interrelationship and clinical significance of increased resistance in the uterine arteries in patients with hypertension or pre-eclampsia or both. *American Journal of Obstetrics and Gynecology* **166**: 601–606

25. Fitzgerald DE, Drumm JE (1977) Non-invasive measurement of human fetal circulation using ultrasound: a new method. *British Medical Journal* **2**: 1450–1451

26. Giles WB, Trudinger BJ, Baird PJ (1985) Fetal umbilical artery flow velocity waveforms and placental resistance: pathological correlation. *British Journal of Obstetrics and Gynaecology* **92**: 31–38

27. Mires G, Dempster J, Patel NB, Crawford JW (1987) The effect of fetal heart rate on umbilical artery flow velocity waveforms. *British Journal of Obstetrics and Gynaecology* **94**: 665–669

28. Gill RW, Trudinger BJ, Garrett WJ, Kossoff G, Warren PS (1980) Fetal umbilical venous flow measured *in utero* by pulsed Doppler and B-mode ultrasound. *American Journal of Obstetrics and Gynecology* **139**: 720–725

29. Kofinas AD, Penry M, Swain M, Hatjis CG (1989) The effect of placental laterality on uterine artery resistance and development of pre-eclampsia and intrauterine growth retardation. *American Journal of Obstetrics and Gynecology* **161**: 1536–1539

30. Erskine RLA, Ritchie JWK (1985) Umbilical artery blood flow characteristics in normal and growth-retarded fetuses. *British Journal of Obstetrics and Gynaecology* **92**: 605–610

31. McParland P (1992) Modern approach to the poorly grown fetus. *Irish Medical Journal* **85**: 88–89

32. Trudinger BJ, Cook CM, Giles WB et al (1991) Fetal umbilical artery velocity waveforms and subsequent neonatal outcome. *British Journal of Obstetrics and Gynaecology* **98**: 378–384

33. Neilson JP (1993) Doppler ultrasound in high-risk pregnancies. In: Enkin MW, Keirse MJNC, Renfrew MJ, Neilson JP (eds) *Pregnancy and Childbirth Module.* Cochrane Database of Systematic Reviews, No. 03889. London: BMJ Publishing

34. Poulain P, Palaric JC, Paris-Liado J, Jacquemart F (1994) Fetal umbilical Doppler in a population of 541 high-risk pregnancies: prediction of perinatal mortality and morbidity. Doppler Study Group. *European Journal of Obstetrics, Gynaecology and Reproductive Biology* **54**: 191–196

35. Devoe LD, Gardner P, Dean C, Faircloth D (1992) The significance of increasing umbilical artery systolic-diastolic ratios in the third-trimester pregnancy. *Obstetrics and Gynecology* **80**: 684–687

36. Zimmermann P, Alback T, Koskinen J, Vaalamo P, Tuimala R, Ranta T (1995) Doppler flow velocimetry of the umbilical artery, uteroplacental

arteries and fetal middle cerebral artery in prolonged pregnancy. *Ultrasound in Obstetrics and Gynecology* 5: 189–197

37. Devine PA, Bracero LA, Lysiliewicz A, Evans R, Womack S, Byrne DW (1994) Middle cerebral to umbilical artery Doppler ratio in post date pregnancies. *Obstetrics and Gynaecology* 84: 856–860

38. Faber R, Viehweg B, Burkhardt U (1995) Predictive value of Doppler ultrasound findings in twin pregnancies. *Zentralblatt für Gynäkologie* 117: 353–357

39. Giles WB, Trudinger BJ, Cook CM, Connelly A (1988) Umbilical artery flow velocity waveforms and twin pregnancy outcome. *Obstetrics and Gynaecology* 72: 894–897

40. Rochelson B, Kaplan C, Guzman E, Arato M, Hansen K, Trunca C (1990) A quantitative analysis of placental vasculature in the third-trimester fetus with autosomal trisomy. *Obstetrics and Gynecology* 75: 59–63

41. Pearce JMF (1992) The application of uteroplacental waveforms to complicated pregnancies. In: Pearce JMF (ed.) *Doppler Ultrasound in Perinatal Medicine*, pp 173–174. Oxford: Oxford University Press

42. Jauniaux E, Ramsay B, Campbell S (1994) Ultrasonographic investigation of placental morphologic characteristics and size during the second trimester of pregnancy. *American Journal of Obstetrics and Gynecology* 170: 130–137

43. Robel R, Ruckhaberle KE, Faber R, Viehweg B (1991) Doppler sonographic examinations of uteroplacental, fetoplacental and fetal haemodynamics and their prognostic value in preterm labour. Journal of Perinatal Medicine 19: 341–350

44. European Association of Perinatal Medicine (1989) Regulation for the use of Doppler technology in perinatal medicine. In: *Consensus of Barcelona,* pp 22–26. Barcelona: Instituto Barcelona

45. Bilardo CM, Campbell S, Nicolaides KH (1988) Mean blood velocity and flow impedence in the fetal descending thoracic aorta and common carotid artery in normal pregnancy. *Early Human Development* 18: 213–217

46. Lingman G, Marsal K (1986) Fetal central blood circulation in the third trimester of normal pregnancy – a longitudinal study; aortic and umbilical blood flow. *Early Human Development* 13: 137–150

47. Griffin D, Bilardo K, Masini L *et al* (1984) Doppler blood flow waveforms in the descending thoracic aorta of the human fetus. *British Journal of Obstetrics and Gynaecology* 91: 997–1002

48. Vyas S, Nicolaides KH, Bower S, Campbell S (1990) Middle cerebral artery flow velocity waveforms in fetal hypoxaemia. *British Journal of Obstetrics and Gynaecology* 97: 797–803

49. Vyas S, Nicolaides KH, Campbell S (1989) Renal artery flow velocity waveforms in normal and hypoxemic fetuses. *American Journal of Obstetrics and Gynecology* 161: 168–172

50. Marsal K, Lindblad A, Lingman G, Eik-Nes SH (1984) Blood flow in the descending aorta: intrinsic factors affecting fetal blood flow, i.e. fetal breathing movements and cardiac arrhythmia. *Ultrasound in Medicine and Biology* 10: 339–348

51. Vyas S, Campbell S, Bower S, Nicolaides KH (1990) Maternal abdominal pressure alters fetal cerebral blood flow. *British Journal of Obstetrics and Gynaecology* 97: 740–742

52. Scherjon SA, Kok JH, Oosting H, Wolf H, Zondervan HA (1992) Fetal and neonatal cerebral circulation: a pulsed Doppler study. *Journal of Perinatal Medicine* 20: 79–82

53. Rowlands DJ, Vyas SK (1995) Longitudinal study of fetal middle cerebral artery flow velocity waveforms preceding fetal death. [Comment in *British Journal of Obstetrics and Gynaecology* 103(8): 852.] *British Journal of Obstetrics and Gynaecology* 102: 888–890

54. Laurin J, Lingman G, Marsal K, Persson PH (1987) Fetal blood flow in pregnancies complicated by intrauterine growth retardation. *Obstetrics and Gynaecology* 69: 895–902

55. Hackett GA, Campbell S, Gamsu H, Cohen-Overbeek T, Pearce JMF (1987) Doppler studies in the growth-retarded fetus and prediction of neonatal necrotising enterocolitis, haemorrhage, and neonatal morbidity. *British Medical Journal* 294: 13–16

56. Laurin J, Marsal K, Persson PH, Lingman G (1987) Ultrasound measurements of fetal blood flow in predicting fetal outcome. *British Journal of Obstetrics and Gynaecology* 94: 940–948

57. Ott W (1993) Placenta praevia. *Ultrasound in Obstetrics and Gynecology* 139: 1493–1494

58. Heinonen S, Ryynanen M, Kirkinen P, Saarikoski S (1996) Perinatal diagnostic evaluation of velamentous umbilical cord insertion: clinical, Doppler, and ultrasonic findings. *Obstetrics and Gynecology* 87: 112–117

59. Dillon EH, Case CQ, Ramos IM, Holland CK, Taylor KJ (1993) Endovaginal ultrasound and Doppler findings after first-trimester abortion. *Radiology* 186: 87–91

60. Dobkin GR, Berkowitz RS, Goldstein DP, Bernstein MR, Doubilet PM (1991) Duplex ultrasonography for persistent gestational trophoblastic tumor. *Journal of Reproductive Medicine* 36: 14–16

61. Long MG, Boultbee JE, Langley R, Newlands ES, Begent RH, Bagshawe KD (1992) Doppler assessment of the uterine circulation and the clinical behaviour of gestational trophoblastic tumours requiring chemotherapy. *British Journal of Cancer* 66: 883–887

62. Thaler I, Weiner Z, Itskovitz J (1992) Renal artery flow velocity waveforms in normal and hypertensive

pregnant women. *American Journal of Hypertension*
5: 402–405

63. Weston MJ, Dubbins PA (1994) The diagnosis of
obstruction: colour Doppler ultrasonography of
renal blood flow and ureteric jets. *Current Opinion
in Urology* 4: 69–74

64. Roobottom CA, Hunter JD, Weston MJ, Dubbins PA
(1995) Hepatic venous Doppler waveforms: changes
in pregnancy. *Journal of Clinical Ultrasound* 23:
477–482

65. Campbell S, Hernandez CJ, Cohen-Overbeek T,
Pearce JMF (1984) Assessment of fetoplacental and

uteroplacental blood flow using duplex pulsed
Doppler ultrasound in complicated pregnancies.
Journal of Perinatal Medicine 12: 261–265

66. Trudinger BJ, Giles WB, Cook CM (1985) Flow
velocity waveforms in the maternal uteroplacental
and fetal umbilical placental circulations. *American
Journal of Obstetrics and Gynecology* 152: 155–163

67. Newnham JP, O'Dea MR, Reid KP, Diepeveen DA
(1991) Doppler flow velocity waveform analysis in
high-risk pregnancies: a randomised control trial.
British Journal of Obstetrics and Gynaecology 98:
956–963

Appendix:
System controls
and their uses

In addition to the basic choice of transducer type and frequency for the examination in hand, there are many other factors on a Doppler ultrasound system which need to be adjusted. Despite the efforts of the manufacturers to automate and simplify things, it is still necessary to adjust continually many of the scan and Doppler parameters during the course of an examination. Is the vessel superficial or deep? Is flow fast or slow, high volume or low volume? Most systems have the option to programme different examination parameters for a variety of examinations. Whilst these allow the basic appropriate settings to be entered, fine adjustments will be required during the course of the examination.

GENERAL PRINCIPLES

Transducer frequency The highest frequency which will achieve the highest resolution consistent with adequate penetration is normally chosen. The Doppler frequency used by any transducer is often 1–2 MHz below the imaging frequency, although some modern equipment may have a wide range of receive frequencies such as 5–10 MHz.

B-mode image This should be set up with relatively low overall gain, so that the image is a little on the dark side as the software tends to allocate colour to darker areas, rather than to areas which contain echoes.

Transmit power The transmit power of the system should be set at the lowest level consistent with an adequate examination, especially obstetric and gynaecological examinations. It is better to start at a medium level and increase the power only after other measures to improve system sensitivity have been tried, such as adjusting colour gate size, removing filters, adjusting the scale/pulse repetition rate.

Update/duplex/triplex In duplex ultrasound there is the ability to acquire and display both imaging and Doppler information either simultaneously, or alternately. Simultaneous display results in degradation of both the image and the spectral display as the computer has to process data from both sources. The update facility allows the operator to set the system to handle either imaging data, or Doppler data. This results in a higher quality of display for the selected mode and it is usually used for acquisition of the best-quality spectral display for analysis. Duplex scanning is of some value in the initial stages of an examination in order to position the sample volume in the area of interest. Triplex mode refers to the simultaneous acquisition, processing and display of colour Doppler, spectral display and imaging information. As with duplex scanning, this requires significant division of processing power and consequent compromise in the quality of the display. Newer systems with more powerful computers will be less prone to these problems.

COLOUR DOPPLER CONTROLS

Colour map Choose one that has good contrast for the identification of aliasing. Maps which grade to white at each end, or to very pale colours, do not give as much information about aliasing as those which have significantly different colours, such as pale green and pale orange. Variance maps were said to register the amount of spectral broadening in the colour map, although this is not easy to appreciate and may, in fact, not be true as this 'variance' seems to reflect the velocity, rather than spectral broadening. Variance maps are most frequently used in cardiological examinations. In addition, colour tags can be put into the scale so that velocities above or below the chosen range can be identified.

Colour gain The colour gain is set to the optimal level. This can be identified by turning up the gain until noise is seen in the colour box and then backing off slightly.

Colour scale The colour scale should be set to levels appropriate for the range of velocities under investigation. It should be remembered that colour Doppler gives information on the mean shift estimates only; the mean velocity in a pixel is only calculated when an angle correction for that pixel is performed. The scale is closely related to the pulse repetition frequency, or sampling rate; this has to be above the Nyquist limit for the frequency shift being measured. If it is set too low then aliasing will occur; this can be removed by increasing the colour scale range. If it is set too high then there will be poor colour sensitivity for slower velocities, resulting in inadequate colour fill-in across the vessel.

Colour inversion This changes the colour map disposition in relation to flow direction, e.g. red for blue, or vice versa.

Colour gate This relates to the size of the colour pixels, a smaller size gives better spatial resolution, whereas a larger size provides better sensitivity at the expense of spatial and sometimes temporal resolution.

Colour baseline The colour baseline can be adjusted to provide a wider range of shifts on one side or the other, depending on the characteristics of the blood flow in the vessel being examined and particularly if the flow is in only one direction.

Colour filters These help remove low-frequency noise and clutter from the image. It is best to set filters at the lowest level compatible with an acceptable image as they also remove low-frequency shift information from the image.

Colour write priority A pixel in the image can display either B-mode imaging information, or colour Doppler information. The colour write priority facility allows the relative priority for these two types of information to be defined. High colour priority results in colour information being displayed in areas which might contain low-intensity imaging information, for instance at the margins of vessels. Alternatively, high imaging priority results in grey-scale information displacing colour information, such as might occur with reverberation artefacts within the vessel lumen amongst the colour Doppler information.

Colour box This defines the volume of tissue from which colour Doppler information will be gathered. It is better to keep the box as small and as superficial as practical, because larger areas take more processing power and time; deeper boxes need slower pulse repetition frequencies. Most systems now allow the direction of the box to be steered but this reduces sensitivity.

Colour persistence This reflects the amount of frame-averaging which occurs. A low level of persistence results in an image which has a fast temporal response but may have a poor signal to noise ratio. A high level of persistence improves the signal to noise ratio by summating data from several frames, but this results in an impaired temporal response, so that pulsatile flow information is dampened.

POWER DOPPLER CONTROLS

Although the power mode is intrinsically simpler than velocity mode, there are still several controls and options which influence the power image.

Power maps Most systems offer a variety of colour maps from which the operator can select according to personal preference, usually a yellow- or magenta-based scale is used for display of power Doppler information. The threshold or sensitivity can be varied; this results in changes in the transparency of the power box. When the power map background is opaque the sensitivity is maximal. Various degrees of increasing translucency are available so that sensitivity can be traded for imaging and anatomical information.

Power gain This is similar to colour gain and amplifies the received Doppler signal. Excessive gain will result in unnecessary noise and artefact in the image.

Scale The energy scale affects the sensitivity of the system for signal intensities of varying strengths: lower scales are more sensitive to lower-intensity signals; on some systems the scales are linked to the filters.

Dynamic range As in spectral Doppler, this affects the range of signal intensities over which the available colour scale is spread and the appearance of the Doppler information on the screen: increasing the dynamic range will tend to increase the amount of colour on the screen.

Power box steering angle Although the power display is much less dependent on angle than the velocity display, there may still be loss of the power signal at 90° because these low Doppler frequencies fall below the motion discrimination filter cut-off level. In most situations, steering the power Doppler box does not have much effect on the display; however, the loss of signal at 90° may be overcome by having a degree of angulation.

Filters Motion discrimination filters are used to filter out excessive signal noise from structures, other than blood, which are moving in the Doppler box. Low filter settings provide more sensitivity but are more prone to flash artefacts, whereas higher filter settings reduce flash artefacts but will also filter out some blood flow information.

SPECTRAL CONTROLS

Spectral gain This affects the receiver gain for the spectral display. As in B-mode imaging, the level should be adjusted in order to give a balanced distribution of grey shades across the displayed spectra.

Spectral dynamic range This can be varied to optimize the display of particular frequency shifts. A narrow dynamic range results in the loss of low-intensity shifts above and below the main shift frequencies. Conversely a wide dynamic range, particularly if associated with a high level of spectral receiver gain, can result in artefactual broadening of the spectra displayed. Further manipulation of the spectral display can be performed by altering the post-processing algorithms in order to emphasize,

279

or suppress, particular frequency shifts. In normal practice a simple linear allocation is most convenient.

Spectral scale Altering the scale affects the pulse repetition frequency and thus the range of shifts which can be registered without aliasing. In practice the scale is adjusted so that the Doppler waveform is displayed without wrap-around, which indicates aliasing. The scale may be displayed with either a KHz scale for frequency shift, or m s^{-1} for velocity. The use of m s^{-1} allows some comparison of different examinations, performed with different transducer frequencies and with different angles of insonation.

Spectral inversion This allows the operator to change the orientation of the display. Many operators prefer to display arterial waveforms above the baseline, even if flow is away from the transducer. However, care is therefore required when assessing the vertebral arteries for reverse flow, or the leg veins for reflux, as errors may occur if spectral inversion is not recognized. Some centres do not allow spectral inversion because of the potential for misinterpretation, particularly in relation to examinations for venous insufficiency.

Spectral sweep speed A medium speed is adequate for most arterial work, with a slower speed for venous flow. A fast sweep speed is useful for acceleration time measurement and waveform analysis, particularly if there is tachycardia.

Angle correction The measurement of the angle of insonation relative to the direction of flow is required in order to convert frequency shift information into velocities in spectral Doppler and mean pixel velocities in colour Doppler. The main direction of flow may not necessarily be parallel to the vessel wall and colour Doppler is useful in precise positioning

of the angle-correction cursor along the line of the jet. The angle of insonation should be less than 60–65° or the errors in velocity calculation become significant.

Gate size This defines the range of depths from which Doppler data are collected. The gate should be positioned within the lumen of the vessel, clear of the walls in order to reduce wall thump. The position of the gate which corresponds to the maximum Doppler shift is located with the use of the colour map and the operator's ears, which are the most sensitive and efficient spectral analyser available and will register when the peak frequency shift is obtained. If an assessment of volume flow is being made, the gate should be wide enough to encompass the entire vessel width so that all the flow contributes to the signal and the time-averaged mean velocity will be most representative. Smaller gates give a cleaner signal, especially with laminar flow, but at the expense of a reduction in sensitivity.

Filters Removal of low-frequency noise and clutter arising from the vessel wall and surrounding tissues contributes to a cleaner signal, but filters should be set as low as is practical, otherwise low-frequency shifts from slow blood flow will be filtered out, which could result in the mistaken impression of absent diastolic flow in arteries, or occlusion in veins. In practice it is best to keep the filters set at the lowest setting and only increase filtration as required during an examination.

Modern systems allow the operator to preset many of these parameters and create different profiles for different types of examination such as veins, carotids, renal, etc. However, it should be remembered that ultrasound is a dynamic examination and the best results will be obtained if the system controls are adjusted to optimum settings for the task in hand, rather than relying on the preset profiles alone.

Index

INDEX